Experimental and Clinical Progress in Cancer Chemotherapy

Cancer Treatment and Research

Wᴵᴸᴸᴵᴬᴹ L McGᵁᴵᴿᴱ, *series editor*

Livingston RB (ed): Lung Cancer 1. 1981. ISBN 90-247-2394-9.
Bennett Humphrey G, Dehner LP, Grindey GB, Acton RT (eds): Pediatric Oncology 1. 1981. ISBN 90-247-2408-2.
DeCosse JJ, Sherlock P (eds): Gastrointestinal Cancer 1. 1981. ISBN 90-247-2461-9.
Bennett JM (ed): Lymphomas 1, including Hodgkin's Disease. 1981. ISBN 90-247-2479-1.
Bloomfield CD (ed): Adult Leukemias 1. 1982. ISBN 90-247-2478-3.
Paulson DF (ed): Genitourinary Cancer 1. 1982. ISBN 90-247-2480-5.
Muggia FM (ed): Cancer Chemotherapy 1. ISBN 90-247-2713-8.
Bennett Humphrey G, Grindey GB (eds): Pancreatic Tumors in Children. 1982. ISBN 90-247-2702-2.
Costanzi JJ (ed): Malignant Melanoma 1. 1983. ISBN 90-247-2706-5.
Griffiths CT, Fuller AF (eds): Gynecologic Oncology. 1983. ISBN 0-89838-555-5.
Greco AF (ed): Biology and Management of Lung Cancer. 1983. ISBN 0-89838-554-7.
Walker MD (ed): Oncology of the Nervous System. 1983. ISBN 0-89838-567-9.
Higby DJ (ed): Supportive Care in Cancer Therapy. 1983. ISBN 0-89838-569-5.
Herberman RB (ed): Basic and Clinical Tumor Immunology. 1983. ISBN 0-89838-579-2.
Baker LH (ed): Soft Tissue Sarcomas. 1983. ISBN 0-89838-584-9.
Bennett JM (ed): Controversies in the Management of Lymphomas. 1983. ISBN 0-89838-586-5.
Bennett Humphrey G, Grindey GB (eds): Adrenal and Endocrine Tumors in Children. 1983. ISBN 0-89838-590-3.
DeCosse JJ, Sherlock P (eds): Clinical Management of Gastrointestinal Cancer. 1984. ISBN 0-89838-601-2.
Catalona WJ, Ratliff TL (eds): Urologic Oncology. 1984. ISBN 0-89838-628-4.
Santen RJ, Manni A (eds): Diagnosis and Management of Endocrine-related Tumors. 1984. ISBN 0-89838-636-5.
Costanzi JJ (ed): Clinical Management of Malignant Melanoma. 1984. ISBN 0-89838-656-X.
Wolf GT (ed): Head and Neck Oncology. 1984. ISBN 0-89838-657-8.
Alberts DS, Surwit EA (eds): Ovarian Cancer. 1985. ISBN 0-89838-676-4.
Muggia FM (ed): Experimental and Clinical Progress in Cancer Chemotherapy. 1985. ISBN 0-89838-679-9.
Higby DJ (ed): The Cancer Patient and Supportive Care. 1985. ISBN 0-89838-690-X.
Bloomfield CD (ed): Chronic and Acute Leukemias in Adults. 1985. ISBN 0-89838-702-7.

Experimental and Clinical Progress in Cancer Chemotherapy

edited by

FRANCO M. MUGGIA

Clinical Director
The Rita and Stanley H. Kaplan Cancer Center
New York University Medical Center
New York, New York, USA

1985 **MARTINUS NIJHOFF PUBLISHERS**
a member of the KLUWER ACADEMIC PUBLISHERS GROUP
BOSTON / DORDRECHT / LANCASTER

Distributors

for the United States and Canada: Kluwer Academic Publishers, 190 Old Derby Street, Hingham, MA 02043, USA
for the UK and Ireland: Kluwer Academic Publishers, MTP Press Limited, Falcon House, Queen Square, Lancaster LA1 1RN, UK
for all other countries: Kluwer Academic Publishers Group, Distribution Center, P.O. Box 322, 3300 AH Dordrecht, The Netherlands

Library of Congress Cataloging in Publication Data

Main entry under title:

Experimental and clinical progress in cancer
  chemotherapy.

  (Cancer treatment and research)
  1. Cancer--Chemotherapy. 2. Antineoplastic agents.
I. Muggia, Franco M. II. Series. [DNLM: 1. Neoplasms--
drug therapy. W1 CA693 / QZ 267 E956]
RC271.C5E97 1985   616.99'4061   84-16698
ISBN 0-89838-679-9

ISBN 0-89838-679-9 (this volume)
ISBN 90-247-2426-0 (series)

Copyright

PRINTED IN THE NETHERLANDS

Contents

Foreword to the series

Where do you begin to look for a recent, authoritative article on the diagnosis or management of a particular malignancy? The few general oncology textbooks are generally out of date. Single papers in specialized journals are informative but seldom comprehensive; these are more often preliminary reports on a very limited number of patients. Certain general journals frequently publish good indepth reviews of cancer topics, and published symposium lectures are often the best overviews available. Unfortunately, these reviews and supplements appear sporadically, and the reader can never be sure when a topic of special interest will be covered.

Cancer Treatment and Research is a series of authoritative volumes which aim to meet this need. It is an attempt to establish a critical mass of oncology literature covering virtually all oncology topics, revised frequently to keep the coverage up to date, easily available on a single library shelf or by a single personal subscription.

We have approached the problem in the following fashion. First, by dividing the oncology literature into specific subdivisions such as lung cancer, genitourinary cancer, pediatric oncology, etc. Second, by asking eminent authorities in each of these areas to edit a volume on the specific topic on an annual or biannual basis. Each topic and tumor type is covered in a volume appearing frequently and predictably, discussing current diagnosis, staging, markers, all forms of treatment modalities, basic biology, and more.

In *Cancer Treatment and Research,* we have an outstanding group of editors, each having made a major commitment to bring to this new series the very best literature in his or her field. Martinus Nijhoff Publishers has made an equally major commitment to the rapid publication of high quality books, and world-wide distribution.

Where can you go to find quickly a recent authoritative article on any major oncology problem? We hope that *Cancer Treatment and Research* provides an answer.

WILLIAM L. MCGUIRE
Series Editor

Preface

As in CANCER CHEMOTHERAPY 1, this volume brings to the reader highlights in three different areas of cancer therapeutics: new concepts and models; drug classes; and clinical settings. Topics were chosen because of their timeliness or probable current impact in cancer treatment. Authors were selected on the basis of their ability to provide a critical overview of specific subjects and their involvement in original work. I shall review the aims of this second volume, and then elaborate on the scope of its contents.

The principal aim of the volumes on cancer chemotherapy in the 'Cancer Treatment and Research' series, as stated in the preface to the first volume, is to assemble in a *concentrated* form selected ingredients of chemotherapeutic progress. These ingredients are to include concepts in therapeutic strategy, pre-clinical studies, development of major classes of compounds, identification of new directions and of landmarks of clinical progress. Thus we do not foresee overlap with series which provide an yearly update of chemotherapy in an encyclopedic manner, or reviews of cancer chemotherapy. Unlike those publications, our volumes are not intended to seek a place in shelves as a reference manual. It is this Editor's hope that persons representing various biomedical disciplines will seek the 'Cancer Treatment and Research' chemotherapy volumes to survey advances in the field at regular intervals. If this aim is fulfilled, one may expect experimental chemotherapists, clinical oncologists of various specialties, and even biomedical scientists working in other fields to follow developments in cancer chemotherapy in these pages. As the series evolves, the Editor's responsibility will be to maintain continuity in objectives and display a wide variety of topics to the readers. Thus the selection also reflects a wish to fulfill these ongoing objectives.

In CANCER CHEMOTHERAPY 1, we reviewed the Goldie-Coldman hypothesis of drug resistance and its impact in treatment strategies, the question of optimal schedule as deducted from animal models, and the relevance of animal models and human tumor cloning assay on drug development. Overview of new drug categories included detailed but concise presentation on the anthracycline antibiotics and the platinum compounds. These reviews will be of interest even to those readers not seeking to be deeply familiar with experimental aspects of cancer chemotherapy. Amino acid depletion as a novel target is presented alongside these successful anticancer drugs. Finally, three clinical conditions which are demonstrating a substantial impact from the application of recent developments in chemotherapy were selected for review. Testicular cancer, gastric cancer and acute myelogenous leukemia each represented major targets for clinical research because of advances in chemotherapy or recent experiences in clinical trials. EXPERIMENTAL AND CLINICAL PROGRESS IN CANCER CHEMOTHERAPY parallels its predecessor by directing its view to analogous aspects of pre-clinical and clinical investigations.

A new class of cytotoxic molecules is introduced in the paper by Johnson and Grollman. These base propenals, which were discovered while investigating the mechanism of action of bleomycin, have interesting structure-activity relationships to be the subject of future investigations. Yesair, on the other hand, describes novel intracellular targets, macromolecular lipids, and carefully documents its possible role in the selectivity of known cytotoxic drugs. Biochemical concepts of alkylating toxicity protection by thiols are presented by Gurtoo and co-workers. Such concepts are making an introduction into the clinical arena, witness symposia which have taken place at the UICC International Cancer Congress in Seattle in August 1982, and at the International Chemotherapy Congress in Vienna in September 1983. It is important especially for clinicians to be aware of modifications which thiols may bring about in the metabolism of chemotherapeutic agents. Finally, Tritton and Hickman describe the cell membrane as a neglected target for anticancer drugs.

Among drug classes we review fluorinated pyrimidines which are in considerable greater development in Japan than in the U.S. Ogawa and co-workers review this area extensively following the opportunity of achieving a global perspective at a recently held International meeting on these drugs in Nagoya, as well as their own substantial experience. Ludlum describes the biochemical interactions of nitrosoureas providing an insight which hopefully will inspire additional work to enhance the selectivity of these compounds so effective in murine tumor systems and so far disappointing in humans. Bridging biochemistry to the clinical experience is the overview by Jackman, Jones, and Calvert on thymidylate synthetase inhibitors. Therapeutic concepts of autologous bone marrow for solid tumors are presented by McVie utilizing the specific example of small cell carcinoma of the lung.

The results obtained are particularly instructive in signaling problems which one should be mindful of, when embarking in similar clinical ventures.

Clinical cancer therapeutics, beyond the paper of McVie dealing with a specific therapeutic approach to small cell lung cancer, is represented by osteosarcoma and by ovarian cancer. Both chapters dissect out the issues in the management of these diseases. Controversies have abounded in interpreting the results achieved with adjuvant chemotherapy of osteosarcoma. Similarly, the contribution of more effective chemotherapies in ovarian cancer have been clouded by many other important prognostic determinants often neglected in reporting of results. Jaffe provides his perspective in osteosarcoma, whereas Beller and Speyer utilize their own clinical experience, resulting from the close alliance of a gynecologist and medical oncologist, in discussing important issues in the assessment of chemotherapy in ovarian cancer.

From this preface, the direction of the chemotherapy volumes should be obvious. There is no one specialist in cancer chemotherapy. The volumes will continue to be targetted to a wide spectrum of biomedical researchers, and to provide an overview of conceptual and actual highlights.

New York   FRANCO M. MUGGIA

List of Contributors

BANSAL, SK, Grace Drug Center, Roswell Park Memorial Institute, Buffalo, NY 14263

BELLER, Uziel, Dept of Ob-Gyn NY U Medical Center, 550 First Avenue, New York, NY 10016

BERRIGAN, MJ, Grace Drug Center, Roswell Park Memorial Institute, Buffalo, NY 14263

CALVERT, AH, Department of Biochemical Pharmacology, Institute of Cancer Research, Block E, Clifton Avenue, Belmont, Sutton, Surrey, U.K. S52 5PX

GROLLMAN, AP, Department of Pharmacological Sciences Health Sciences Center, SUNY-Stony Brook, Stony Brook, NY 11794

GURTOO, HL, Grace Drug Center, Roswell Park Memorial Institute, Buffalo, NY 14263

HICKMAN, JA, CRC Experimental Chemotherapy Corp, University of Aston, Birmingham BY7 ET, United Kingdom

HIPKENS, JH, Grace Drug Center, Roswell Park Memorial Institute, Buffalo, NY 14263

JACKMAN, AZ, Department of Biochemical Pharmacology, Institute of Cancer Research, Block E, Clifton Avenue, Belmont, Sutton, Surrey, U.K. S52 5PX

JAFFE, N, Department of Pediatrics, U of Texas, M.D. Anderson Hospital and Tumor Institute, Houston, 6723 Bertner Avenue, Houston, TX 77030

JOHNSON, F, Department of Pharmacological Sciences Health Sciences Center, SUNY-Stony Brook, Stony Brook, NY 11794

JONES, TR, Department of Biochemical Pharmacology, Institute of Cancer Research, Block E, Clifton Avenue, Belmont, Sutton, Surrey, U.K. S52 5PX

KOSER, P, Grace Drug Center, Roswell Park Memorial Institute, Buffalo, NY 14263

XIV

LOVE, J, Grace Drug Center, Roswell Park Memorial Institute, Buffalo, NY 14263

LUDLUM, DB, Department of Medicine, The Albany Medical College, Albany, NY 12208

MARINELLO, AJ, Grace Drug Center, Roswell Park Memorial Institute, Buffalo, NY 14263

McVIE, JG, Netherlands Cancer Institute, Plesmanlaan 21, 1066 CS, Amsterdam, The Netherlands

OGAWA, M, Cancer Chemotherapy Center, Japanese Foundation for Cancer Research, 1-37-1, Kami Ikebukuro, Toshima-ku, Tokyo 153

PAVELIC, Z, Grace Drug Center, Roswell Park Memorial Institute, Buffalo, NY 14263·

SHARMA, SD, Grace Drug Center, Roswell Park Memorial Institute, Buffalo, NY 14263

SPEYER, JL, NYU Medical Center, 550 First Avenue, Suite 4J, New York, NY 10016

STRUCK, RF, Southern Research Institute, Birmingham, AL 35255

TONG, WP, Department of Medicine, The Albany Medical College, Albany, NY 12208

TRITTON, TR, Department of Pharmacology, University of Vermont College of Medicine, Burlington, VT 05045

YESAIR, DW, Biomolecular Products Inc, PO Box 347, Byfield, MA 01922

1. Cytotoxic base propenals from DNA

FRANCIS JOHNSON and ARTHUR P. GROLLMAN

1. INTRODUCTION

While investigating the mechanism of action of bleomycin, we discovered that the action of this antibiotic on DNA leads to strand-scission and the formation of four nucleoside-derived base N-propenals [1]. Production of these substances (*1a–1d*) is consistent with a mechanism of strand-scission involving radical abstraction of a hydrogen atom from the C-4′ position of deoxyribose [1, 2].

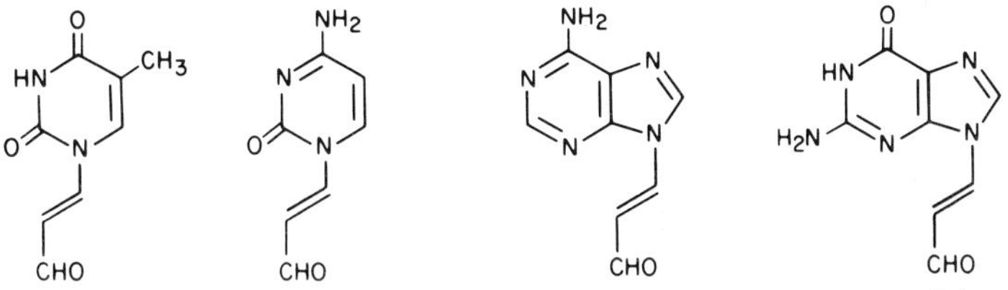

Figure 1a-d

The base N-propenals proved to be novel compounds whose chemical and biological properties had not been reported. Based on their apparent structural similarity to acyclovir [3], these compounds were tested for antiviral activity. Surprisingly, several proved cytotoxic to the host cell used for the antiviral assay. We pursued this serendipitous observation and subsequently showed that the thymine- and adenine-N-propenals were highly cytotoxic to a variety of tumor cells in culture [4].

These initial observations stimulated a search for related active substances. Accordingly, we synthesized [5] a family of compounds with the deoxynucleoside/nucleoside structure represented by *2* (Figure 2). This series was based on the rationale (a) that a sugar residue would enhance cellular uptake

F.M. Muggia (ed.), Experimental and Clinical Progress in Cancer Chemotherapy
© *1985, Martinus Nijhoff Publishers, Boston. ISBN 0-89838-679-9. Printed in the Netherlands.*

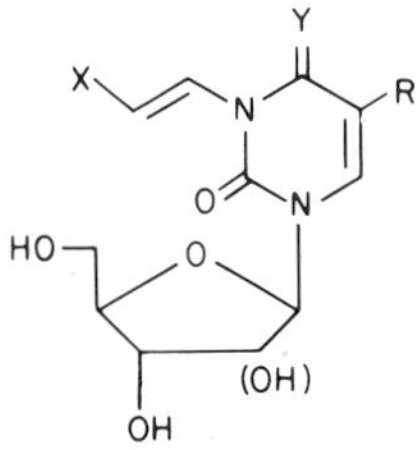

Figure 2

of the compound and provide better site-direction to the molecule and (b) that the position of the reactive and presumably toxiphoric propenal group would not be critical for biological activity. Both suppositions proved to be correct.

The cytotoxicity of several of the base propenals derived from DNA was comparable to that reported for bleomycin. Since bleomycin reacts with DNA to release base propenals [1], these substances may be responsible for the cytotoxic properties of the antibiotic. In this respect, an analogy may be drawn to the action of cyclophosphamide in which the cytotoxic aldehyde, acrolein, is postulated to be responsible, in part, for the cytotoxic actions of the drug [6]. In this case, the drug, rather than DNA, is the source of the toxic substance.

The antitumor properties of bleomycin have generally been attributed to inhibition of DNA synthesis and/or strand-scission. However, many aspects of bleomycin cytotoxicity, including blockage of cells in the G-2 phase of the cell cycle [7], bacteriocidal effects at concentrations of bleomycin that do not affect DNA synthesis [8] and selective toxicity to the skin and lungs in humans [9], are not satisfactorily accounted for by this hypothesis. We have, therefore, suggested [4] that that cytotoxic base propenals which can inactivate essential macromolecules and are generated in the cell nucleus, may be responsible for the therapeutic and toxic properties of bleomycin. In support of this proposal, we found that base N-propenals react readily with SH and NH$_2$ groups under physiological conditions [1, 5]. For example, compund 1a reacts with β-mercaptoethanol to form the products shown below (Figure 3):

In this chapter, we review the origin of the base propenals and their relationship to our current understanding of the mechanism of action of bleomycin. We also discuss the chemical reactivity of these compounds with emphasis on their reactions with functional groups found in enzymes and other biological molecules. We outline structure activity studies as they relate to the design of other base propenals and, finally, review the biological properties of these cytotoxic compounds with particular reference to the mechanism of toxicity of bleomycin.

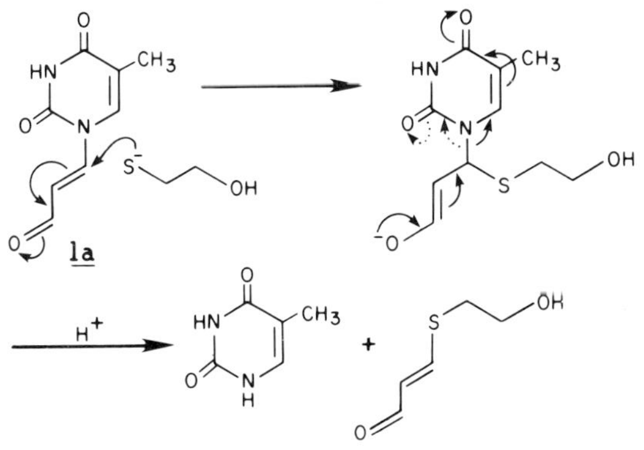

Figure 3

2. ORIGIN OF BASE N-PROPENALS

The bleomycins bind to DNA and cause strand-scission in a reaction requiring Fe(II) and oxygen [10–12]. Strand-scission is accompaned by the simultaneous release of free bases [13, 14] and formation of a series of base propenals, represented generically by *1* (Scheme 1). The *trans*-propenal group is attached to the heterocyclic base at the position previously occupied by the deoxyribose residue [1]. In the presence of thiols, *a* is degraded to form β-thio-substituted propenals. Steam distillation of the (acidified) reaction mixture produces malondialdehyde [15], a compound originally considered to be a primary product of DNA degradation [16, 17].

Bleomycin modifies DNA in several ways. Alkali-labile apurinic and apyrimidinic sites may arise in the absence of strand-scission [18]. When strand-scission occurs, the oligodeoxynucleotides formed are found to contain O-phosphoglycolate residues at the 3′ termini [1] and phospho-monoesters at the 5′ termini [18].

Previously [1, 2], we outlined a detailed mechanism to explain formation of the base-propenals from bleomycin and DNA. Scheme I shows one sequence leading to the formation of *1* and a second pathway which accounts for the formation of free heterocyclic bases. The initial steps in this series of reactions almost certainly involves reduction of molecular oxygen by Fe(II)-BLM to form the hydroperoxy derivative of Fe(II)-BLM [19]. If DNA is omitted from the reaction and Fe(II)-BLM is present in excess, oxygen is reduced at a rate of 5000 atom/min [20]. When excess Fe(II) is not present, the initial Fe(II)-BLM complex undergoes transformation *in situ* to form 'activated' bleomycin (BLM*) [21]. BLM* may also be produced by treating Fe(II)-BLM with hydrogen peroxide.

The life-time of BLM* seems to be very short. The complex undergoes self-degradation but is stabilized in the presence of DNA. The structure of

SCHEME 1

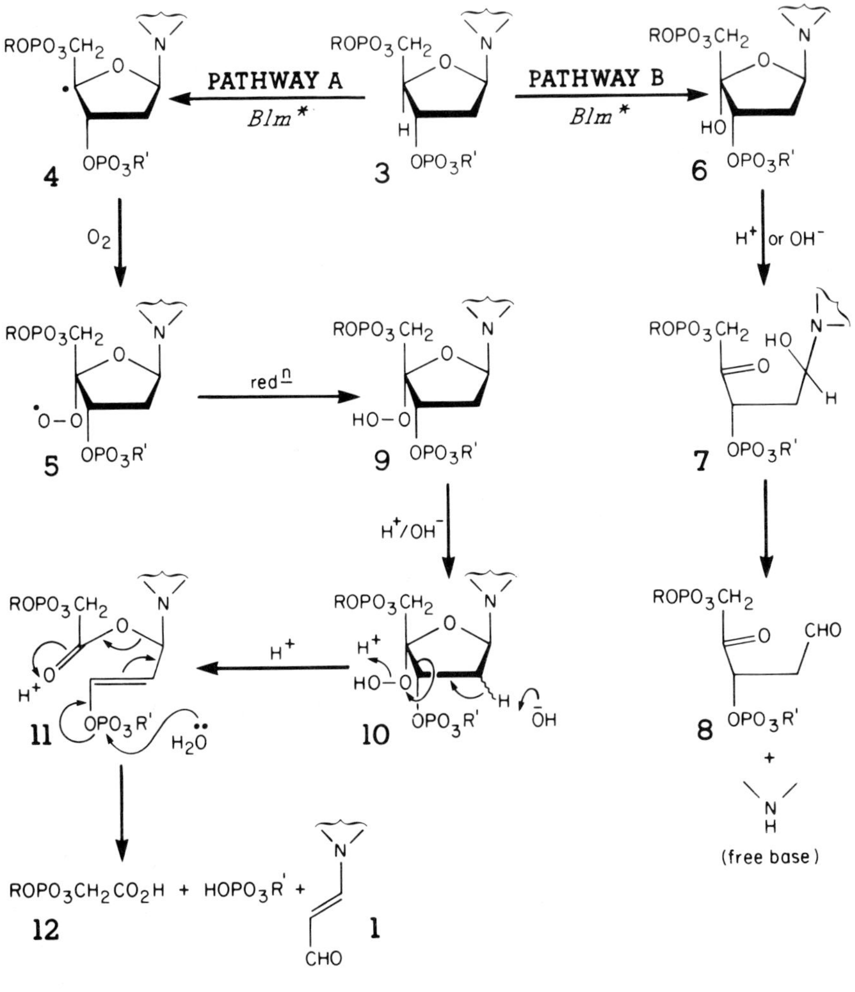

N⁓ = nucleotide base; R, R' = residual polynucleotide chains; Blm^* = "activated" bleomycin

BLM* has not been established but it is thought that the iron is bound to one or possibly two oxygen atoms [21].

In the presence of additional oxygen, BLM* reacts with DNA to produce base propenals. In its absence neither base propenals nor malonaldehyde are detected [22]. However, the same quantity of free heterocyclic bases is produced whether or not additional oxygen is present. Thus, diminished formation of base-propenals is not accompanied by a corresponding increase in the amount of free bases released. This important observation renders it unlikely that a common intermediate, such as the C-4′ radical, could serve as a source both of the free heterocyclic bases and the base propenals, as proposed by Wu *et al.* [23]. Nevertheless, both types of product appear to originate from attack at the C-4′ position of deoxyribose. Thus, Pathways A and B must arise at an earlier point in the reaction sequences.

The simplest mechanistic explanation of these results is that BLM* behaves dichotomously in its reaction at C-4′. The active complex may either produce radical *4* at C-4′, leading by oxygen capture to the base propenals via hydroperoxide *9* (Pathway A) or cause the insertion of a single oxygen atom (Pathway B) to form intermediate *6*. Available data suggest that BLM* is homogeneous [21], but it is possible that BLM* consists of two (or more) species, each giving rise to a different product.

The source of the electron or hydrogen atom necessary to accomplish the reduction of *5* in Pathway A is not apparent. It may be derived from bleomycin, thereby inactivating the antibiotic and accounting for the failure of bleomycin to act as a true catalyst (or enzyme) [20, 24]. Postulation of a caged radical at C-4′ would explain the failure of radical scavengers to inhibit DNA degradation [25, 26]. The possibility that BLM* presents an oxygen radical species in close proximity to DNA and reacts in some manner as to preclude scavenger intervention, has also been postulated by Rodriguez and Hecht [27].

The fragmentation reaction whereby *9* leads to *11* is a well-established reaction of aliphatic tertiary hydroperoxides [28] and is known to proceed by an acid-catalysed mechanism. The proton required for this reaction may be derived from the adjacent phosphate residue. Wu *et al.* [23] reported that proton abstraction at C-2′ is highly stereospecific. This observation is in accord with the mechanism proposed (*10→11*) since stereospecificity is a necessary requirement for a concerted reaction mechanism [29]. The overall scheme shown in Pathway A is supported by our earlier studies [1] on the rate of formation of the base propenals and is in agreement with the work of Burger *et al.* [22] who showed kinetically that two equivalents of O_2 are necessary for the formation of malonaldehyde (base propenal) derived from DNA.

With regard to the release of free bases, Pathway B is essentially identical to that recently proposed by Wu *et al.* [23]. As shown, this mechanism leads to the formation of alkali-labile sites, postulated generically as *8* (or its double hemi-acetal form). Isotope exchange studies [23] provide convincing evidence for the formation of a carbonyl group at C-4′. In contrast to Pathway A, DNA strand-scission does not occur when the bases are released.

Considered in a catalytic sense [20, 24], the reactions of BLM* with DNA display dual character. Single oxygen insertion (Pathway B) leads to products by a mechanism similar to that of the cytochrome oxidases. On the other hand, formation of base propenals, a reaction which involves an intermediate hydroperoxide (Pathway A), reflects the character of hydroperoxidases.

3. CHEMICAL REACTIVITY AND STRUCTURE-ACTIVITY RELATIONSHIPS

Our earlier observation that base propenals react with β-mercaptoethanol led to the recognition that these compounds are electrophiles which readily undergo addition-elimination in the presence of thiol or primary amino groups [1, 5]. The heterocyclic bases behave as excellent leaving groups, a property that seems not to have been widely recognized. At physiological pH, the rates of reaction of base propenals vary considerably, proceeding rapidly with β-mercaptoethanol or glutathione and slowly with primary amines such as β-aminoethanol [5]. It is probable that base propenals also form Schiff bases or cyclic amino-acetals.

Many aliphatic and aromatic aldehydes, especially those with a, β-unsaturation or which contain two aldehyde groups, are biologically active [30, 31]. a, β-unsaturated aldehydes readily undergo 1,4-addition reactions with nucleophiles and appear to exert biological activity by reacting with sulfhydryl, amino or possibly hydroxyl groups at a critical site. In effect, these substances behave as potentially reversible alkylating agents. Unsaturated aldehydes also may enter into 1,2-addition reactions to form diadducts; this mechanism includes crosslinking reactions and condensations with amino groups to yield Schiff bases.

Base propenals undergo 1,4-addition to form an intermediate anion, expelling the β substituent X (the heterocyclic base) to yield a more stable, a, β-unsaturated aldehyde (Pathway 1). This reaction differs from that observed with simple unsaturated aldehydes [31] where the intermediate anion is protonated (Pathway 2). At a biological site, the product could undergo crosslinking reactions by 1,2- (or 1,4-) addition provided that another nucleophile (e.g. an amino group) is available. Pathway 1 may not be thermodynamically reversible because of increased resonance energy effects in the conjugated system of the product (see Figure 4).

In effect, base propenals are masked forms of malonaldehyde. As such they are more reactive than malonaldehyde which tends to exist in aqueous solution as the highly stabilized anion $[O \doteq HC \doteq CH \doteq CH \doteq O]^-$. Thus, base propenals will form adducts under physiological conditions with simple nucleophiles such as glutathione, provided that the nucleophilic group is sterically accessible.

Based on these considerations, we carried out a limited structure-activity study of the base propenals by varying the nature of the heterocyclic base,

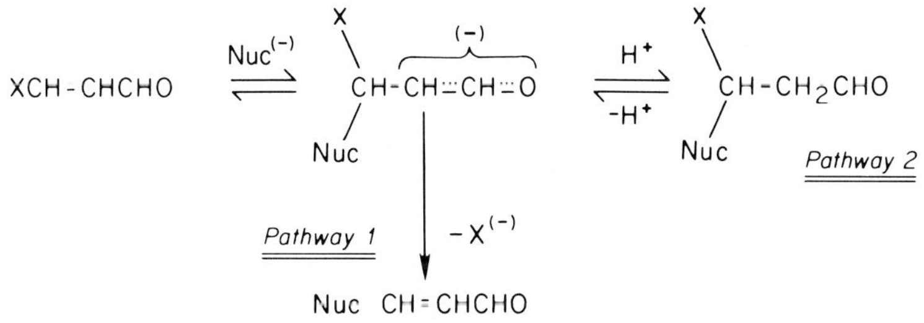

$$XCH-CHCHO \rightleftharpoons \begin{array}{c} X \\ \backslash \\ CH-CH \dot= CH \dot= O \\ / \\ Nuc \end{array} \xrightleftharpoons[-H^+]{H^+} \begin{array}{c} X \\ \backslash \\ CH-CH_2CHO \\ / \\ Nuc \end{array}$$

Nuc$^{(-)}$ $^{(-)}$ *Pathway 2*

Pathway 1 $-X^{(-)}$

Nuc CH=CHCHO

Figure 4

replacing the aldehyde group with other electron-withdrawing groups or altering the nuclear position of the three-carbon side chain. A series of nucleoside derivatives was prepared, in part, based on the expectation that introduction of a ribosyl or deoxyribosyl residue should provide site-direction to the molecule and that either N-1 or N-3 could serve as a point of substitution by the propenal moiety.

A number of compounds were synthesized and tested for their cytotoxic properties and ability to inhibit DNA, RNA and protein synthesis in HeLa cells. The structure-activity relationships established by these experiments [5] may be summarized as follows:

In the pyrimidine series, transposition of the propenal group from N-1 to N-3 increases the inhibitory effect, and compounds substituted at C-5 in the uracil nucleus exhibit reduced capacity to inhibit DNA synthesis ($CH_3 > H > F > CF_3 > CH_2OH$). Changes in the aldehyde group reduce ($COCH_3$), or abolish (CN), inhibition of macromolecular synthesis.

In the nucleoside series, those compounds having a 2'-deoxyribosyl group are highly cytotoxic and show markedly increased inhibition of DNA synthesis in HeLa cells. Compounds containing ribosyl or arabinosyl groups in place of deoxyribose show reduced ability to inhibit DNA synthesis. Replacement of the aldehyde group with an acetyl group reduces but does not abolish inhibitory activity whereas the related nitrile is inactive. The latter result emphasizes the need for a carbonyl group in the side chain.

The rates of reaction of *1a* and *13* with glutathione were similar [5]; and identical results were noted with aminoethanol. These data indicate that any differences between *1a* and *13* in biological activity are not related to chemical reactivity and suggests that the deoxynucleoside structure is responsible for the observed site-directive effects (Figure 5).

In summary, we draw the following tentative conclusions concerning structure-activity relationships: The location of the N-propenal group does not appear to be a crucial determinant of biological activity but 3-N-propenals are better inhibitors than those substituted at N-1. The presence of a 2'-deoxyribose moiety at N-1 in this series substantially enhances biological activity and increases selectivity of the compound, as measured by inhibi-

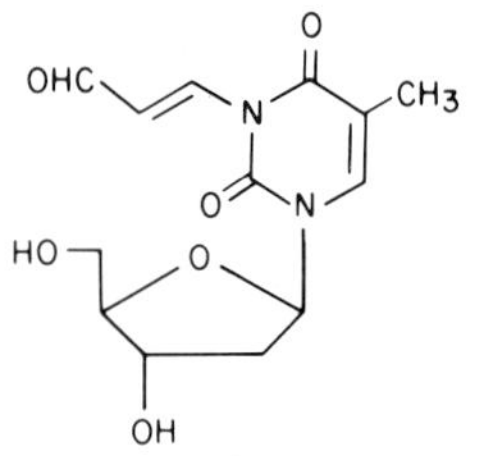

8

13

Figure 5

tion of incorporation of ^{3}H-thymidine into DNA. Biological activity, represented by inhibition of DNA synthesis and cytotoxicity, is optimized in
compound *13* in which a *trans*-propenal group is located at N-3 and the
sugar residue is 2′-deoxyribose. Significant changes in the aldehyde function
or substitution of cytosine or guanine for thymine or uracil markedly reduce
or abolish bioilogical activity. The site-directing properties of the deoxynucleoside residue suggests the design of new drugs in which toxiphores other
than propenals are attached to nucleoside or deoxynucleoside moieties.

4. CYTOTOXIC EFFECTS AND INHIBITION OF MACROMOLECULAR SYNTHESIS

The cytotoxic effects of the base propenals may be relevant to several
aspects of cancer chemotherapy. Thymine N-propenal (*1a*) and adenine N-
propenal (*1c*), substances derived by degrading DNA with bleomycin, are
highly cytotoxic, raising questions as to their possible involvement in the
cellular toxicity of this antibiotic. These compounds inhibited growth of
HeLa cells by 50% at concentrations of 1–2 µM while the IC_{50} for the cytosine (*1b*) and guanosine (*1d*) analogs were 15 and 25 µM, respectively [5].
Cytotoxicity was also determined by a procedure in which HeLa cells were
exposed to the inhibitor then tested for their ability to form colonies. The
IC_{50} for *1a* in this assay was 10 µM. Compounds *1a* and *1c* inhibited macromolecular synthesis in HeLa cells by 50% at somewhat higher concentrations than those which blocked cell growth. Both compounds showed selective inhibition of DNA synthesis, an effect which preceded inhibition of
RNA and protein synthesis in HeLa cells [4].
    Thymidine N-propenal (*13*), the most active of the deoxynucleoside pro-
penals tested, is considered a prototype for this series. This compound inhibited cell growth in cultures of L-1210 leukemia cells (1.6 µM), Lewis lung
carcinoma (5.9 µM), B-16 melanoma (4.2 µM) and human colon carcinoma
(5.0 µM) [4]. Inhibition of growth of L-1210 leukemia cells was not reversed
by the addition of deoxynucleosides. The IC_{50} for compound *13* in the

colony-forming assay was $1 \mu M$; the compound was also effective against L-1210 leukemia in mice [4].

Thymidine N-propenal did not affect uptake of ^{3}H-thymidine into HeLa cells but blocked the subsequent conversion of thymidine to TTP at concentrations of $< 1.0 \mu M$. The reduction product, thymidine N-propenol, was inactive, indicating the importance of the aldehyde moiety. Several enzymes are involved in converting thymidine to TTP in HeLa cells; one of these, thymidine kinase (pyrimidine deoxyribonucleoside kinase), is competitively inhibited by compound *13* ($K_1 = 5.1 \mu M$). The structural specificity observed is comparable with that of other inhibitors of this enzyme which, through conversion to their phosphorylated derivatives, act as selective inhibitors of viral replication [32].

5. BASE PROPENALS AND THE TOXICITY OF BLEOMYCIN

Damage to DNA is frequently implicated in discussions of the cytotoxic effects of this antibiotic [9, 11, 33, 34]. Nevertheless, a direct relationship between these phenomena has not been established. As noted in the introduction to this review, certain biological effects of bleomycin are not satisfactorily accounted for on the basis of DNA damage. For example, most drugs that inhibit DNA synthesis exhibit their effects almost exclusively during the S phase of the cell cycle [34–36] while bleomycin, inhibits cell growth during G_2 phase near the S-G2 boundary [cf. 7, 34]. In synchronized cultures, mitotic and G_2 phase cells are killed effectively by bleomycin; nondividing cells are even more sensitive. Cells treated in G1 and S phase appear to recover fully from bleomycin damage. Selective effects of base propenals on proteins involved in mitotic functions could acount for these effects, including reports [8, 37] in which cell killing by bleomycin occurs at concentrations of drug which do not inhibit DNA synthesis.

There is general agreement that therapeutic concentrations of bleomycin preferentially inhibit DNA synthesis in culture cells. Inhibition of macromolecular synthesis by bleomycin in HeLa cells [38] is quantitatively and qualitatively similar to those observed in cells treated with base propenals [4]. Based on the reaction mechanism outlined in Scheme 1, stoichiometric amounts of base propenals may be formed for each mole of bleomycin involved in strand scission. These substances, presumably liberated during strand scission of DNA, could react with DNA polymerase, a sulfhydryl-containing nuclear enzyme which is known to be sensitive to the effect of reactive aldehydes [31, 39] and aldehyde-related substances [40].

Pulmonary fibrosis is an important toxic effect of bleomycin in man [9]. This pathology has been reported to occur with certain other antitumor drugs [41]. We postulate that liberation of base propenals and their subsequent reaction with proteins or enzymes initiates this pathological process. An enzyme (bleomycin hydrolase) has been described [42] which inactivates bleomycin in various organs and is absent from lung and skin, insuring that higher concentrations of the antibiotic [42, 43] and, therefore, base propenals, would accumulate in these tissues.

Although most of the cytotoxic effects of bleomycin can be fully explained on the basis of intranuclear generation of cytotoxic base propenals, DNA damage may contribute to the cellular toxicity of the drug. Breaks, gaps, deletions and other chromosomal abberations have been reported in bleomycin-treated cells [34]. It is also known that the oligodeoxynucleotide fragments produced by the action of the antibiotic are resistant to the effect of certain intracellular phosphatases and are inactive as template for the DNA polymerase of E. coli [44]. Bleomycin-induced damage to DNA can apparently be repaired [cf. 34] but even under such conditions, cells do not always survive [7], suggesting that effects other than strand scission are involved. More studies are required to determine if the effects of bleomycin on chromosomes are related to cell killing or other cytotoxic properties of the drug.

ACKNOWLEDGEMENTS

The authors are grateful to Dr. Masaru Takeshita and Dr. Radhakrishna Pillal for many helpful discussions during the preparation of this paper. We are also indebted to Ms. Jeneane Dunn for expert assistance in preparing this manuscript.

Studies described in this review were supported, in part, by Grant CH-240 from the American Cancer Society and Grant CA 17395 from the National Institutes of Health.

REFERENCES

1. Giloni L, Takeshita M, Johnson F, Iden C, Grollman AP: Bleomycin-induced strand-scission of DNA: Mechanism of deoxyribose cleavage. J Biol Chem 256:8606–8615, 1981.
2. Takeshita M, Grollman AP: A molecular basis for the interaction of bleomycin with DNA. In: Hecht S (ed), Bleomycin: Chemical, Biochemical and Biological Aspects. 207–221, 1979, Springer-Verlag, New York.
3. Elion GB, Freeman PA, Fyfe JA, deMiranda P, Beauchapm L, Schaeffer HJ: Selectivity of action of an antiherpetic agent, 9-(2-hydroxyethoxymethyl)guanine. Proc Natl Acad Sci 74:5716–5720, 1977.
4. Takeshita M, Johnson F, Pillal KMR, Grollman AP: Base propenals from DNA: their

origin and cytotoxic properties. Cancer Res 1984 (in press).

5. Johnson F, Pillal KMR, Grollman AP, Tseng L, Takeshita M: Synthesis and biological activities of a new class of cytotoxic agents: N-(3-Oxoprop-1-enyl)-substituted pyrimidines and purines. J Med Chem 1984 (in press).

6. Alarcon RA, Meinhofer J: Formation of the cytotoxic aldehyde acrolein during *in vitro* degradation of cyclophosphamide. Nature (London), 233:250–252, 1971.

7. Barranco SC: A review of the survival and cell-kinetics and effects of bleomycin. In: Carter SK, Crooke ST, Umezawa H (eds), Bleomycin: Current Status and New Developments. pp 81–90, 1978, Academic Press, New York.

8. Cohen S, I, J: Synthesis and the lethality of bleomycin in bacteria. Cancer Research 36:2768–2774, 1976.

9. Chabner B: Bleomycin. In: Chabner BA (ed), Pharmacologic Principles of Cancer Treatment. W.B. 377–386, Saunders Phildelphia, 1982.

10. Takeshita M, Grollman AP: Interaction of bleomycin with DNA. In: Wever G (ed), Advances in Enzyme Regulation. 18:673–683, 1980, Pergamon Press.

11. Haidle CW, Lloyd RS: Bleomycin. In: Hahn FE (ed), Antibiotics: Mechanism of Action of Antieukaryotic and Antiviral Compounds. Vol. V:124–254, 1979, Springer-Verlag, New York.

12. Burger RM, Peisach J, Horwitz SB: Mechanisms of bleomycin action: *in vitro* studies. Life Sciences 28:715–727,1981.

13. Haidle CW: Fragmentation of deoxyribonucleic acid by bleomycin. Mol Pharmacol 7:645–652, 1971.

14. Haidle CW, Weiss KK, Kuo MT: Release of free bases from deoxyribonucleic acid after reaction with bleomycin. Mol Pharmacol 9:531–537, 1972.

15. Gutteridge JMC: Identification of malondialdehyde as the TBA-reactant formed by bleomycin-iron free radical damage to DNA. FEBS Lett 105:278–282, 1979.

16. Muller WEG, Yamazaki Z, Breter HJ, Zahn RK: Action of bleomycin on DNA and RNA. Eur J Biochem 31:518–525, 1972.

17. Kuo MT, Haidle CW: Characterization of chain breakage in DNA induced by bleomycin. Biochim Biophys Acta 335:109–114, 1974.

18. Burger RM, Peisach J, Horwitz SB: Stoichiometry of DNA strand-scission and aldehyde formation by bleomycin. J Biol Chem 257:8612–8614, 1982.

19. Burger RM, Peisach J, Blumberg WE, Horwitz SB: Iron-bleomycin interactions with oxygen and oxygen analogues. Effects on spectra and drug activity. J Biol Chem 254:10906–10912, 1979.

20. Caspary WJ, Niziak C, Lanzo DA, Friedman R, Bachur NR: Bleomycin A_2: A ferrous oxidase. Mol Pharmacol 16:256–260, 1979.

21. Burger RM, Peisach J, Horwitz SB: Activated bleomycin: a transient complex of drug, iron and oxygen that degrades DNA. J Biol Chem 256:11636–11644, 1981.

22. Burger RM, Peisach J, Horwitz SB: Effects of O_2 on the reactions of activated bleomycin. J Biol Chem 257:3372–3375, 1982.

23. Wu JC, Kozarich JW, Stubbe J: Mechanism of free base formation from DNA by bleomycin. A proposal based on site-specific tritium release from poly (dA-dU). J Biol Chem 258:4694–4697, 1983.

24. Povirk LF: Catalytic release of deoxyribonucleic acid bases by oxidation and reduction of an iron-bleomycin complex. Biochemistry 18:3989–3995, 1979.

25. Sausville EA, Stein RW, Peisach J, Horwitz SB: Properties and products of the degradation of DNA by bleomycin and iron (II). Biochemistry 17:2746–2754, 1978.

26. Ishida R, Takahashi T: Increased DNA chain breakage by combined action of bleomycin and superoxide radical. Biochem Biophys Res Commun 66:1432–1438, 1975.

27. Rodriguez LO, Hecht SM: Iron (II)-bleomycin. Biochemical and spectral properties in the

12

presence of radical scavengers. Biochem Biophys Res Commun 104:1470–1476, 1982.

28. Deno NC, Billups WW, Kramer KE, Lastomusky RR: The rearrangement of aliphatic primary, secondary and tertiary hydroperoxides in strong acid. J Org Chem 35:3080–3082, 1970.

29. Grob CA, Scheiss PW: Heterocyclic fragmentation. A class of organic reactions. Angew Chemie Int Ed 6:1–15, 1967.

30. Schauenstein E, Esterbauer H: Formation and properties of reactive aldehydes. In: Submolecular Biology and Cancer. CIBA Foundation Symposium 67:225–244, 1979.

31. Schauenstein E, Esterbauer H, Zollner H: Aldehydes in Biological Systems: Their Natural Occurrence and Biological Activities. Pion Press, London, 1977.

32. Smith RA, Sidwell RW, Robins RK: Antiviral mechanisms of action. Ann Rev Pharmacol Toxicol 20:259–284, 1980.

33. Umezawa H: Bleomycin in Antibiotics III: Mechanism of Action of Antimicrobial and Antitumor Agents. Corcoran JW, Hahn FE (ed). Springer-Verlag, New York, pp 21–33, 1975.

34. Vig BK, Lewis R: Genetic Toxicology of Bleomycin. Mutation Research 55:121–145, 1978.

35. Madoc-Jones H, Mauro F: Site of action of cytotoxic agents in the cell life cycle. In: Sartorelli AC, Johns DG (eds), Antineoplastic and Immunosuppressive Agents. 38/1:205–219, 1974.

36. Hoffman J Post J: The effect of antitumor drugs in the cell cycle. In: Zimmerman TM, Padilla GD, Cameron IL (ed), Drugs and the Cell Cycle. Academic Press, New York, pp 219–247, 1973.

37. Tobey RA: Arrest of Chinese hamster cells in G_2 following treatment with the anti-tumor drug bleomycin. J Cell Physiol 79:259–265, 1972.

38. Takeshita M, Horwitz SB, Grollman AP: Bleomycin, an inhibitor of vaccinia virus replication. Virology 60:455–465, 1974.

39. Suzuki K, Miyaki M, Umeda M, Nishimura M, Ono T: Differential inactivation of DNA polymerases α and β by aldehyde compounds. Biochem Biophys Res Comm 100:1626–1633, 1981.

40. Sugimoto Y, Suzuki H, Yamaki H, Nishimura T, Tanaka N: Mechanism of action of 2-crotonyloxymethyl-4, 5, 6-trihydroxyxycyclohex-2-eone, a SH inhibitory antitumore antibiotic, ant its effect on drugresistant neoplastic cells. J Antibiotics 35:1222–1230, 1982.

41. Weiss RB, Muggia FM: Cytotoxic drug-induced pulmonary disease: update 1980. Am J Med 68:259–266, 1980.

42. Umezawa H, Takeuchi T, Hori S, Sawa T, Ishizuka M, Ichikawa T, Kanal T: Studies on the mechanism of the antitumor effect of bleomycin on squamous cell carcinoma. J Antibiot 25:409–420, 1972.

43. Lazo JS, Humphreys CJ: Lack of metabolism as the biochemical basis of bleomycin-induced pulmonary toxicity. Proc Nat Acad Sci 80:3064–3068, 1983.

44. Niwa O, Moses RE: Synthesis by DNA Polymerase I on bleomycin-treated deoxyribonucleic acid: A requirement for Exonuclease III. Biochemistry 20:238–244, 1981.

2. Lipid Macromolecules as Chemotherapeutic Target

DAVID W. YESAIR

SUMMARY

The macromolecular lipids were discovered in 1962 when they were found to complex with the antineoplastic phthalanilide drugs. These lipids are distributed ubiquitously in mammalian tissues, principally in the nucleoplasm of the cell and are found also in *E. coli B* and a parasite, *Anaplasma marginale*. The extent of the complex formation between the phthalanilides and the macromolecular lipids relate to both therapy and toxicity of the drugs. At low phthalanilide intracellular concentrations, there was extensive inhibition of both DNA and protein but minimal chemotherapeutic response. Lipid and RNA synthesis was inhibited at therapeutic intracellular concentrations of drugs.

The macromolecular lipids were shown to complex with those antineoplastic drugs which intercalate with DNA; for example, doxorubicin and the amino-anthraquinones. These drugs, which are not cross-resistant to the phthalanilides, complex with the macromolecular lipids from phthalanilide resistant cells whereas binding of cross-resistant drugs was not possible. In addition, the association constants for the chemotherapeutically inactive aminoanthraquinones were an order of magnitude less than that found for the *in vivo* active compounds. The macromolecular lipids bind the polyamines; spermine, spermidine and the diamines, histones and polyvalent cations. The binding characteristics of the macromolecular lipids from multiple sources indicate that the lipids are not all equivalent in binding diverse groups of chemotherapeutic agents, polyamines and cations and that multiple binding regions can be present on the lipids from a specific source of lipid.

The most striking physical and chemical characteristics of the macromolecular lipids are its large molecular weight, $> 15,000$; ultraviolet and fluorescent chromophor; a glycerol phosphonate/phosphate backbone, cytosine

F.M. Muggia (ed.), Experimental and Clinical Progress in Cancer Chemotherapy
© *1985, Martinus Nijhoff Publishers, Boston. ISBN 0-89838-679-9. Printed in the Netherlands.*

and possibly guanine constituents as well as hexoses and amino acids. These components provide a hydrophilic region which complement the fatty acid hydrophobic region.

A unique structure has been proposed for the macromolecular lipids, based upon the elemental and component analyses, molecular weight and the competitive displacement amoung the polyamines and the chemotherapeutic drugs. An important feature of this proposed structure is the diversity that it can have with respect to size, molecular organization of the components and binding of a variety of compounds. The potential diversity in its structure is compatible with the conclusion that the molecular lipids from different tissues and organisms are not identical, yet have many similarities.

A functional role for the macromolecular lipids in the expression of genetic material has been proposed. Specific macromolecular lipids may be synthesized *de novo* within the nucleoplasm of the nucleus during the transition from the repressed chromatin to active chromatin. These lipids then effect a shift in the interactions among DNA, histones, acidic protein and polyamines. Eventually the transcribed RNA interacts with the 'coded' macromolecular lipid, which is then transported from the nucleus to the cytoplasm.

This proposed role of the 'coded' macromolecular lipids in the regulation of gene expression, the unique structure of the macromolecular lipids and their specificity for binding polyamines and drugs indicate that these lipids represent a new mechanism for drug discovery. Several classes of drugs are discussed in terms of their potential for binding with the macromolecular lipids.

INTRODUCTION

Discovery of the Macromolecular Lipids

The terephthalanilides (Figure 1) were a new class of antineoplastic agents in 1962 [1] and were highly active against animal leukemias [2–6]. In clinical trials early toxic symptoms such as oculomotor paralysis and thrombophlebitis limited the clinical evaluation of this group of compounds against human neoplasms [7, 8]. These early clinical toxic responses were followed by delayed and/or chronic renal toxicity in humans [9]. The toxic responses that were observed in humans were also demonstrated in animals [9].

The initial method of analysis for the terephthalanilides in tissues required extraction of drug with ethanolic levulinic acid and subsequent chromatographic separation of the drug from biological contaminants on DEAE cellulose [10]. When this method was used for analysis of the terephthalan-

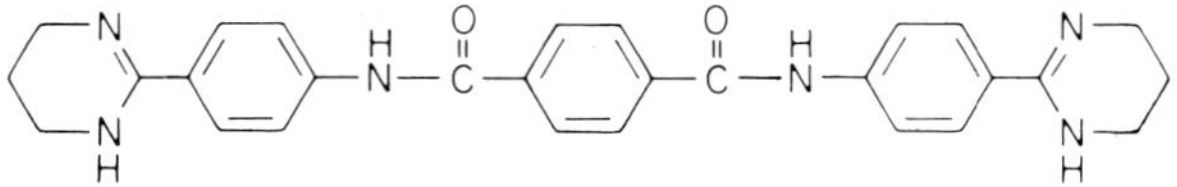

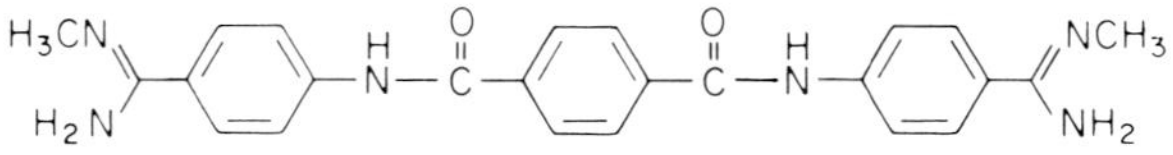

NSC 53313

4',4''-Bis (N'-methylamidino) Terephthalanilide

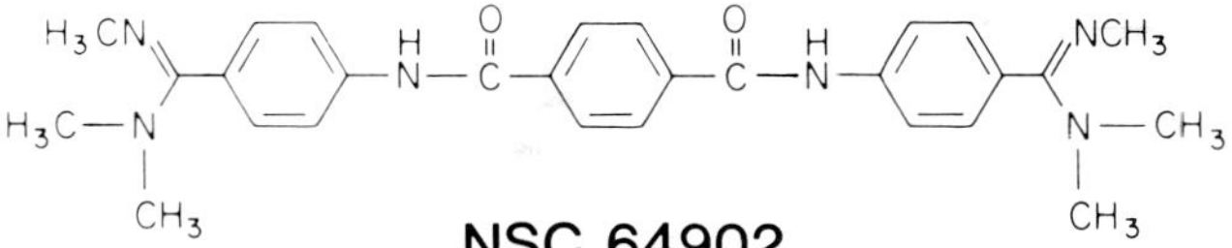

NSC 64902

4',4''-Bis (trimethylamidino) Terephthalanilide

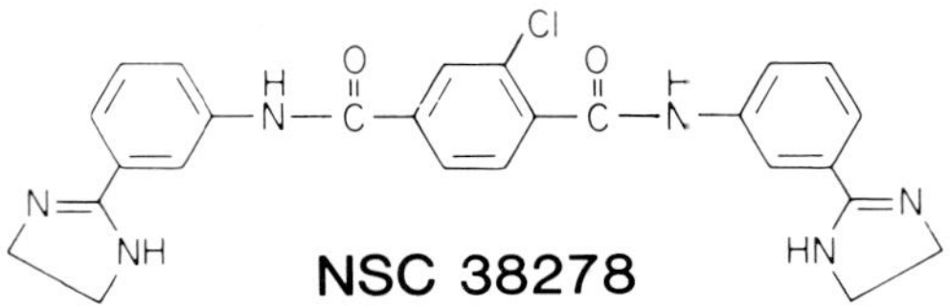

NSC 38278

2-chloro-3',3''-Di 2-imidazolin-2-yl) Terephthalanilide

NSC 57153

4',4''-Bis (1,4,5,6-tetrahydro-2-pyrimidinyl) Terephthalanilide

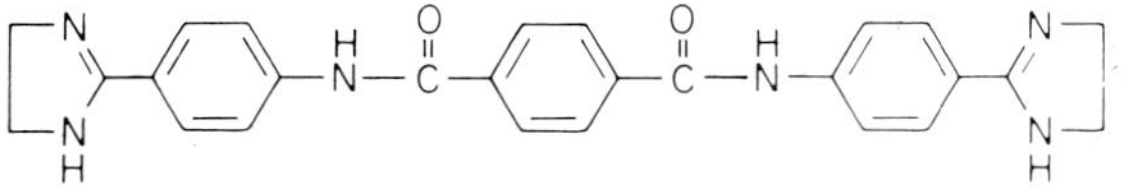

NSC 35843

4',4''-Di (2-imidazolin-2-yl) Terephthalanilide

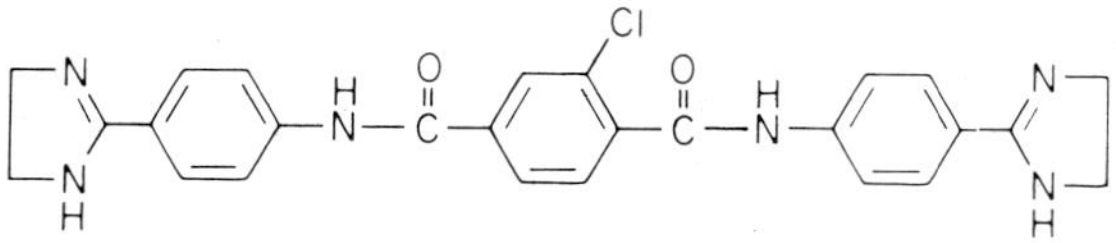

NSC 38280

2-chloro-4',4''-Di(2-imidazolin-2-yl) Terephthalanilide

Figure 1. Structures of the substituted phthalanilides.

ilides in ocular motor muscle, optic nerve and brain in order to define the
basis for the ocular motor paralysis, the alcoholic levulinic acid extraction
of these tissues solubilized considerable quantities of lipid. The extracted
lipid prevented the subsequent chromatographic separation of drug from
contaminants. When the lipid-extraction procedure of Folch *et al.* [11] was
used, the phthalanilides, which stayed in the aqueous phase in the absence
of tissues, partitioned to the nonaqueous phase and were associated with
lipid (see page 1360 of reference 12). These findings were totally unexpected
and especially noteworthy since muscle, nerve and brain were equivalent in
binding the drug to lipid and since protein [10] and nucleic acid [13–16]
were known to bind the terephthalanilides.

Hirt and Berchtold [1] first described the substituted phthalanilides as
'phosphatide blockers'. These investigators employed a simple biophysical
model: lecithin (phosphatidyl choline) dissolved in carbon tetrachloride
promotes the transport of cationic dyes from an aqueous solution into the
lipid phase. They showed that the phthalanilides maximally inhibited dye
transfer when at least two strongly basic groups are connected by several
coplanar rings and by carbonamide groups. Subsequently, many known
lipids (Table 1) [17, 18] were evaluated for their ability to form complexes
with the substituted phthalanilides NSC 57153, NSC 38280, and
NSC 35843. Those lipids, which formed complexes with the substituted

Table 1. Ability of known lipids to form complexes with the substituted phthalanilides

Phosphalipids	Complex formed
Phosphatidic acid	Yes
Phosphatidyl choline	No
Phosphatidyl serine	Yes
Phosphatidyl ethanolamine	No
Phosphatidyl inositol	Yes
Phsophatidyl glycerol	Yes
Diphosphatidyl glycerol	Yes
Sphingomyelin	No

Other Lipids	
Cerebroside	No
Ganglioside	No
Sulfatide	Yes
Taurocholate	Yes
Palmitic acid	No
Retinoic acid	No
Tripalmitin	No
Cholesterol	No

phthalanilides, required approximately 2 to 3 moles of lipid per mole of drug indicating an ionic interaction between the anionic groups of the lipid and the cationic groups of the substituted phthalanilides. These complexes can be dissociated by cations, protons and by the zwiterionic phosphatidyl choline [17].

These findings strongly implied that the known lipids may be the complexing species when the substituted phthalanilides were extracted from tissues into chloroform-methanol solutions. However, later studies which define the physical and chemical characteristics of the complexing lipid from tissues and leukemic cells [17–24] proved unequivocally that the binding lipid was a new class of macromolecular phospholipid which was ubiquitous in all tissues.

Ubiquitous Distribution and Intracellular Localization of the Macromolecular Lipids

The substituted phthalanilides were first shown to complex with lipids from brain, optic nerve and ocular motor muscle *in vitro* [12]. Were such complexes obtained from tissues and tumors of animals and humans when the drug was administered intravenously? As shown in Table 2, all tissues and tumors with the exception of red blood cells contained the macromolecular

Table 2. Extraction of substituted phthalanilide — macromolecular lipid complexes from normal tissues, tumors and microorganisms

Species[a]	Normal tissues	Tumors	Microorganisms
		Animals[b]	
Human	Liver	L1210	*Escherichia coli* B
Mouse	Kidney	L1210/MTX	*Anaplamsa marginale*
Rat	Heart	L1210/araC	
Dog	Muscle	P388	
Monkey	Gastrocnemius	P815	
Chick Embryo	Ocular	Dunning	
	Spleen	L1210/NSC 60339	
	Lung	P388/NSC 60339	
	G.I. Tract	P388/VCR	
	white blood cells	P388/VLB	
	Bone Marrow		
		Humans	
		Acute myeloblastic leukemia (AML)	
		Acute lymphocytic leukemia (ALL)	
		Various solid tumors	

[a] The drug was administered intravenously to the species except for chick embryo.
[b] The tumor cell lines are either resistant or sensitive to the listed agent.

lipids [9, 21–26]. In addition, the macromolecular lipids were found in two microorganisms and in chick embryos at 3 days of incubation. The lipids of chick embryos increased in absolute amount up to 21 days of incubation. However, the concentration of extractable drug-lipid complexes in heart, liver, kidney and brain decreased with age (12 to 21 days of incubation) indicating that the macromolecular lipids are associated with rapid growth as well as with adult tissues. The egg prior to incubation does not have any drug-binding capacity. These findings indicate a *de novo* synthesis of the macromolecular lipids which would be similar to the *de novo* synthesis of the known phospholipids in the chick embryo [27].

Another important feature of the macromolecular lipids may relate to the long retention of the terephthalanilides by selected body tissues. Humans, who received the last dose of NSC 60339 which is the base of NSC 38280 (Figure 1) 64 and 164 days prior to death, had considerable quantities of drug in heart, pectoral and oculomotor muscles and kidney. The other tissues showed little or no drug at these time periods, but drug was extracted as a complex from these tissues at shorter times following administration of the drug to both humans and animals [21]. These differences among tissues in their retention of drug by the macromolecular lipids may indicate differences in these lipids among tissues. In this context differences were especially noteworthy in the macromolecular lipids from terephthalanilide-sensitive and -resistant leukemic tumors [20, 23–25]. The drug-lipid complexes from the resistant tumors were more hydrophobic than those from sensitive tumors [23, 24], effluxed faster from the cell [23–25] and had a higher molecular weight [20].

Since the macromolecular lipids were ubiquitous in their distribution among tissues and tumors, we evaluated the intracellular distribution of these lipids [23]. This aspect was evaluated by several different methods. Leukemic cells were first treated with the phthalanilides *in vivo* and the macromolecular lipid and drug complexes were extracted from the cell fractions at 0.5 and 24 hours after administration of drug. By a second method, the cells were first fractionated into their cellular fractions, the lipids were extracted and the drug-lipid complexes were formed in the organic extract. Either method demonstrated that the nuclear and, to a lesser extent, the mitochondrial fractions contained the macromolecular lipids. Microsomes, which contain the greatest percentage of the cellular lipids, had minimal concentrations of the macromolecular lipids. Some unpublished studies with my colleague (Dr. Paul Baronowsky) have shown that the macromolecular lipid was primarily extracted from the extended chromatin rather than the condensed chromatin fraction of the nucleus. In a subsequent and preliminary report [28], the majority of the binding of drug occurred with the lipids which were extracted from the nuclei and, to a lesser extent, from

CAIN QUINOLINIUMS

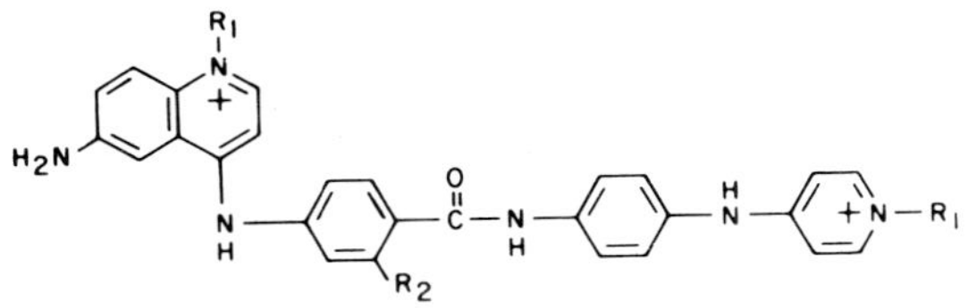

NSC 114347 $R_1 = -CH_3$, $R_2 = -NH_2$

NSC 113089 $R_1 = -CH_2CH_3$, $R_2 = -H$

CARBANILIDE

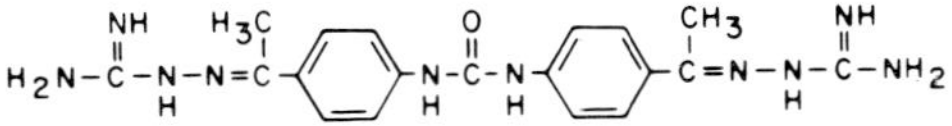

NSC 109555

AMINOANTHRAQUINONES

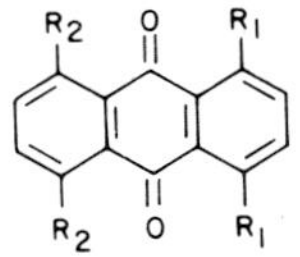

COMPOUND	R_1	R_2
NSC 287513	$-NH(CH_2)_2NH(CH_2)_2OH$	– H
NSC 279836	$-NH(CH_2)_2NH(CH_2)_2OH$	– OH
NSC 281246	$-NH(CH_2)_2NH_2$	– H
NSC 281249	$-NH(CH_2)_2NH(CH_2)_2NH(CH_2)_2OH$	– H
NSC 278467	$-NH(CH_2)_3NH(CH_2)_2OH$	– H
NSC 279837	$-NH(CH_2)_2$ N⟨ ⟩NH	– H

DOXORUBICIN
ADRIAMYCIN

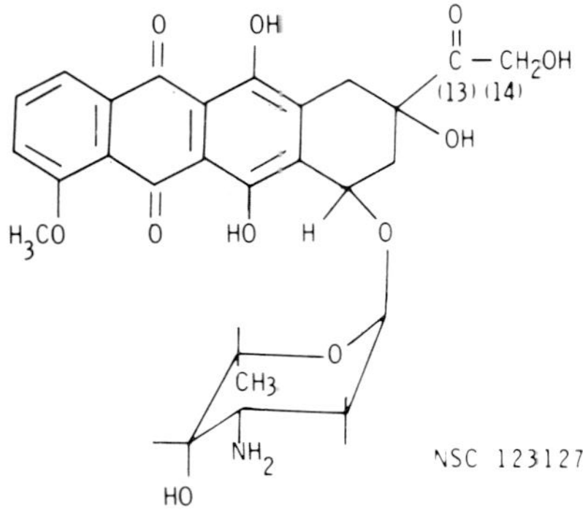

NSC 123127

Figure 2. Antineoplastic drugs which complex with the macromolecular lipids from various tissues and tumors.

SPERMINE

$H_2NCH_2CH_2CH_2NHCH_2CH_2CH_2CH_2NHCH_2CH_2CH_2NH$

SPERMIDINE

$H_2NCH_2CH_2CH_2NHCH_2CH_2CH_2CH_2NH_2$

PUTRESCINE

$H_2NCH_2CH_2CH_2CH_2NH_2$

CADAVERINE

$H_2NCH_2CH_2CH_2CH_2CH_2NH_2$

Figure 3. Natural products which complex with macromolecular lipids isolated from tumor cells.

mitochondria of phthalanilide-sensitive and -resistant L1210 cells and doxorubicin (NSC 123127) -sensitive and -resistant P388 cells. Further fractionation of the nuclei from both NSC 60339 and NSC 123127 cell-types demonstrated that approximately three times more drug was bound by lipids from the nucleoplasm than from the nuclear envelopes. In this case, the nuclei and nuclear envelopes were examined by electron microscopy to assure their homogeneity. The drugs which were complexed with the extracted lipids from these cellular fractions [28] were NSC 38280 (Figure 1), NSC 113089 (Figure 2), NSC 287513 (Figure 2), doxorubicin (NSC 123127, Figure 2), and spermine (Figure 3).

Therapy and Toxicity of Phthalanilides and Their Binding to Macromolecular Lipids

The ubiquitous distribution of the macromolecular lipids and their primary localization in the nucleoplasm and mitrochondria of leukemic cells may indicate that these lipids have a role in the therapeutic response of those drugs which are extracted as macromolecular lipid complexes.

The antileukemic phthalanilide, NSC 60339 which is the base of NSC 38280 (Figure 1) is taken up by P388 lymphocytic leukemic cells growing in culture [23–25]. The uptake was related to the extracellular concentration of drug and the length of exposure to drug (Table 3) [24]. As shown in Figure 4, the concentration of the extracted macromolecular lipid-bound phthalanilide was correlated significantly with the chemotherapeutic response. Further, the retention and efflux of lipid-bound phthalanilide, NSC 60339, was correlated with the sensitivity (retention), resistance and cross-resistance (efflux) of many animal tumors [23, 25]. In addition, many phthalanilides were active against *Escherichia coli* [16, 29, 30]. Drug-lipid complexes were

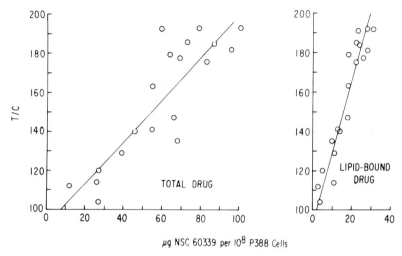

Figure 4. The relationship of chemotherapy (T/C) and the concentration of total and lipid-bound NSC 60339 in P388 leukemic cells.

extracted from *E. coli B* after treatment with the phthalanilide, NSC 60339 [25]. The treatment schedule of 30 μg NSC 60339 per ml for 90 minutes caused the cessation of growth. However, when the treated microbial cells were diluted and plated onto agar, colonies appeared. This indicates that this concentration of NSC 60339 was bacteriostatic and perhaps that the phthalanilide-lipid complexes could efflux from the cell. These results

Table 3. Relationship of uptake and chemotherapeutic effect of NSC 60339 to its extracellular concentration and its duration of exposure of P388 cells growing in culture

μg NSC 60339 pr ml medium	Time hr.	μg NSC 60339/10⁸ Cells		Average growth inhibition [a]	T/C [b]
		Total	Bound drug		
1	18	12	7	21	112
2	18	25	15	37	117
5	18	60	25	69	144
8	18	72	45	70	185
16	18	107	76	82	191
40	4	50	29	—	134
20	8	61	35	—	152
14	12	61	40	—	168

[a] Growth inhibition was obtained by dividing the difference in total cells (control minus treated) by the change in the number of control cells during the 18-hr. growth period (control cells at 18 hr. minus control cells at 0 hr.) multiplied by 100.

[b] Average T/C for inocula of 10^6 and 10^5 cells, each into 10 BDF$_1$ female mice.

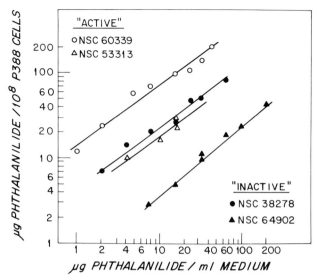

Figure 5. Comparative uptake of 'active' and 'inactive' terephthalanilide congeners by P388 leukemic cells treated *in vitro* for 18 hours.

were similar to those for the phthalanilide-resistant and -cross resistant tumors.

The terephthalanilides, NSC 38278 and 64902 (Figure 1) that are inactive in affecting chemotherapy *in vivo* do complex with the macromolecular lipids and are similar in characteristics to their *in vivo* active congeners, NSC 60339 and NSC 53313, respectively. The uptake of these inactive terephthalanilides by P388 cells growing *in vitro* was comparable to the active congeners when the extracellular concentrations of the inactive congeners were five to eight times that of the active drugs (Figure 5) [31]. Comparable chemotherapy with these 'active' and 'inactive' terephthalanilides was demonstrated after first exposing the leukemic cells *in vitro* and bioassaying the treated cells *in vivo*. Chemotherapy *in vivo* with the 'inactive' terephthalanilides was not possible at nontoxic doses, noting that the 'inactive' terephthalanilides were at least five times more toxic than the 'active' congeners *in vivo*. Thus the inactive terephthalanilides do not produce sufficiently high drug levels in the tumor cells at doses tolerated by the host.

Some effort has been made to minimize the toxic effects of the phthalanilides without sacrificing chemotherapeutic activity. Burchenal and coworkers [32, 33] showed that the acute and chronic activity of several phthalanilides can be prevented by complexing the phthalanilides with sulfonic and phosphoric compounds, but all these agents, except suramin, also blocked the antileukemic activity of the phthalanilides in mice. It was subsequently demonstrated [34] that the administration of suramin does not affect the uptake of the terephthalanilide, NSC 57153 (Figure 1) in P815 cells but does result in lower drug concentrations in the kidney and liver of tumor bearing mice. The terephthalanilides are complexed primarily with the macromolecular lipids in these tissues [21, 22] as in P388 cells. Since suramin is not deposited in any particular tissue, it probably enhances the excretion of the terephthalanilide as a suramin complex before deposition of NSC 57153 as a lipid complex in tissues.

The Biochemical Effects of the Phthalanilides Binding to the Macromolecular Lipids

Biochemical studies have indicated that DNA, RNA, protein and lipid syntheses were inhibited after phthalanilide treatment of leukemia cells either in cell culture or in BDF$_1$ mice [12, 14, 30, 35–37]. In addition, at high concentrations, NSC 57153 and NSC 60339 (Figure 1) inhibited oxidative phosphorylation in mitochondria of tissues from animals [38, 39].

In studies with P388 cells exposed to NSC 60339 for 18 hours *in vitro* [24], the degree of inhibition of biosynthetic pathways was compared with intracellular concentration of drug and with chemotherapy (Figure 6).

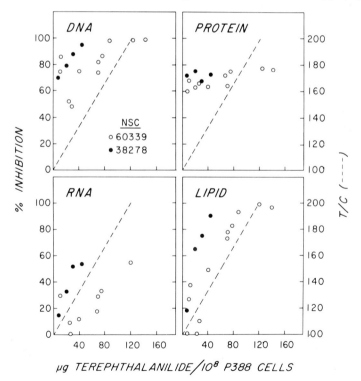

Figure 6. Inhibition of biosynthetic processes in P388 cells by 'active' NSC 60339 and 'inactive' NSC 38278 as related to chemotherapeutic response.

The incorporation of thymidine into DNA and valine into protein was strongly inhibited at low intracellular drug concentrations of both 'active' and 'inactive' phthalanilides. Further increases in drug concentration did not significantly increase the 60 to 70% inhibition of valine incorporation into protein whereas inhibition of thymidine incorporation into DNA reached the >95% level at about 80 $\mu g/10^8$ P388 cells for the 'active' NSC 60339 and at about 40 $\mu g/10^8$ P388 cells for the 'inactive' NSC 60339. In spite of the extensive inhibition of nucleic acid and protein synthesis at the low (<20 $\mu g/10^8$ cells) intracellular concentrations of phthalanilide, the chemotherapeutic response was minimal. Uridine incorporation into RNA and acetate incorporation into lipid were not significantly inhibited at these low intracellular drug concentrations but were inhibited at higher drug concentrations. The inhibition of both RNA and lipid synthesis was greater with the 'inactive' phthalanilide, NSC 38278 than with the 'active' NSC 60339. The drugs in both cases were extracted primarily as drug-lipid complexes, and of the drug taken up by the cells, the percentage of 'inactive' NSC 38278 as lipid complex (ca 90%) was higher than the 'active' NSC 60339 (ca 60%) [24, 31]. Since there are multiple binding regions on the macromolecular lipids [19], one might anticipate qualitative differences in the binding of the 'inactive' NSC 38278 and the 'active' NSC 60339 at low intracellular drug concentrations, i.e., nonsaturation of the bound macromolecular lipids. Any qualitative differences in binding by these two congeners may contribute to the differences that are seen in the biochemical effects.

The lipid content and composition of cell nuclei and intranuclear fractions have been described for a variety of tissues [40–50]. Frenster [44] and Rose *et al.* [49] have shown that the chromatin fraction, active in RNA synthesis, is rich in phospholipids. They have suggested that phospholipids along with nonhistone protein may function as derepressors by affecting the histone-DNA interaction [49]. We have suggested [12, 24, 51] that histones may interact with the macromolecular lipids which complex with the phthalanilides and may be displaced by phthalanilides. In this regard, the chemotherapeutic and biochemical data in Figure 6 may be interpreted with reference to the phthalanilides affecting a phospholipid-histone-DNA equilibrium within the nucleoplasm of the nucleus. Substantial inhibition of DNA and protein synthesis occurs at drug concentrations which do not depress lipid and RNA synthesis or result in cell death (Figure 6). Therefore, these inhibitions must be reversible. An explanation of these findings at low drug concentrations is that new macromolecular lipid is synthesized to effect the histone-DNA equilibrium towards a histone-macromolecular lipid complex and the transcription of DNA. At high drug concentrations, the synthesis of macromolecular lipids is inhibited, thus maintaining the repressed state, i.e., a histone-DNA complex and a macromolecular lipid-drug complex. Gellhorn *et al.* [35] postulated that the depression of lipid biosyn-thesis may be the primary mechanism of antileukemic action of the phthal-anilides.

BINDING CHARACTERISTICS OF THE MACROMOLECULAR LIPIDS

Cancer Chemotherapeutic Drugs
When the terephthalanilides were first demonstrated to complex with lipids, a large number of these structurally related compounds were evaluated for their potential binding with macromolecular lipids which were isolated from tumor cells and normal tissues. Representatives of the phthalanilides, which were synthesized by several groups [1, 15, 16, 52–55], are shown in Figure 1. Phthalanilide congeners, which were active or inactive *in vivo*, were shown to bind with the macromolecular lipids from several sources [17–26, 28, 31, 34, 51, 56], including leukemic cells which were resistant and cross-resistant to the phthalanilides [17, 25] and resistant to many other conventional agents [25, 28].

When highly purified macromolecular lipids were obtained from both phthalanilide sensitive and resistant cell lines, we found substantial differ-ences in the drug-binding characteristics among the lipids from these cell lines [20]. Briefly, a type of macromolecular lipid from the resistant line, designated A_r, did not bind the phthalanilides (Table 4). Further, this same lipid-type did not bind those chemotherapeutic agents which were cross-resistant with the phthalanilides, NSC 38280, for example, a terephthalanil-ide, NSC 35843 (Figure 1), Cain quinoliniums, NSC 114347 and NSC 113089 [52–55] (Figure 2), and a carbanilide (NSC 109555) (Figure 2). Macromolecular lipids which did complex with these drugs noted above were also isolated from resistant lines, designated B_r, and from sensitive lines, designated B_s. The resistant lipid, B_r, bound two to three moles of these drugs per mole of lipid with a K_m of approximately 1 µM. The lipid B_s from the sensitive-tumor line had two binding regions, a high affinity (K_m of 4 to 6 µM) region which bound 1 to 2 moles of drug per mole of lipid and a low affinity region (K_m greater than 10 µM) which bound 2 to 6 moles of drug per mole of lipid. Also shown in Table 4 the anthracycline glycoside, doxorubicin, NSC 123127 (Figure 2) and several aminoanthraqui-nones [57, 58] (Figure 2), which are not cross-resistant with the terephthal-anilides, did bind to the resistant lipid A_r [19]. However, the specificity of the binding of A_r with these agents was lacking in comparison to lipids B_r and B_s. For example, more than 30 moles of doxorubicin, NSC 123127, were bound per mole of lipid A_r and the binding of NSC 123127 was not competitively displaced by spermine as is the case for lipids B_r and B_s. Another feature of the binding specificity of macromolecular lipids is the

26

Table 4. Drug saturation of the macromolecular lipids from L1210 leukemic tumors

Tumor type	NSC 38280 Resistant				NSC 38280 Sensitive			
Lipid type	Lipid A$_r$		Lipid B$_r$		Lipid B$_s$			
Binding regions	1		1		1		2	
Drug	Drug Bound[a]	Km (µM)	Drug Bound	Km (µM)	Drug Bound	Km (µM)	Drug Bound	Km (µM)
NSC 38280	0		3.4	0.9	1.2	3.9	5.7	68
(Cross resistant with NSC 38280 resistant cells)								
NSC 35843	0		3.0	0.9	1.4	6.0	3.5	83
NSC 113089	0		2.9	0.9	2.0	2.1	4.1	13
NSC 114347	0		2.3	0.9	1.1	4.1	2.2	27
NSC 109555	0		2.9	3.2	1.5	5.5	3.7	74
(Active against NSC 38380 resistant cells)								
NSC 123127	32	4.2	3.7	0.2	3.3	2.9	11.5	7
NSC 287513	10	6.1	1.6	0.2	2.5	2.3	5.3	19
NSC 279836	47	8.5	6.4	0.2	8.3	2.0	88	68
NSC 281246	23	4.1	8.2	6.1	7.0	2.7	100	95
(Inactive against NSC 38280 resistant and sensitive cells)								
NSC 281249	41	15	13.2	19	29	20	NS[b]	
NSC 278467	NS		2.8	7.6	5.2	10	NS	
NSC 279837	NS		8.6	16	3.1	13	NS	

[a] Drug bound (mol/mol lipid) at saturation.
[b] NS, not saturable at the highest drug concentration.

differential binding between 'active' and 'inactive' aminoanthraquinones (Figure 2 and Table 4). In this instance, the relative K_m for the binding regions was approximately an order of magnitude greater for the 'inactive' series, i.e., less tightly bound in comparison to the 'active' series and in many instances saturation of the macromolecular lipids with the 'inactive' series was not possible. Such differences in binding among the 'active' and 'inactive' aminoanthraquinones to the macromolecular lipids, if coupled with differences in their toxicity *in vivo*, and in their uptake by tumor cells, may be similar to the findings for the 'active' and 'inactive' terephthalanilides [31].

It was noted earlier that macromolecular lipids were isolated from doxorubicin-sensitive and -resistant P388 cells and that these lipids complexed with a number of cancer chemotherapeutic drugs and spermine. It would be interesting to speculate whether or not a macromolecular lipid, similar to A_r from NSC 38280-resistant cells, could be isolated from doxoribicin-resistant P388 cells and to evaluate whether or not the isolated lipid would bind doxorubicin and those drugs which are cross-resistant with doxorubicin. If such lipids were present in doxorubicin resistant P388 cells, would their chemical and physical characteristics be similar or different to the characteristics of the macromolecular lipid isolated from NSC 38280 sensitive and resistant cells?

The macromolecular lipids, isolated from phthalanilide-sensitive and -resistant L1210 cells, were shown to be similar in their chemical and physical characteristics [20] yet differed in their binding of several types of cancer chemotherapeutic drugs [20, 25, 28]. The macromolecular lipid that was isolated from dog brain bound many of these same agents [17, unpublished results], and the chemical and physical characteristics of the lipid from brains of dogs [17] were similar to those of L1210 cells [20]. The binding characteristics of the Cain's quinolinium, NSC 113089, to lipid extracts of tissues from rats would further indicate that the macromolecular lipids are similar but not equivalent from different sources [59].

As shown in Table 5, the amount of extractable lipid which bound NSC 113089 ranged from approximately 300 nmol bound/gram of skeletal muscle to 1100 nmol bound for liver. The dissociation constant (K_D) of the NSC 113089-lipid complex, calculated from double reciprocal plots of the saturation data, was the same regardless of lipid-tissue source. Increasing acidity caused displacement of NSC 113089 from the lipid extract (Table 5). Half discplacement of the drug occurred at the same pH regardless of tissue source, and near complete drug displacement was achieved with all extracts at approximately pH 1. These findings for tissues from rats would be comparable to that found for the macromolecular lipids from various L1210 cells and brain of dogs.

The displacement of NSC 113089 from these lipids, extracted from several tissues of rats with polyamines or calcium ions, showed some differential effects (Table 6, Figure 7). For example, spermine caused the maximum (100%) displacement of NSC 113089 from lipid extracts from kidney but only 48% displacement from liver. The displacement of NSC 113089 by spermine ranged from 70 to 80% for heart and skeletal muscle. When the amount of spermine required for half displacement of total displaceable drugs is calculated from the displacement plots (Figure 7), it is seen that approximately 1 to 2 moles of spermine is required per mole of drug. When spermidine and calcium ions were the displacing agent, the amount of NSC 113089 displaced was either less or equivalent to spermine. However, the amount of displacing agent needed was two to three times greater than spermine.

The binding characteristics of the macromolecular lipids from multiple sources indicate that the lipids are not all equivalent in binding cancer chemotherapeutic drugs, polyamines and cations and that multiple binding regions can be present on lipids from a specific source of lipid. Whether

Table 5. Binding of NSC 113089 to lipids extracted from tissues of rat

| Tissue | Drug bound at saturation | | K_D μM | Maximum proton displacement % | Half drug displacement pH |
	Lipid phosphorus (nmol/μmol)	Tissue (nmol/gram)			
Liver	33.0	1110	1.4	98	3.7
Kidney	24.1	780	1.5	90	3.8
Heart	28.2	610	1.6	100	3.6
Skeletal muscle	31.9	330	1.4	84	3.5

Table 6. Displacement of NSC 113089 from lipids extracted from tissues of rat

Displacing agent	Kidney	Liver	Heart	Skeletal muscle
Maximum amount NSC 113089 displaced (%)				
Spermine	100	48	71	78
Spermidine	62	49	59	84
Calcium ions	86	80	82	77
Agent drug ratio at half of maximum amount NSC 113089 displaced				
Spermine	1.1	1.1	1.4	1.8
Spermidine	2.5	2.5	2.5	3.3
Calcium ions	2.9	2.5	2.4	2.7

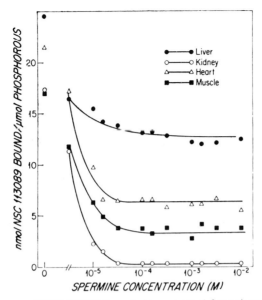

Figure 7. Displacement of NSC 113089 from lipids, extracted from tissues of rat by increasing concentrations of spermine.

such postulated sites are common to a single macromolecular lipid or are on different lipids must await further fractionation, purification and characterization of the lipids from multiple sources.

Polyamines, Histones and Polyvalent Cations
It has been shown that the polyamines, spermine and spermidine and several cations, e.g., calcium and protons can displace part or all of the quinolinium, NSC 113089, that is bound to lipids which are extracted from several sources of tissues from rat [58]. Further, spermine was shown to competitively displace several cancer chemotherapeutic drugs from lipids extracted from phthalanilide-sensitive L1210 cells and to both competitively and noncompetitively displace the same drugs for the drug-lipid complexes from phthalanilide-resistant cells [20].

In a paper to be published [56], we have characterized the binding of polyamines to lipids from phthalanilide-sensitive and -resistant L1210 cells. There are two saturable polyamine-binding affinities for each lipid type. The first has low to moderate capacity with high affinity and the second a three to twenty-five fold greater capacity with a lower affinity. The latter has been summarized in Table 7 for the various types of macromolecular lipids which have been described for the phthalanilide-resistant and -sensitive L1210 cells [20]. In comparing the B lipids from sensitive and resistant lipids, approximately 2 moles of the polyaminen, spermidine, putrescine and cadaverine are bound per mole of lipid whereas the same lipids bind approximately one mole of spermine. The Michaelis constants, which define the association of each polyamine with each lipid, shows that the lipids, B_s and B_r, have approximately the same affinity (range from 3.7 to 10.7 µM) for the four polyamines and have an order of magnitude greater affinity for the polyamines than lipid A_r.

The specificity of the binding region for spermine on these macromolecular lipids has been further evaluated [56]. As shown in Table 8, spermine was competitive with itself on a molar basis which demonstrates the accessibility of the binding region of the lipids for displacement of spermine. In comparison spermidine, putrescine and cadaverine, which have similar binding affinities, were poor displacers of spermine which indicates that the singular binding region for spermine differed from the multiple binding regions for these three polyamines with one possible exception. For lipid A_r,

Table 7. Saturation of macromolecular lipids isolated from leukemic cells with polyamines [56]

Polyamine	Parameter	Macromolecular lipids [a]		
		B_s	B_r	A_r
[14C] Spermine	Bound [b]	1.1	0.6	0.65
	Km (µM)	8.7	3.7	66
[14C] Spermidine	Bound	1.8	1.9	1.0
	Km	4.6	6.9	93
[14C] Putrescine	Bound	2.1	1.7	3.9
	Km	5.4	3.7	526
[14C] Cadaverine	Bound	1.8	1.9	8.5
	Km	7.7	10.7	417

[a] There are two binding regions on each macromolecular lipids but only region 2 (higher capacity and lower affinity) is described in this review.
[b] Mole polyamine bound per mole lipid at saturation.

Table 8. Displacement of spermine from the macromolecular lipids by polyamines [56]

Polyamine	Molar ratio of polyamine for 50% displacement of spermine / Macromolecular lipid		
	B_s	B_r	A_r
Spermine	1.1	0.9	0.9
Spermidine	18.2	19.6	1.7
Putrescine	42.5*	49.5*	6.1*
Cadaverine	50.2*	47.2*	5.0*

* Determined by extrapolation of the displacement curves.

1.7 moles of spermidine were required to displace 1 mole of spermine which would be consistent with a similar binding region for these two polyamines. Further, the relatively poor displacing ability of the diamines, putrescine and cadaverine in comparison to the triamine, spermidine in displacing spermine may indicate that the macromolecular lipids have at least three binding regions for polyamines.

This multiplicity in binding regions on the macromolecular lipids is also indicated from the competitive displacement of these polyamines by several cancer chemotherapeutic drugs (Table 9). The terephthalanilide, NSC 38280, which is bound in excess of 3 moles/mole of lipid, is easily displaced in a competitive manner by spermine whereas the reverse, i.e., displacement of spermine by NSC 38280 is comparatively difficult but competitive. In general NSC 38280, in comparison to the other three cancer drugs, is a poor displacing agent for all the polyamines. Doxorubicin, NSC 123127, on the

Table 9. Displacement of polyamines from the macromolecular lipids by cancer chemotherapeutic drugs [20, 59]

Displacing agent	Compound	Ratio of Km* for displacing agent: compound / Macromolecular lipids	
		B_s	B_r
	NSC 38280	6.8	44.4
	NSC 112089	6.9	9.2
	NSC 287513	2.4	35.5
Spermine	NSC 123127	1.3	16.5
NSC 38280		1.4	8.5
NSC 113089		1.7	18.3
NSC 287513		5.1	28.8
NSC 123127	Spermine	26.8	109.3
NSC 38280		1.4	5.3
NSC 113089		4.2	8.4
NSC 287513		7.7	15.2
NSC 123127	Spermidine	7.3	32.7
NSC 38280		2.7	34.2
NSC 113089		13.0	68.9
NSC 28713		13.4	112.9
NSC 123127	Putrescine	20.4	112.5
NSC 38280		3.3	7.4
NSC 113089		4.3	12.3
NSC 287513		10.8	12.8
NSC 123127	Cadaverine	23.6	20.2

* The greater the ratio, the greater the ability of the displacing agent to competitively displace the compound.

other hand, is an excellent displacer of the polyamines spermine, putrescine and cadaverine that are bound to the macromolecular lipids B_s and B_r. Doxorubicin does not show the same degree of displacement for spermidine. Similar comparison for the other drugs provide the same conclusion, i.e., there are different binding regions for the antineoplastic drugs and polyamines. However, there must be some overlap in their juxtaposition.

In discussing a potential role for the macromolecular lipids in the derepression of nucleic acid transcription [12, 24, 51], we have postulated an interaction among these lipids and histones. Some unpublished studies with my colleague, Dr. Richard Taylor, have demonstrated that histones are some of the best displacers of spermine from the macromolecular lipids. For example, Histone III-S, which is rich in lysine, displaced approximately 10 times its molar ratio of spermine whereas those histones II and VIII-S, which are enriched in arginine, displaced less than 2 times their molar ratio of spermine. Since spermine binds to these macromolecular lipids on a 1:1 molar ratio, and in order to account for the displacement ratios noted above, the histones must interact in a concerted manner with multiple moles of the macromolecular lipids.

The relative effectiveness of cations to displace cancer chemotherapeutic drugs or spermine from the macromolecular lipids from several sources has provided a data base which may be useful in defining the various binding regions on the macromolecular lipids. The displacement of drugs from macromolecular lipids by protons demonstrated that the pK for the binding regions was approximately 3.5 for many sources of the macromolecular lipid [17, 59]. These findings indicate that an ionizable group, common to all lipids, was responsible for the binding of the drugs.

Calcium ions were equivalent to protons in the displacement of NSC 57153 (Figure 1) from a terephthalanilide-lipid complex isolated from brain [17]. In comparison much higher concentrations of other cations were required to displace equivalent amounts of drug, for example, 5 times greater concentrations of magnesium ions and 150 to 200 times greater concentrations of sodium and potassium ions. The wide variations in the effectiveness of cations to displacement drugs from crude drug-lipid complexes [17] were also found for purified macromolecular lipids complexed with spermine (Table 10) [60].

In considering the displacement of spermine from the macromolecular lipids by cations, there is approximately one mole of spermine bound per mole of macromolecular lipids (Table 7) [56]. If the affinity between the lipid and spermine requires the four nitrogens of spermine, then approximately 6 to 8 moles of the cations, Al^{3+}, $Fe^{2+, 3+}$, Rn^{2+} and $Sn^{2+, 4+}$ were required to displace spermine from the phthalanilide sensitive lipid B_s. The Km affinity of B_r for spermine is greater than lipid B_s and one generally finds that a greater number of moles of these cations are required to displace spermine from lipid B_r in comparison to lipid B_s. In addition, displacement by cations of spermine from lipid A_r requires a smaller mole ratio than for lipids B_r and B_s, most likely due to the lower affinity of spermine for lipid A_r (Table 7) [56].

There is a definite difference between the various metals in their ability to displace spermine from the lipids. This displacing ability is not simply a function of charge or atomic size. Many factors may influence the formation of complex ions and coordination compounds, for example, the hybridization of orbitals, the formation of polydentate groups, and the nature of the coordinating group.

Chemotherapeutic Drugs Other Than Antineoplastic Drugs
The spacial arrangement of the various groupings on the antineoplastic drugs (Figure 1 and 2) corresponds to the basic groups of the polyamines (Figure 3). The macromolecular lipids have multiple binding regions for

Table 10. Relative effectiveness of cations to displace spermine from the macromolecular lipids, isolated from terephthalanilide sensitive and resistant L 1210 cells

Cations	Mole ratio of displacing cations to spermine		
	B_s	B_r	A_r
Li^+	> 1000	> 1000	560 [a]
Na^+	> 1000	> 1000	820 [a]
Mg^{2+}	320 [a]	> 1000	132
Al^{3+}	6	6	0.5
K^+	> 1000	−	−
Ca^{2+}	162	154	36
Cr^{3+}	19	58	8
Mn^{2+}	90	280 [a]	38
$Fe^{2+, 3+}$	7	7	1
Co^{2+}	210 [a]	> 1000	55
Ni^{2+}	330 [a]	> 1000	103
Cu^{2+}	55	86	11
Zn^{2+}	117	350 [a]	82
Sr^{2+}	> 1000	> 1000	110
Ru^{2+}	7	43	5
Ag^+	> 1000	> 1000	103
Cd^{2+}	35	420 [a]	92
$Sn^{2+, 4+}$	8	15	7
Hg^{2+}	> 1000	> 1000	> 1000
Tl^{3+}	25	68	0.1
Pb^{2+}	17	36	9
Bi^{3+}	22	10	0.8

[a] Extrapolated for 50% displacement.

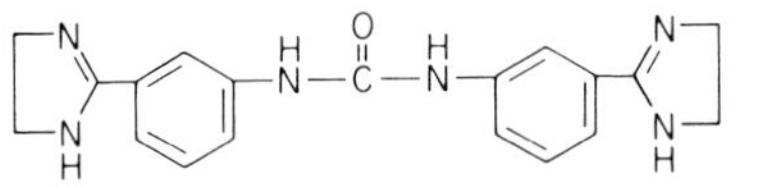

34

IMIDOCARB

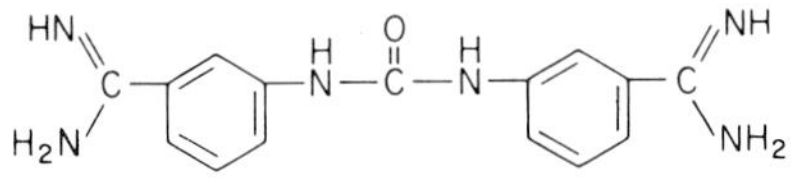

AMICARBALIDE

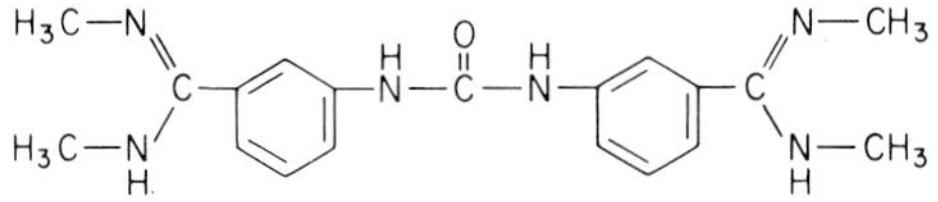

DIOXALATE

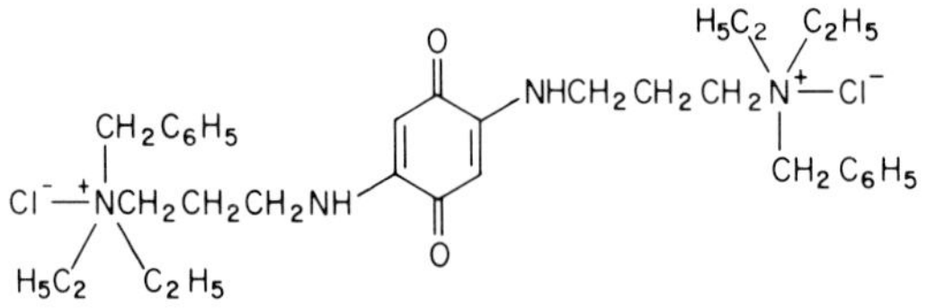

MYTOLON

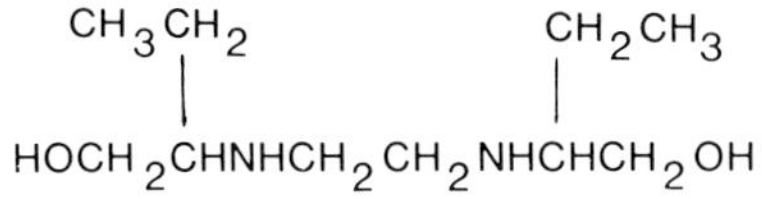

ETHAMBUTOL

Figure 8. Chemotherapeutic drugs which complex with the macromolecular lipids.

both classes of compounds, and the relative juxtaposition of the binding regions results in competitive interactions among the compounds.

Amicarbolide and imidocarb (Figure 8) are also cationic compounds with antileukemic, tuberculostatic and antitrypanosomal activities and were developed from the phthalanilides [61, 62]. The spacial arrangement of imidocarb, which is active against *Anaplasma marginale* [63], compares closely to the polyamine spermidine (Figure 3). In collaboration with my colleague, Ms. Marianne Callahan, and Dr. C. A. Nichol of Burroughs Wellcome, we showed that imidocarb, amicarbalide and dioxalate will complex with a macromolecular lipid from *Anaplasma marginale*. In comparing the relative effectiveness of various agents in displacing imidocarb from a partially purified macromolecular lipid from *Anaplasma marginale* (Table 11), spermidine was the best agent being twice as effective as spermine. Further, spermidine displaced 100% of the lipid-bound imidocarb whereas spermine displaced a maximum of 70 to 80%. These interactions may be important since these polyamines can reverse *in vivo* the trypanocidal activity of both amicarbalide and imidocarb [64, 65]. Spermine blocked cures at a dose of 100 mg/kg, spermidine at 300 mg/kg and putrescine was ineffective at 500 mg/kg. This disparity in the effectiveness among the polyamines to displace imidocarb from the macromolecular lipid and block cures *in vivo* may relate to differences in the macromolecular lipids from *Anaplasma marginale* and from *Trypanosoma brucei*. For example, in comparing the displacement of imidocarb from macromolecular lipids extracted from several tissues of rats and beef cattle by these polyamines, spermine, however, was the better displacing agent.

In defining the nature of the imidocarb binding capacity of the extracted macromolecular lipids from tissues of both beef cattle and rats, one again would conclude that the macromolecular lipids from many sources were not all equivalent. In Table 12, it is seen that the binding capacity varies extensively among the tissues as well as between the same tissue from different animal species. The effectiveness of the displacing agents also varies among the tissues and animal species.

Two trypanocidal agents, amicarbalide and dioxalate (Figure 8), which bind to the macromolecular lipid from *Anaplasma marginale* and to tissue lipids, were shown to be relatively ineffective in displacing imidocarb. Their

Table 11. Characteristics of imidocarb-lipid complexes from *Anaplasma Marginale* [a]

	nMole of Imidocarb Bound
Per μmole of Phospholipid Phosphorus	20
Per gm of *Anaplasma Marginale*	420
	Moles of agent required for displacing one mole of bound imidocarb
Hydrogen ions	34 ($\cong$ pK 4.5)
Calcium ions	410
Spermine	14
Spermidine	6

[a] These studies were sponsored by Dr. C.A. Nichol of Burroughs Wellcome and were carried out in collaboration with Ms. Marianne Callahan, presently at Lipid Specialties, Inc., Danvers, Massachusetts.

structural similarity would have presupposed a greater effectiveness in the displacement of imidocarb if a similar binding region on the lipid were involved. Therefore, in considering these data and similar data for active and inactive phthalanilides, we must anticipate that these compounds are binding to different regions of the macromolecular lipids.

The antiparasitic agents, imidocarb, amicarbalide and dioxalate, bind to the macromolecular lipids from many sources and show structural similarities to the terephthalanilides and the polyamines. The aminoanthraquinones, NSC 287513 and NSC 279836, contain a structural grouping in the R_1 position (Figure 2) which is similar to the antituberculosis agent, ethambutol (Figure 8). Ethambutol was shown to bind with the macromolecular lipids isolated from the terephthalanilide sensitive and resistant L1210 leukemic cells. The specificity of the binding was not defined but the preliminary binding characteristics would indicate both a low affinity and high capacity for the interaction of ethambutol with these macromolecular lipids.

The skeletal muscle relaxant Mytolon, benzoquinonium chloride (Figure 8), possesses a structure which is similar to the phthalanilide (Figure 1) and the Cain's quinoliniums (Figure 2). These drugs have net positive charges at both ends of the molecule with a separation of about 20 Å, alternating hydrophobic-hydrophilic areas, and a planar configuration. Since the benzoquinonium chloride may be affecting the nerve network either peripherally or centrally, we evaluated the potential for Mytolon to complex with the

Table 12. Characteristics of the imidocarb-macromolecular lipid complexes[a]

Tissues	nmole bound per µmole of phospho lipid phosphorus	Binding capacity nmole/ gm tissue	Molar ratio displacing agent: Imidocarb					
			H^+	Ca^{2+}	Spermine	Spermidine	Amicarbalide	Dixalate
Beef								
Kidney	62	1200	32	44	3	9	—	—
Liver	44	1500	36	57	5	7	194	2
Heart	33	760	74	82	2	23	—	—
Muscle	24	220	16	283	21	24	—	—
Rat								
Kidney	14	430	18	576	1	—	63	—
Liver	14	520	3	431	1.6	—	18	—
Heart	18	500	8	29	1.4	—	40	—
Muscle	33	300	1	69	1.1	—	67	—

[a] See footnote a of Table 11.

macromolecular lipids from brains of dogs. Benzoquinonium did form a lipid complex comparable to the phthalanilide-lipid complexes from brains of dogs. However, the significance of this complex formation may relate more to its toxicity rather than its pharmacological properties if the two properties can be separated experimentally.

In summary chemotherapeutic agents that have a planar structure, that have alternating hydrophobic-hydrophilic regions and that have electron-deficient regions at the ends of the molecule, have the potential to complex with macromolecular lipids. The specificity of the interaction among the agents and these lipids will need to be defined in more detail since the macromolecular lipids have multiple binding regions and are not equivalent among tissues. This multiplicity in binding regions and in the physical/chemical characteristics of the lipids from different sources may be utilized not only as an *in vitro* drug screen for predicting activity *in vivo* but also for the design of new and more efficacious drugs.

PHYSICAL AND CHEMICAL CHARACTERISTICS OF THE MACROMOLECULAR LIPIDS

Physical Characteristics

The partitioning characteristics were similar for macromolecular lipids isolated from dog brain [17], P388 cells [25] and L1210 cells [20]. The polarity of the organic solvent mixture had to accommodate both hydrophobic and hydrophilic regions. A biphasic solvent system, composed of chloroform, methanol and water, permitted the macromolecular lipid to partition into the organic phase. The lipids were not soluble in any one of these solvents alone. If a more nonpolar solvent were substituted for chloroform, such as trichlorotrifluoroethane, the macromolecular lipids partitioned into the aqueous rich phase. This amphoteric characteristic of the macromolecular lipids appears to promote a unilamellar packing of the molecules at the surface-air interface, similar to what is observed for phosphatidyl choline. Therefore, rather stable foams were formed whenever the lipid containing solvents were shaken.

The infrared spectrum of the lipid from dog brain [17] and L1210 cells is consistent with the interpretation that the lipid contains ester groups ($1740\ cm^{-1}$) and primary carbon-hydrogen linkages ($-CH_2-$, $2930\ cm^{-1}$, CH_3-, $2960\ cm^{-1}$, $-CH=CH-$, $3030\ cm^{-1}$) as would be found in fatty acids. There is a strong absorption at $3400\ cm^{-1}$ indicating the presence of some OH and/or NH groups and a weak absorption at $1640\ cm^{-1}$ indicating an amide functional group. The lipid also contained some functional oxygen (1050, 1230 and $1460\ cm^{-1}$) probably of phosphorus [17, 66, 67]. X-ray fluorescence analyses also demonstrated that the lipids contained a trace of sulfur but were negative for cations such as magnesium, calcium, sodium, etc.

The molar absorptivity of the ultraviolet absorbance (270–275 nm) ranges from about 1000 to 7000 depending upon the source of the lipid [17, 20]. Similar variations were found in the yield of fluorescence for the various sources of lipids [19, 20]. This probably relates to a variable number of similar absorbing groups per macromolecular lipid molecule.

In our earliest studies, we proposed that the lipids which associated with the terephthalanilides were macromolecular [17]. We based our hypothesis on the facts that acid displacement of drug from lipid degrades the lipid and yields four subfractions whose molar ratio of glycerol, fatty acids, phosphorus and nitrogen varied widely [17] and whose aggregate molecular weight was greater than 10,000. We have demonstrated the macromolecular characteristics of purified lipids using exclusion chromatography on controlled pore glass (CPG-10, 2650 Å) Porasil Ax(60x) and Sephadex (LH20). In a more recent study [20], the macromolecular lipids from terephthalanilide-sensitive and -resistant L1210 cells had a molecular weight range of 15,800 for macromolecular weight lipid B_s to 20,600 for lipid A_r as defined by polyacrylamide gel electrophoresis (PAGE). Molecular weight determinations by high pressure gel permeation chromatography (HPGPC) were consistently lower than those found with PAGE, presumably due to the inconsistencies in comparing a natural macromolecule to rigid and linear polystyrene molecular weight standards in HPGPC analysis. Therefore, we have chosen the PAGE molecular weight of 15,800 for the macromolecular lipid B_s in our subsequent comparisons.

Chemical Characteristics

The elemental analyses for the purified macromolecular lipid from phthalanilide-sensitive L1210 cells are seen in Table 13. The lipid contained about

Table 13. Elemental analyses of macromolecular lipid from phthalanilide-sensitive L 1210 cells

Element	Weight (%)
Carbon	56.89
Hydrogen	8.49
Nitrogen	1.04
Oxygen	19.46 [a]
Phosphorus	3.25
Sulfur	Trace ($<0.2\%$)
Total	89.03

[a] This represents the minimum value, since there was phosphorus in the sample.

1 % nitrogen which was low for a normal phospholipid such as phosophatidyl choline or phosophatidyl serine. The phosphorus content of 3.25 % was
high for a common phospholipid except cardiolipin, but the latter does not
contain nitrogen. We found a trace of sulfur both by wet chemistry techniques and by X-ray fluorescence. The carbon and hydrogen percentages are
partially represented by fatty acids. The fatty acids were the usual ones
— 11 % palmitic (16:0), 56 % stearic (18:0), 11 % oleic (18:1), 9 % linoleic
(18:2), 2 % linolenic (18:3) and about 5 % arachidonic (20:4). The oxygen
content represents the minimal amount due to the presence of phosphorus.

Component analysis of the hydrolyzed macromolecular lipids confirmed
the presence of glycerol, sugars and nitrogenous material [20]. Amino acid
analysis demonstrated that the ultraviolet absorbing amino acids were insufficient to account for the ultraviolet absorbing species in the hydrolysate.
The principal amino acids were serine (57%), glutamic acid (5%), glycine
(7%) and tyrosine (7%).

In collaboration with Dr. Edgar Lederer [19], several volatile derivatives
were obtained after acetylation, silylation or methylation of the acid or base
hydrolyzed macromolecular lipids. Phosphorus containing ions were identified in the high resolution mass spectra of the acetylated hydrophilic fraction (Table 14). The predominant species at m/z 95 and 109 had an oxygen
phosphorus ration of 3:1 which would indicate a phosphonate rather than a
phosphate grouping. Other evidence would also suggest a stable carbon
phosphorus linkage, for example, the ultraviolet absorbing species and phosphorus were not chemically hydrolyzed by base or acid. It is well known
that the glycerol ether phospholipids are chemically more stable [68]. Furthermore, a carbon phosphorus bond is much more stable than a carbon
oxygen phosphorus bond [69]. The carbon phosphorus containing phospholipids have been termed phosphonolipids [70] and have been widely

Table 14. Phosphorus containing ions in the high resolution mass spectrum of the acetylated
hydrophilic fraction

| Relative intensity | m/z | | Elemental composition |
	Found	Calculated	
1.0	80.97399	80.97415	H_2O_3P
0.4	81.98253	81.98198	H_3O_3P
4.9	94.99016	94.98980	CH_4O_3P
6.9	109.00501	109.00545	$C_2H_6O_3P$
0.4	138.00753	138.00819	$C_3H_7O_4P$
0.3	155.01045	155.01093	$C_3H_8O_5P$
3.3	169.02621	169.02658	$C_4H_{10}O_5P$

found in nature [71–79] and in mammalian tissues [80, 81]. Thus, we propose that the ultraviolet absorbing components might be covalently bonded to glycerol phosphonate via an ether linkage. The high resolution mass spectrometry data of the volatile derivatives of the hydrolyzed macromolecular lipids support this thesis.

High resolution mass spectrometry studies were performed on both the acetylated and methylated hydrophilic fractions that were obtained from hydrolyzed macromolecular lipids. The corresponding fatty acids or methylated fatty acids represented the major components of the lipophilic fraction. The elemental composition – the calculated m/z for the probable elemental composition did not differ from the observed m/z by more than 0.001 – of most fragments in both the acetylated and methylated hydrophilic fractions, which were volatile at temperature less than 150 °C, contained three moles of nitrogen. The probable structures and fragmentation patterns of the methylated hydrophilic components are shown in Figure 9. Similar interpretations of the high resolution mass spectra of the acetylated hydrophilic components are consistent with the nitrogen containing component being cytosine (Figure 10). In addition, one also finds fragments which correspond to the phosphonate ions that were noted in Table 14.

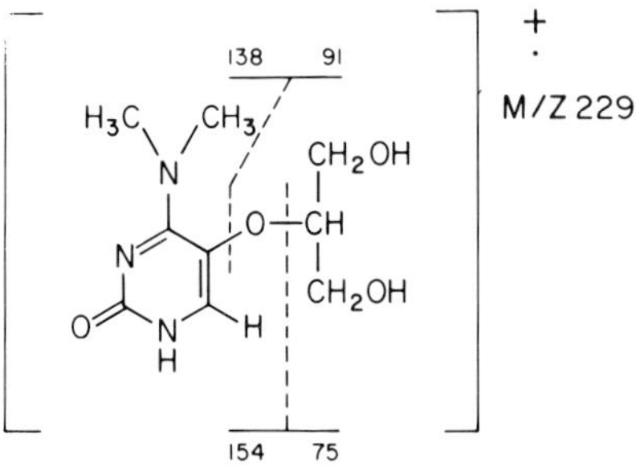

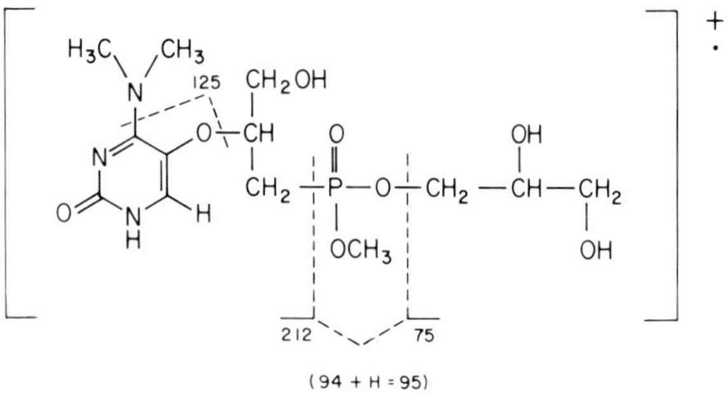

Figure 9. Probable structure and fragmentation pattern of the methylated hydrophilic components.

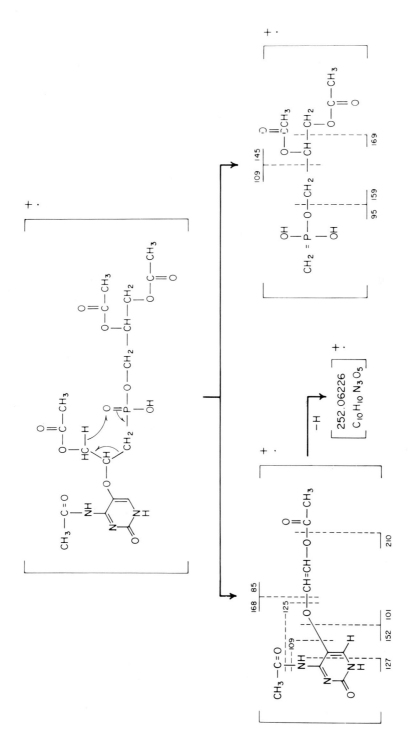

Figure 10. Probable structure and fragmentation pattern of the acetylated hydrophilic components.

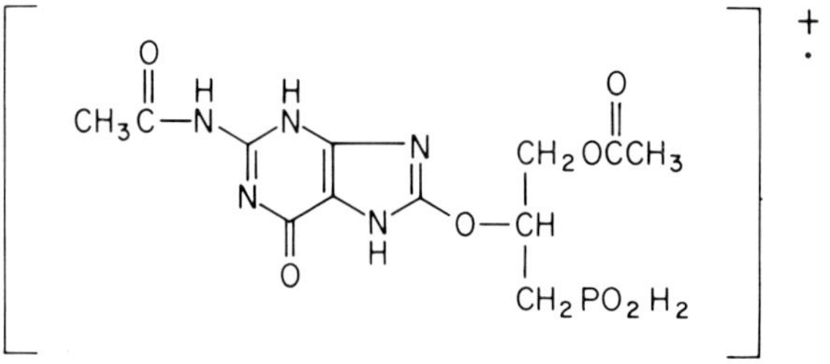

Figure 11. Proposed structure for the m/z 373 ion found in the high resolution mass spectrum of the acetylated hydrophilic fraction.

Ions at m/z 373 and 331 were observed in the acetylated hydrophilic fraction at temperatures greater than 150 °C and may arise from thermal decomposition. The 42 atomic mass units difference may represent the 373 ion minus a ketene radical. An elemental compositoin of $C_{12}H_{16}N_5O_7P$ would approximate the observed 373.09603 mass. Since several ninhydrin positive components are present in the hydrophilic fraction that cannot be separated from phosphorus, it is tempting to propose a guanine type structure for this fragmentation ion (Figure 11).

INNOVATIVE CONCEPTS CONCERNING THE MACROMOLECULAR LIPIDS

In proposing a structure and function for the macromolecular lipids at this embryonic state of knowledge, I hope that it will stimulate interest in the experimental evaluation of the concepts and in the use of macromolecular lipids for the discovery of new drugs.

Structure

The elemental and component analyses of the macromolecular lipids (Table 13) [17, 20] can be interpreted in terms of a structure. The number of mole-

Figure 12. Structural characteristics of the macromolecular lipid B_s. The atoms have the following colors: phosphorus atom is yellow; carbon atom is black; hydrogen atom is white; oxygen atom is red; and nitrogen atom is blue. (a) A top view showing the proposed glycerol-phosphonate/phosphate backbone of the macromolecular lipid. (b) A side view showing the esterification of fatty acids to the hydroxyl grouping on the glycerol phosphonate/phosphate backbone. The fatty acid shown is oleic acid whereas the other straight rods would represent the saturated fatty acids. (c) A top view showing the hydrophilic region of the macromolecular lipids which contains covalently-bound purine/pyrimidine bases, hexoses and a tetrapeptide. (d) A top view showing the binding of polyamines to the macromolecular lipid B_s; namely, one mole of spermine and two moles of spermidine and putrescine. (e) A top view showing the three binding regions for Adriamycin (Doxorubicin, NSC 123127). One molecule of Adriamycin is shown bound to the lower spermidine binding region. (f) A top view showing the three binding regions for the amino-anthraquinone, NSC 287513. One molecule is shown bound to the lower spermidine binding region.

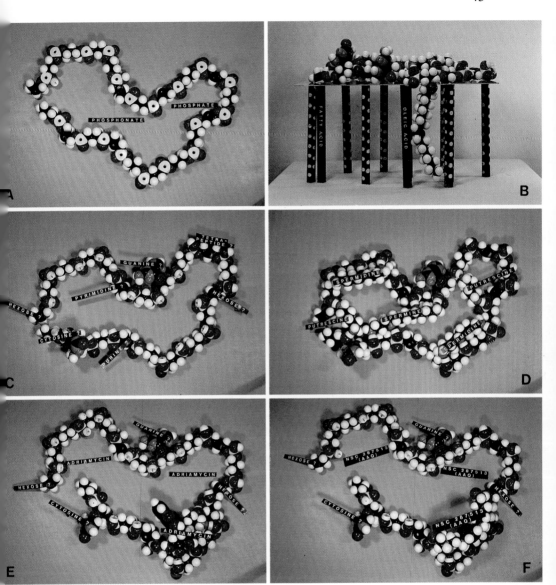

44

cules of each component that is estimated for the macromolecular lipid B_s is shown in Table 15. If we assume a glycerol phosphonate and glycerol phosphate backbone similar to cardiolipin, then the backbone contains approximately 16 to 18 glycerols connected by phosphonate and phosphate (Figure 12a). The β-carbon of the connecting glycerol moiety and the a and β carbons of the terminal glycerols in the backbone contain approximately 19 to 21 free hydroxyl functional groups. This number of hydroxyl groups is inadequate to accommodate 15 to 16 molecules of fatty acid, 3 to 4 amino acids, several other nitrogenous compounds, e.g., cytosine and guanine that account for the 6 to 9 molecules of nonamino acid nitrogen and 1 or 2 hexoses. The esterification of the fatty acids to this glycerol phosphonate/phosphate backbone results in a hydrophobic plane (Figure 12b). The hydrophilic plane (side view and upper region of Figure 12b and top view in Figure 12c) is represented by the phosphonate and phosphate groups of the backbone and the polar constituents, namely, bases, sugars and amino acids. The amino acids are represented by a tetrapeptide in order to accommodate a protein positive test and the inadequate number of glycerol hydroxyl groups noted earlier.

This proposed structure for the macromolecular lipid has accounted for the components listed in Table 15 with the exception of carbon and hydrogen and, to a lesser extent, with oxygen. A summation of these elements in

Table 15. Composition of the macromolecular lipid-B_s* isolated from L 1210 cells

Atom or component	Molecular weight	Composition range (%)	Range of estimated number of atoms or components per Lipid B_2
Carbon	12	56.1 –56.9	738–749
Hydrogen	1	8.1 – 8.5	1280–1341
Oxygen	16	19.5 (Minimum)	183 (Minimum)
Nitrogen	14	0.83– 1.04	9–12
Phosphorus	31	0.19– 3.25	1–17
Amino Acids	119 [a]	2.8	3–4
Hexose	180	1.8	1–2
Glycerol	92	2.1	3–4
Fatty Acids	283 [b]	28.3	15–16
Glycerol phosphonate [c]	156	13.1 [c]	13 –14

* Estimate of molecular weight by PAGE is 15,800.

[a] This molecular weight is an average for those principal amino acids that were obtained from acid hydrolysis of the lipids.

[b] This molecular weight is the average for those fatty acids which were found in the hydrolysis of the macromolecular lipid.

[c] Glycerol phosphonate was not identified but is estimated from the total sugar analysis (17.0%) minus that found for glycerol (12.1%) and hexose (1.8%).

the fatty acids, the glycerol phosphonate/phosphate backbone and the hydrophilic species, namely, the purine/pyrimidine bases, amino acids and hexoses, will account for approximately 50% of the 740 carbon atoms per B_s macromolecular lipid, 53% of the 1300 hydrogen atoms and 80% of the minimal 183 oxygen atoms. The net difference in these three elements indicates that approximately one-third of the molecular weight of the B_s macromolecular lipid remains an unknown but whose composition is primarily C, H and O.

The macromolecular lipids, which were isolated from brains of dogs [17] and from leukemic cells [20], possessed some ultraviolet-visible absorption (Figure 13) and fluorescence (Figure 13). The chromophores have not been identified [17, 20]. The tyrosine and the purine/pyrimidine bases of the lipid cannot totally account for this absorption. In addition, the chromophores may relate to the unaccounted fraction of the B_s macromolecular lipid noted previously.

There are relatively few naturally occurring biological materials which are enriched in C, H and O and which are themselves a chromophore. Several examples are listed in Table 16. Vitamin D has a UV absorption maximum

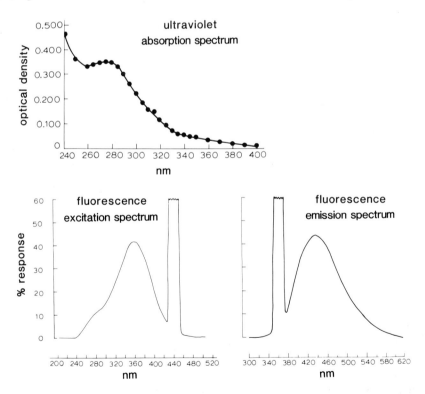

Figure 13. Ultraviolet absorption and fluorescence-spectra of purified macromolecular lipid B_s.

approximating that found in the lipids. The fluorescence characteristics of vitamin D show excitation and emission maxima that are higher than those found for the lipid. However, this may reflect differences in the milieu which will greatly effect fluorescence. Further, the extinction coefficient of vitamin D ranged from 450 to 490 which indicates that approximately 17 molecules of vitamin D might be associated with each mole of the macromolecular lipid. This number correlates with the 14 molecules that would be needed to account for the unidentified fraction of the B_s macromolecular lipid.

Vitamin D_3 undergoes metabolic alteration to yield 1,25-dihydroxy $D_3[1,25(OH)_2-D_3]$ which is the biologically active species [82]. Biochemical and autoradiographic evidence indicates that like other steroid hormones, such as estradiol and testosterone, $1,25(OH)_2-D_3$ functions at the molecular level within the nucleus by modulating genetic expression [83–87]. If $1,25(OH)_2-D_3$ were associated with the macromolecular lipids, there are relatively few sites for reacting a hydroxyl group of the $1,25(OH)_2-D_3$ molecule to the macromolecular lipid. The only apparent reaction is the formation of a phosphoric ester grouping. The possibility that $1,25(OH)_2-D_3$ or any of the candidates listed in Table 16 might be covalently linked to the macromolecular lipid will help to define the function of these lipids within the nucleus.

Obviously, further studies will be necessary to define the exact chemical structure of the macromolecular lipid. Nevertheless, the proposed structure, as shown in Figure 12, does provide some insight into the binding characteristics of the macromolecular lipids to both polyamines (Figure 12d) and to drugs (Figures 12e and 12f). The polyamines, spermine, spermidine and putrescine appear to bind to different regions on the macromolecular lipid, primarily by ionic and hydrogen bonding interactions. It is proposed that the interactions are between the nitrogen of the polyamines and the phos-

Table 16. Potential candidates for the unidentified chromophore(s) in the macromolecular lipid B_s

Candidate	Elemental composition	Absorption maxima (nm)	$E^{1\%}$ 1 cm	Fluorescence (nm)	
				Excitation	Emission
Vitamin A	$C_{20}H_{30}O$	325	1835	327	510
Vitamin D	$C_{27}H_{44}O$	265	450–490	390	480
Vitamin E	$C_{29}H_{50}O_2$	294	70	295	340
Vitamin K_1	$C_{31}H_{46}O_2$	245, 248, 264, 271 and 329	425, 426, 419, 420 and 348	None	
β-Estradiol	$C_{18}H_{24}O_2$	280	2,120	285	330
Testosterone	$C_{19}H_{28}O_2$	238	16,800	None	

phonate/phosphate groupings of the macromolecular lipid. It should be noted that the spacing of $-NHCH_2CH_2CH_2NH_2$ in spermine and spermidine requires a $-O_3PCH_2CH_2CH_2PO_3-$ glycerol phosphonate spacing in the macromolecular lipid whereas the spacing of $-NHCH_2CH_2CH_2CH_2NH-$ requires a $-O_3POCH_2CH_2CH_2OPO_3-$ arrangement of a typical cardiolipin type glycerol phosphate group.

In placing the polyamines on the macromolecular lipids, we took into account the relative effectiveness of the polyamines in displacing the cancer chemotherapeutic drugs. For example, one mole of spermine will displace approximately three moles of Adriamycin (Figure 12e) and aminoanthraquinone (Figure 12f), and *vice versa*. Thus, in order to accommodate this 1:3 mole ratio for spermine:drug displacement, the binding regions for spermine must result in a conformational change in the lipid (Figures 12c and 12d) to prevent the interaction of the drugs with the lipids (Figures 12e and 12f). This conformational change may be due to spermine bridging the luminal space of the two halves of the lipid. Doxorubicin and aminoanthraquinones were also excellent displacers of the polyamines, putrescine and cadaverine but did not show the same degree of displacement for spermidine. In this instance, we have projected the bridging of the diamines across the luminal space to be similar to spermine. On the other hand, spermidine is viewed to bind to specific regions along the backbone of the macromolecular lipid. The displacement of spermidine by these drugs (Figures 12e and 12f) might, therefore, be more difficult.

The functional groups of the Adriamycin (doxorubicin, NSC 123127) molecule which closely matches the spermidine binding region on the macromolecular lipid are the hydroxyl and amino groups of daunosamine and the 13-carbonyl and 14-hydroxyl of the aglycone moiety. The quinone regions of the aglycone moiety may further enhance the binding by hydrogen bonding with the purine/pyrimidine bases and tetrapeptide which are near the binding regions – compare Figures 12c and 12e.

In comparing the relative binding of the aminoanthraquinones (Figure 2) [20], NSC 287513 showed the lowest number of moles bound per mole of the macromolecular lipids. The spacial arrangement of the amino and hydroxyl groupings on the two side arms of NSC 287513 appear to interact with the phosphoric groupings in the vicinity of the spermidine binding regions – compare Figures 12c and 12f. In considering the binding of 7 to 8 moles of the active aminoanthraquinones, NSC 279836 and NSC 281246, to the B_s macromolecular lipid (Figure 2) [20], the backbone phosphoric groupings cannot accommodate this number of molecules. Therefore, one might anticipate an association between two phosphoric groupings with one arm of the aminoanthraquinone and the other arm may interact with the yet unidentified chromophoric groups of the macromolecular lipids. The inactive aminoanthraquinones, NSC 281249, NSC 278467 and NSC 279837, whose affinity are an order of magnitude less than the active series, may only employ one arm of the compound in its interaction with the macro-molecular lipid.

In proposing a structure for the macromolecular lipid, we have utilized the following information:

— molecular weight estimates
— elemental and component analyses
— hydrophobic/hydrophilic characteristics
— binding of polyamines and drugs
— the competitive displacement among these binding components

An important feature of this type of structure is the diversity that it can have, with respect to its size, molecular organization of the components and binding of a diverse array of compounds, e.g., polyamines, drugs and cations. The potential diversity in its structure is compatible with the conclusion that the macromolecular lipids from different tissues and organisms are not identical and yet is compatible with the many similarities that were found for the macromolecular lipids from diverse sources. If the lipids contain different components that are intimately involved in the expression of genetic material, then the macromolecular lipid will have an important role in the growth and maintenance of the cell.

Function
In proposing a functional role for the macromolecular lipids in the expression of genetic material, we have take into account the following considerations:

— ubiquitous distribution of the macromolecular lipids
— nucleoplasm localization of the lipids
— binding of drugs to effect biochemical processes
— binding of polyamines and histones
— the macromolecular lipid may contain compounds; for example, vitamin D that initiate genetic expression
— chromatin fraction, active in RNA synthesis, is rich in phospholipids

It is now well established that interphase chromatin in the eukaryotic cell nucleus is organized into repeating subunits or nucleosomes [88]. The nucleosome is composed of a well protected nucleosome core and a nuclease sensitive linker region of variable length. The core fragment of 146 base pairs of double stranded DNA is wrapped around a globular histone bead containing two each of the histones H2A, H2B, H3 and H4 which are known as the histone octamer. The linker region interacts with heterogeneous histone fraction H1 which appears to be in close contact with the histone octamer. The high mobility group, nonhistone acidic proteins are located near the end of the DNA associated with the histone octamer and at this location may take the place of H1. The nucleosome provides only a first level of organization of the DNA. Inside the cell the nucleosomes are further compacted culminating in a beaded structure having a diameter of 250–300 Å. Most important is the absolute requirement for the presence of histone H1 for its formation.

In describing the ultrastructure of actively transcribing chromatin [88], there is a general agreement that the beaded nucleosomal structures are absent from highly active gene regions. It appears that the reversible transition from the beaded structures to uniform fibers is caused by an unfolding of the polysome filament rather than by histone depletion. In this regard, chromatin fractions, which are active in RNA synthesis, are rich in phospholipids [44, 49] which may play a role in this unfolding and in affecting the histone DNA interactions [49].

A number of interesting features have been described with respect to the active gene regions. DNase I sensitivity, as a property of active gene regions, has been correlated with the undermethylation of DNA and, in particular, the demethylation of the nucleotide sequence, CCGG [88, 89]. In the eukaryotic cells, the primary transcript ends as mature messenger RNA (mRNA) which is methylated [90]. Once the mature fully processed eukaryotic mRNA is formed, selective transport of the mRNA from the nucleus to the cytoplasm must take place so as to allow function.

Many studies have demonstrated the importance of polyamines in growth, in stabilizing nucleic acids, and in stimulating protein synthesis [91]. The complexity of the effects has made it nearly impossible to identify definitively any specific step as the primary site of action of the polyamines *in vivo*. However, it is clear that these compounds are physiologically important, and in this context we have attempted to integrate the polyamines in our proposed function for the macromolecular lipids.

The proposed functional role for the macromolecular lipids is shown in Figure 14. The chromatin contains the repressed methylated DNA, histones and acidic proteins. We have chosen to associate polyamines with the acidic proteins in order to effect any potential histone-acidic protein interaction. The repressed chromatin contains very little lipid material whereas active chromatin contains a considerable quantity of phospholipid. Therefore, we have proposed that the 'coded' macromolecular lipids ('C'/MML) are synthesized *de novo* within the nucleoplasm of the nucleus during the transition from the repressed chromatin to active chromatin.

Active chromatin contains the same quantities of DNA, histone and nonhistone protein as the repressed chromatin. Therefore, in order to transcribe

50

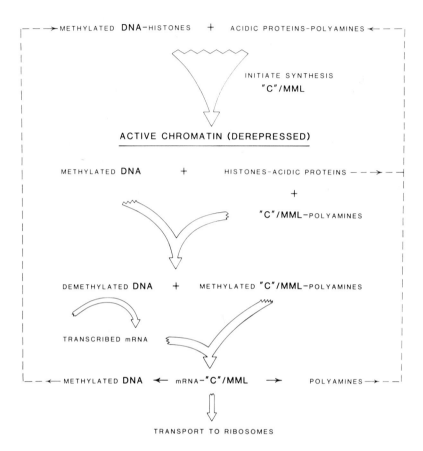

Figure 14. Proposed function of 'coded' macromolecular lipids ('C'/MML).

the DNA, we propose a realignment in the interactions among the various components. If the 'coded' macromolecular lipids ('C'/MML) had a greater binding affinity for the polyamines than the acidic proteins, we might anticipate a shift in the interactions to affect the histone-acidic protein and 'C'/MML-polyamine associations. Since a demethylation of the methylated DNA has to occur prior to transcription, and yet there has to be conservation of the methyl group, we have proposed a transfer of the methyl grouping from DNA to 'C'/MML. The methyl group is located primarily on the cytosine of DNA and a cytosine moiety has been characterized in the macromolecular lipid. Once the DNA has been transcribed, the messenger RNA (mRNA) may have the opportunity to interact with the 'C'/MML. The methyl group of the 'C'/MML might be transferred back onto the DNA and/or the mRNA and the displaced polyamine can affect the histone-acidic protein interactions which will reestablish the initial state of the repressed chromatin. The mRNA-'C'/MML species could then be transported from the nucleus to the cytoplasm.

In support of this proposed function for the macromolecular lipids, we have demonstrated that these lipids are located within the nucleoplasm of the nucleus and specifically were found to the greatest extent in the active chromatin fraction. Drugs which tightly bind to the 'C'/MML result in a marked inhibition of DNA and protein synthesis. Such drug interactions with the 'C'/MML would, in effect, shift the associations to a repressed state for chromatin. The synthesis of a coded macromolecular lipid to effect an initial shift in the associations among the nucleosome components is a reasonable hypothesis, especially since the macromolecular lipid has many similar binding characteristics to DNA for histones, polyamines and acidic proteins. Further, the 'C'/MML has a unique chemical composition which might mimic the DNA structure.

Discovery of New Drugs

An important feature of the proposed structure for the macromolecular lipids is the diversity that it can have with respect to its size and molecular organization of the components. The macromolecular lipids are not identical from different tissues and organisms, yet are sufficiently similar to complex with a diverse array of compounds, e.g., polyamines, drugs, and cations. Most striking is the multiple binding sites on the macromolecular lipids. It is this feature which may be exploited in the discovery of new drugs as well as in using specific drugs in combination. For example, doxorubicin (NSC 123127) and the terephthalanilide (NSC 38280) bind to the macromolecular lipid of tumor cells with approximately the same affinity, and based upon their comparative displacement of the polyamines, these compounds would not be expected to bind to the same regions on the macromolecular lipid.

Another example is the binding of imidocarb by the macromolecular lipids from *Anaplasma* and the ineffective displacement of imidocarb by comparable structures, specifically amicarbalide and dioxalate. Further, the 'inactive' phthalanilides, in comparison to their active congeners, bind to the macromolecular lipids yet elicit quantitative differences in their inhibition of protein and nucleic acid synthesis. Overall, the specificity of the binding and the location of the binding site of the drug on the macromolecular lipids will elicit different biochemical effects.

The National Cancer Institute has selected approximately 280 Decision Network 2A compounds for further chemotherapeutic evaluation. In reviewing this list of compounds, I selected approximately twelve on the basis of structure (Table 17) which have the potential for complexing with the macromolecular lipids. Several compounds are especially intriguing: NSC 356894 contains a spermidine moiety which might interact with the spermidine binding region (see Figure 12) as well as a guanidine group which is sufficiently distant from the spermidine moiety to interact with the spermine binding regions of the macromolecular lipid; NSC 296961 has some antineoplastic activity and has been extensively studied as a radioprotective compound, identified as WR2721 or Gammaphos [92–94]. To date the mechanism of action of WR2721 has not been defined, but if this compound interacts with the macromolecular lipid, one might anticipate the inhibition of protein and nucleic acid synthesis like the phthalanilides [24] to affect its radioprotective nature.

Table 17. NCI decision network 2A compounds which have the potential for binding to the macromolecular Lipids

DN 2A Compounds	Chemical name(s)
NSC 143057	4,6–Quinolinediamine, N4,N4'–1,6–hexanediyl–bis 2–methyl–, dihydrochloride
NSC 143969	9H–Fluoren–9–one, 2,7–bis[2–(diethylamino)ethoxyl]–, dihydrochloride Tilorone hydrochloride
NSC 219733	1,6–Hexanediamine, N,N'–di–9–acridinyl–
NSC 238146	4,6–Quinolinediamine, N4N4'–1,6–hexanediyl–bis 2–methyl–, tetraacetate
NSC 246112	Hydrazinecarbothioamide, 2–[(5–amino–4–methyl–1–isoquinolinyl)methylene]–, hydrochloride (2:3)
NSC 247561	1,3–Propanediamine, N,N–dimethyl–N'–(1–nitro–9–acridinyl)–, dihydrochloride Ledacrine
NSC 296961	2–(3–Aminopropylamino)ethyl thiophosphate WR–2721
NSC 301739	9,10–Anthracenedione,1,4–dihydroxy–5,8–bis((2–((2–hydroxyethyl)amino)ethyl)amino)–, dihydrochloride Mitoxantrone hydrochloride
NSC 329680	Sulfamic acid, 1,7–heptanediyl ester
NSC 337766	9,10–Anthracenedicarboxaldehyde,bis(4,5–dihydro–1H–imidazol–2–yl hydrazone), dihydrochloride Bisantrene hydrochloride
NSC 356894	Heptanamide, 7–[(aminoiminomethyl)amino]–N–[2–[[4–[(3–aminopropyl)amino]butyl]amino]–1–hydroxy–2–oxoethyl]– 15-Deoxyspergualin
NSC 522843	Phenanthridinium, 3,8–diamino–5–ethyl–6–phenyl–, chloride Ethidium chloride

In a recent study [95] polyamines were shown to reverse *in vivo* the anti-tumor activity of bleomycin. The mechanism of this reversal is unknown, but the authors pointed out that bleomycin contains a structural region which resembles, to some extent, the natural polyamines. In this regard, this structural region of bleomycin contained a terminally charged tertiary sulfur group. The substitution of tertiary alkyl sulfur groups in the polyamine type drugs noted in this reveiw may lead to useful chemotherapeutic agents. Israel, Rosenfield and Modest [96] synthesized a series of linear aliphatic triamines and tetramines as homologs of the naturally occurring polyamines. The notable feature of the *in vivo* active homologs is the number of carbon atoms between the nitrogens, e.g., $H_2NCH_2CH_2CH_2NH(CH_2)_9NH_2$. This compound, may be binding with two polyamine binding regions along the backbone of the macromolecular lipid.

The macromolecular lipids appear to have a binding affinity for polyvalent cations. The dihydroquinone system of the anthracycline drugs doxorubicin (NSC 123127) and daunomycin (NSC 82151) chelates with polyvalent cations, e.g., Fe^{3+}, Cu^{2+} and Mg^{2+} [97, 99]. These cations will release the anthracyclines from a DNA-anthracycline complex [98, 99]; yet metal chelates of the anthracycline drugs will enhance their chemotherapeutic effectiveness [100]. Such metal chelates may enhance the stability of the anthracycline-macromolecular lipid complex (see Figure 12e). Cis platinum compounds are effective antitumor agents [101]. It has been suggested that their primary target is DNA [102–104] to affect an inhibition of DNA [105] and RNA [106] synthesis in eukaryotic systems. However, it is equally plausible that these compounds may elicit the observed effects by complexing with the macromolecular lipids.

When we reviewed the literature on the mode of action of the 8-aminoquinoline and schizontocide antimalarials, we noted that there were many similarities in the biochemical effects among these antimalarials and the experimental phthalanilide antineoplastic agents. The antimalarials concentrate within the parasites [107], inhibit DNA synthesis [108, 109], and most interact with DNA [110, 111] while some do not [112]. Chloroquine inhibits equally the incorporation of the precursors of DNA, RNA and protein into *P. knowlesi* indicating that its primary action site is not at DNA [113]. The postulated binding site is planar and lipophilic having hydrogen binding groups separated by approximately 4 angstroms from a negatively charged acidic group [114, 115]. It is interesting to note that spermine and several antimalarials enhance the rate of clathrin polymerization [116, 117]. A review of the spatial arrangement of the various groups in the clinically evaluated and experimental antimalarial drugs shows some relationship to the naturally occurring polyamines (Figure 15). The similarities in the biochemical effects of antimalarials and the phthalanilides and their resem-

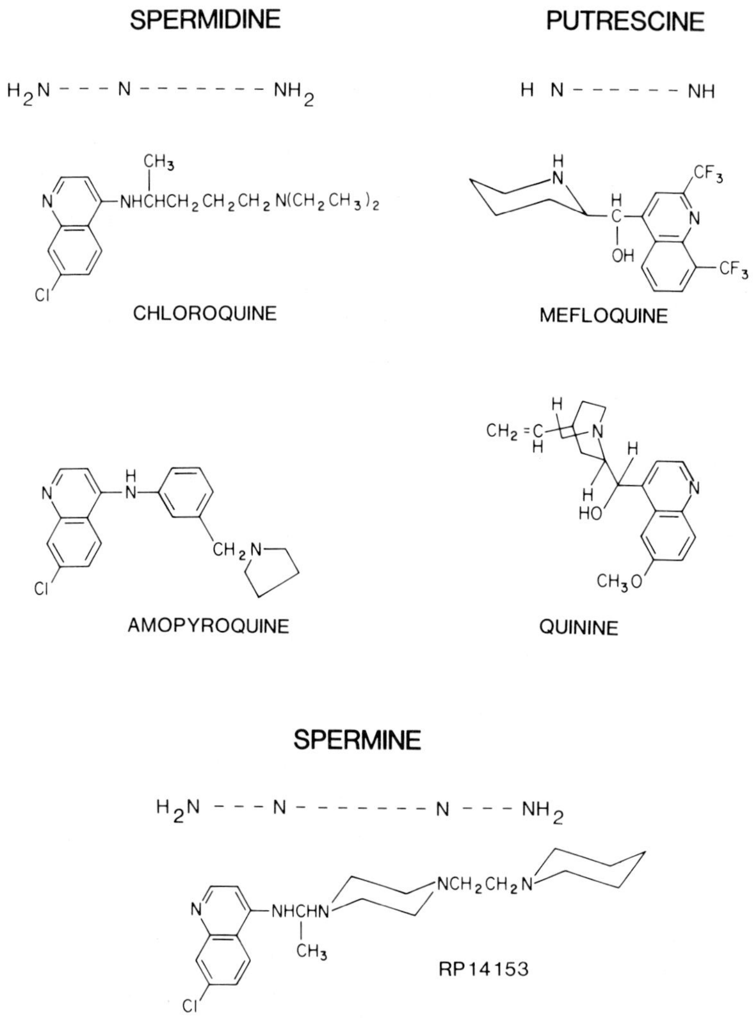

Figure 15. Structural relationships between antimalarials and polyamines.

blance to the polyamines indicate that the antimalarials may bind to the macromolecular lipids of *Plasmodium* sp. and compete with normal substrates.

Regulation of gene expression in eukaryotes and prokaryotes is a fascinating topic in molecular biology with interesting implications for differentiation and for many areas of biology, for example, oncology, virology and parasitology. The proposed role of the 'coded' macromolecular lipid in the regulation of gene expression, the unique structure of the macromolecular lipid and its specificity for the binding of polyamines and drugs indicate that these lipids represent a new mechanism for drug discovery.

ACKNOWLEDGMENT

I would like to pay tribute to the knowledge, skill and dedication of my collaborators whose names are given in the various references. I cannot adequately express my indebtedness to these colleagues. I wish to thank Ms. Erieta Nichols, Ann White and Eleanor Donham for their excellent assistance in typing the manuscript, and Mr. Philip Schepis for drawing the figures. Dr. J. A. R. Mead, Project Officer of NCI Contracts NO1-CM-33727, NO1-CM-53849 and NO1-CM-87163, has supported these studies, and I am especially grateful for his photographic assistance. Lastly, I wish to thank my colleagues at Arthur D. Little, Inc. for their review of the manuscript and, especially, Dr. Alan Branfman who, in addition, provided input into the section on new drug discovery.

REFERENCES

1. Hirt R, Berchtold R: Biophysical studies with synthetic lecithin as a road to new chemotherapeutic agents. Cancer Chemotherap Rep 18:5–7, 1962.
2. Burchenal JH, Lyman MS, Purple JR, Coley V, Smith S, Bucholz E: Therapeutic combination and resistant studies on certain imidazolin phthalanilide derivatives in mouse leukemia. Cancer Chemotherap Rep 19:19–29, 1962.
3. Pittillo RF, Bennett LL, Jr, Short WA, Tomisek AJ, Dixon GJ, Thomson JR, Laster WR, Jr, Trader M, Mattil L, Allan P, Bowdon B, Schabel FM, Jr, Skipper HE: Preliminary studies of some terephthalanilides – A new class of antitumor drugs. Cancer Chemotherap Rep 19:41–53, 1962.
4. Schepartz SA, Wodinsky I, Leiter J: Phthalanilides – A new group of potential antitumor agents. Cancer chemotherap Rep 19:1–3, 1962.
5. Venditti JM, Goldin A, Kline I: Studies on the effectiveness of 4′, 4″-Di (2.Imidazolin-2-yl) terephthalanilides against mouse leukemia L1210 and resistant variants. Cancer Chemotherap Rep 19:5–11, 1962.
6. Law LW: Studies of inhibitory effects of terephthalanilide derivatives against several variants of leukemia L1210. Cancer Chemotherap Rep 19:13–18, 1962.
7. Louis J: Coordinated phase I studies for cooperative chemotherapy groups. Cancer Chemotherap Rep 16:99, 1962.
8. Oettgen HF, Clifford P, Burchenal JH: Malignant Lymphoma involving the jaw in African children: Treatment with 2-Chloro-4′, 4″-2-Imidazolin-2-yl terephthalanilide dihydrochloride. Cancer Chemotherap Rep 27:45–54, 1963.
9. Kensler CJ, Palm PE, Day HM, Battista SP, Rogers WI, Yesair DW, Wodinsky I: Toxicity of Antileukemic Agents with special reference to phthalanilide derivatives. Cancer Res 25:1622–1667, 1965.
10. Rogers WI, York IM, Kensler CJ: Physiological disposition studies of 4′, 4″-Bis(2-Imidazolin-2-yl) terephthalanilide. Cancer Chemotherap Rep 19:67–74, 1962.
11. Folch J Lees M, Sloane Stanley GH: A simple method for the isolation and purification of total lipides from animal tissues. J Biol Chem 226:497–509, 1957.
12. Kensler CJ: Chemotherapeutic activity of phthalanilide derivatives: An approach to anticodic therapy? Cancer Res 23:1353–1363, 1963.

13. Sivak A, Rogers WI, Kensler CJ: Phthalanilide Interaction with Nucleic Acids. Biochem Pharmacol 12:1056–1058, 1963.
14. Sivak A, Rogers WI, Wodinsky I, Kensler CJ: Studies on the formation of phthalanilide-deoxyribonucleic acid complexes and their relationship to chemotherapeutic activity. Cancer Res 25:902–909, 1965.
15. Rauen HM, Haar H, Unterberg W: Coplanare Heterooligobasen (Phthalanilide) und ihr Cytostatischer Wirkungsmechanimus. Arzneimittel Forschg 16:533–541, 1966.
16. Rauen HM, Noroth K, Unterberg W: Coplanare heterooligobasen (Phthalanilide) hochaktive cytostatica. Experientia (Basel) 21:300–304, 1965.
17. Yesair DW, Rogers WI, Funkhouser JT, Kensler CJ: Purification and characterization of Phthalanilide-lipid complexes from tissues. J Lipid Res 7:492–500, 1966.
18. Gaudio LA, Yesair DW, Taylor RF: Cancer chemotherapeutic drug binding to macromolecular lipids from L1210 leukemia cells and to known lipids. Proc Amer Assoc Cancer Res 21:18 (Abstract 70), 1980.
19. Yesair DW, Lederer E, Kensler CJ: New macromolecular lipids from L1210 leukemic cells. Proc Amer Assoc Cancer Res 13:45 (Abstract 178), 1972.
20. Taylor RF, Teague LA, Yesair DW: Drug binding macromolecular lipids from L1210 leukemia tumors. Cancer Res 41:4316–4323, 1981.
21. Palm PE, Rogers WI, Yesair DW, Kensler CJ: Studies on the delayed toxicity of phthalanilides and other compounds. Tox Appl Pharm 7:494 (Abstract 50), 1965.
22. Rogers WI, Yesair DW, Kensler CJ: Physiologic disposition of 4′, 4″-Bis (1,4,5,6-Tetrahydro-2-Pyrimidinyl) teraphthalanilide and 4-(1,4,5,6-Tetrahydro-2-Pyrimidinyl)-4′-(p-(1,4,5,6-Tetrahydro-2-Pyrimidinyl)Phenyl) carbamoylbenzanilide in dogs, monkeys, rats and mice. J Pharm Exptl Therap 152:139–150, 1966.
23. Yesair DW, Kohner FA, Rogers WI, Kensler CJ: Relationship of Phthalanilide-lipid complexes to uptake and retention of 2-Chloro-4′, 4″-Di (2-Imidazolin-2-yl) terephthalanilide (NSC 60339) by sensitive and resistant P388 leukemia cells. Cancer Res 26:202–207, 1966.
24. Yesair DW, Rogers WI, Baronowsky PE, Wodinsky I Thayer PS, Kensler CJ: Relationship of uptake and binding of an antileukemic phthalanilide to its biochemical and Chemotherapeutic effects on P388 lymphocytic leukemia cells. Cancer Res 27:314–321, 1967.
25. Yesair DW, Hofook C: The retention of efflux of phthalanilide (NSC 60339)-lipid complexes by sensitive or resistant murine tumor cells and Escherichia coli B. Cancer Res 28:314–319, 1968.
26. Yesair DW, Levins P, Caragay A, Shuck D, Funkhouser J: Identification of metabolites of 2-Chloro-4′,4″-Di (2-Imidazolin-2-yl) terephthalanilide (NSC 60339) from Cancer Patients with High resolution mass spectrometry. Proc Amer Assoc Cancer Res 10:101 (Abstract 402), 1969.
27. Hevesy GC, Levi HB, Rebbe OH: The Origin of the phosphorus compounds in the embryo of the chicken. Biochem J 32:2147–2155, 1938.
28. Taylor RF, Gaudio LA, Yesair DW: The intracellular localization of cancer chemotherapeutic drug binding macromolecular lipids in leukemia cells, 20th interscience conference on antimicrobial agents and chemotherapy. New Orleans (Abstract 27), 1980.
29. Thayer PS, Gordon HL: Protection of Escherichia coli against the growth-inhibiting effects of terephthanilides by purines, pyrimidines and amino acids. Cancer Chemother Rep 19:55–57, 1962.
30. Pine MJ, Harzewski E, Wissler FC: Action of the phthalanilide drugs on Escherichia coli, Cancer Res 23:932–937, 1963.
31. Yesair DW, Thayer PS, Kensler CJ: Comparative Studies of drug uptake, viability, and biosynthetic capabilities of P388 cells treated with 'active' or 'inactive' terephthalanilides. Ann N Y Acad Sci 172:635–666 (Article 18), 1971.

32. Burchenal JH, Adams HH, Lancaster S, Hirt R: Selective Antagonism of toxicity but not antileukemic effect of terephthalanilides by suramin. Fed Proc 24:443 (Abstract 1745), 1965.

33. Burchenal JH, Gregg VC, Lancaster SP, Hirt R, Berchtold R, Hischer R, Balsiger R: Prevention by Sulfonic and Phosphoric analogs of the terephthalanilide inhibition of leukemic P815Y *in vitro*. Cancer Res 25:469-471, 1965.

34. Yesair DW, Wodinsky I, Rogers WI, Kensler CJ: The effect of suramin-phthalanilide complexes on the chemotherapeutic activity and Toxicity of 4',4''-Bis (1,4,5,6-Tetrahydro-2-Pryimidinyl) terephthalanilide (NSC 57153). Biochem Pharmacol 17:305-313, 1968.

35. Gellhorn A, Wagner M, Rechler M, Koren Z, Benjamin W: The effect of a phthalanilide derivative on lipid metabolism in L1210 leukemia Cells. Cancer Res 24:400-408, 1964.

36. Jondorf WR, Spector A, Chaiken SJ: The effect of two carcinostatic Agents on the chemically induced stimulation of amino acid incorporation in a mammalian system. Biochem Biophys Res Commun 20:787-792, 1965.

37. Ochoa M, Jr, Gellhorn A, Benjamin WB: Phthalanilide inhibition of protein synthesis in a cell-free L1210 mouse ascites leukemia system. Cancer Res 24:480-484, 1964.

38. Rogers WI, Sattinger SA, Kensler CJ: Studies on the effects of 4',4''-Bis (1,4,5,6-Tetrahydro-2-Pyrimidinyl) terephthalanilide Dihydrochloride on oxidative phosphorylation in mitochondria of rat kidney and liver. Biochem Pharmacol 15:1225-1233, 1966.

39. Pine MJ, DiPaolo JA: The antimitochondrial action of 2-chloro-4',4''-Bis (2-Imidazolin-2-yl) Terephthalanilide and methylglyoxal bis (Guanylhydrazone). Cancer Res 26:18-25, 1966.

40. Altmann FP, Hampson SE, Chayen R: Phospholipids in formalin extracts of nuclei isolated from sheep lungs. Nature 202:1215-1216, 1964.

41. Biezinski JJ, Spaet TH: Phospholipid content of subcellular fractions in adult rat organs. Biochim Biophys acta 51:221-226, 1961.

42. Chayen J Gahan PB, Lacour LF: The Nature of a Chromosomal phospholipid. Quart J Microscop Sci 100:279-284, 1959.

43. Chayen J, Gahan PB, Lacour LF: The masked lipids of nuclei. Quart J Microscop Sci 100:325-337, 1959.

44. Frenster JH: Nuclear polyanions as De-repressors of Synthesis of Ribonucleic Acid. Nature 206:680-683, 1965.

45. Getz GS, Bartley W: The intracellular distribution of fatty acids in rat liver. The fatty acids of intracellular compartments. Biochem J 78:307-312, 1961.

46. Gurr MI, Finean JB, Hawthorne JN: The Phospholipids of Liver-cell fractions. The phospholipid composition of the liver-cell nucleus. Biochim biophys acta 70:406-416, 1963.

47. Levine C, Chargaff E: Phosphatide composition in different liver cell fractions. Exptl Cell Res 3:154-162, 1952.

48. Rees KR, Rowland GF, Varcoe JS: The metabolism of Isolated rat-liver nucleoli and other subnuclear fractions. The active site of amino acid incorporation in the nucleus. Biochem J 86:130-136, 1963.

49. Rose HG, Frenster JH: Composition and Metabolism of Lipids within repressed and active chromatin of interphase lymphocytes. Biochim Biophys Acta 106:577-591, 1965.

50. Stoneburg CA: Lipids of the cell nuclei. J Biol Chem 129:189-196, 1939.

51. Yesair DW, Kensler CJ: The Phthalanilides.. In: AC Sartorelli, DG Johns (eds), Antineoplastic and immunosuppressive agents. Handbuch der experimental Pharmacologie, Vol. XXXVIII/2, pp 820-828, Springer Verlag, New York, 1975.

52. Atwell GJ, Cain BF: Potential antitumor agents V.Bisquaternary salts. J Med Chem 10:706-713, 1967.

53. Cain BF, Atwell GJ, Seelye RW: Potential antitumor agents. X. Bisquaternary salts. J Med

58

Chem 12:199–206, 1969.

54. Atwell GJ, Cain BF: Potential Antitantitumor agents. 13. Bisquaternary salts. J Med Chem 16:673–678, 1973.
55. Atwell GJ, Cain BF: Potential antitumor agents. 15. Bisquaternary Salts. J Med Chem 17:930–934, 1974.
56. Taylor RF, Yesair DW: Interactions of cancer chemotherapeutic drugs and macromolecular lipids from L1210 leukemia cells, XIth International congress of biochemistry, Toronto, Canada (Abstract 12–6–H23), 1979.
57. Johnson RK, Zee-Cheng RKY, Lee WW, Acton EM, Henry DW, Cheng CC: Experimental antitumor activity of aminoanthraquinones. Cancer Treat Rep 63:425–439, 1979.
58. Zee-Cheng RKY, Cheng CC: Antineoplastic agents. Structure-activity relationship study of bis (substituted aminoalkylamino)-anthraquinones. J Med Chem 21:291–294, 1978.
59. Yesair DW, Callahan M, McComish MF, Taylor RF: Binding of the Cain quinolinium, NSC 113089, to rat tissue lipid extracts. Cancer Biochem Biophys 3:163–168, 1979.
60. Yesair DW, Taylor RF: Pharmacological implications of the interaction of heavy metals with novel macromolecular lipids. Drug Metab Rev 13:517–533, 1982.
61. Schmidt G: Über die trypanocide wirksamkeit von terephthalaniliden. Experientia 21:276–277, 1965.
62. Schmidt G, Hirt R, Fischer R: Babesicidal effect of basically substituted carbanilides. I. Activity against Babesia rodhaini in mice. Res Vet Sci 10:530–533, 1969.
63. Roby TO, Mazzola V: Elimination of the Carrier State of bovine anaplasmosis with imidocarb. Am J Vet Res 33:1931–1933, 1972.
64. Bacchi CJ, Nathan HC, Hutner SH, Duch DS, Nichol CA: Negation of trypanocidal drug cures by polyamines. In: Nelson JD, Grassi C (eds), Current chemotherapy and infectious diseases. Vol. 2, p 1119–1121. The American society for microbiology, Washington D.C., 1980.
65. Bacchi CJ, Nathan HC, Hutner SH, Duch DS, Nichol CA: Prevention by polyamines of the curative effect of amicarbalide and imidocarb for Trypanosoma brucei infections in mice. Biochem Pharmac 30:883–886, 1981.
66. Baer E, Stanacev NZ: Phosphonolipids. I. Synthesis of a phosphonic Acid Analogue of cephalin. J Biol Chem 239:3209–3214, 1964.
67. Baer E, Stanacev NZ: Phosphonolipids. V. Synthesis of phosphonic acid analogues of L-α-Lecithins. J Biol Chem 240:3754–3759, 1965.
68. Thompson GA, Jr, Kapoulos UM: In: Lowenstein JM, (ed),Methods in enzymology,lipids. Academic Press, New York, 1969, Vol. XIV, p 668.
69. Aalbers JA, Bieber LL: A method for quantitative determination of phosphonate phosphorus in the presence of organic and inorganic phosphates. Anal Biochem 24:443–447, 1968.
70. Kittredge JS, Roberts E: A carbon-phosphorus bond in nature, Science 164:37–42, 1969.
71. Hayaski a, Matsuura F: Isolation of a new sphingophosphonolipid containing galactose from the viscera of Turbo cornutus. Biochim Biophys Acta 248:133–136, 1971.
72. Shelburne FA, Quin LD: Isolation of 2-(Methylamino) Ethylphosphonic acid from the proteinaceous residue of a sea anemone. Biochim Biophys Acta 148:595–597, 1967.
73. Quin LD: The Presence of Compounds with a carbon-phosphorus bond in some marine invertebrates. Biochem 4:324–330, 1965.
74. Smith JD, Law JH: Phosphonic acid metabolism in Tetrahymena. Biochem 9:2152–2157, 1970.
75. Kittredge JS, Hughes RR: The occurrence of α-Amino-β-Phosphonopropionic acid in the zoanthid, Zoanthus sociatus, and the celiate, Tetrahymeana pyriformis. Biochem 3:991–996, 1964.

76. Bridges RG, Ricketss J: Formation of a phosphonolipid by larvae of the housefly, Musca domestica. Nature 211:199–200, 1966.
77. de Koning AJ: Isolation of 2-Aminoethylphosphonic acid from phospholipids of the abalone (Haliotis midae). Nature 210:113, 1966.
78. Kennedy KE, Thompson GA, Jr: Phosphonolipids: Localization in surface membranes of tetrahymena. Science 168:989–991, 1970.
79. Liang CR, Rosenberg J: The biosynthesis of the carbon-phosphorus bond in tetrahymena. Biochim Biophys Acta 156:437–439, 1968.
80. Alhadeff JA, Daves GD, Jr: Occurrence of 2-Aminoethylphosphonic acid in human brain. Biochem 9:4866–4869, 1970.
81. Alhadeff JA, Daves GD, Jr: 2-Aminoethylphosphonic Acid: distribution in human tissues. Biochim Biophys Acta 244:211–213, 1971.
82. DeLuca HF: The vitamin D system in the regulation of calcium and phosphorus metabolism. Nutrition Reviews 37:161–193, 1979.
83. Spencer R, Charman M, Lawson DEM: Stimulation of intestinal calcium-binding protein mRNA synthesis in the nucleus of vitamin D-deficient chicks by 1,25-Dihydroxycholecalciferol. Biochem J 175:1089–1094, 1978.
84. DeLuca HF: Some new concepts emanating from a study of the metabolism and function of vitamin D. Nutrition reviews 38:169–182, 1980.
85. Brumbaugh PF, Haussler MR: Specific binding of $1a$,25-Dihydroxycholecalciferol to nuclear components of chick intestine. J Biol Chem 250:1588–1594, 1975.
86. Price PA, Baukol SA: 1,25-Dihydroxyvitamin D_3 increases synthesis of the vitamin K-dependent bone protein by osteosarcoma cells. J Biol Chem 255:11660–11663, 1980.
87. DeLuca HF, Schnoes HK: Vitamin D: Recent advances. Ann Rev Biochem 52:411–439, 1983.
88. Igo-Kemenes T, Horz W, Zachau HG: Chromatin. Ann Rev Biochem 51:89–121, 1982.
89. Doerfler W: DNA methylation and gene activity. Ann Rev Biochem 52:93–124, 1983.
90. Nevins JR: The Pathway of Eukaryotic mRNA formation. Ann Rev Biochem 52:441–466, 1983.
91. Tabor CW, Tabor H: 1,4-Diaminobutane (Putrescine), Spermidine and spermine. Ann Rev Biochem 45:285–306, 1976.
92. Yuhas JM, Proctor JO, Smith LH: Some pharmacologic effects of WR2721: Their role in toxicity and radioprotection. Radiation Res 54:222–233, 1973.
93. Davidson DE, Grenan MM, Sweeney TR: Biological characteristics of some improved radioprotectors. In: Brady LW (ed),Radiation sensitizers. Their use in the clinical management of cancer. Masson publishing, USA, pp 309–320, 1980.
94. Gaugas JM: Mechanisms of In Vitro cytotoxicity of S-2-(3-Aminopropylamino) ethyl phosphorothioic acid. Adv Polyamine Res 3:441–449, 1981.
95. Nathan HC, Bacchi CJ, Sakai TT, Rescigno, D, Stumph D, Hutner SH: Bleomycin-induced life prolongation of mice infected with Trypanosoma brucei brucei EATRO IIO. Trans Roy Soc Trop Med Hyg 75:394–398, 1981.
96. Israel M, Rosenfield JS, Modest EJ: Analogs of spermine and spermidine I. Synthesis of polymethylenepolyamines by reduction of cyanoethylated, a, ω-Alkylenediamines. J Med Chem 7:710–716, 1964.
97. Yesair DW, McNitt S, Bitman C: Proposed mechanism for the reductive glycosidic clearage of daunomycin (NSC 82151) and adiamycin (NSC 123127). In: Ullrich V, Roots I, Hildebrandt A, Estabrook RW, Conney AH (eds), Microsomes and drug oxidation, p 688–697, Pergamon press, N.Y., 1977.
98. Calendi E, DiMarco A, Reggiani M, Scarpinato B, Valentini L: On physico-chemical interactions between daunomycin and nucleic acids. Biochim Biophys Acta 103:25–31, 1965.
99. Fishman MM, Schwartz I: Effect of divalent cations on the daunomycin-deoxyribonucleic

60

acid complex. Biochem Pharmacol 23:2147-2153, 1974.

100. Yesair DW, Bittman L, Schwartzbach E: Pharmacodynamic significance of metal chelates of the anthracyline drugs NSC 82151 and NSC 123127. Proc Amer Assoc Cancer Res 15:72, 1974.

101. Roberts JJ, Thomas AJ: The mechanism of action of antitumor platinum compounds. Prog Nucleic Acid Res Mol Biol 22:71-133, 1979.

102. Munchausen LL: The chemical and biological effects of cis-dichlorodiammine platinum (II), An antitumor agent, on DNA. Proc Nat Acad Sci 71:4519-4522, 1974.

103. Scovell WM, Kroos LR: Cis-diamminedichloroplatinum (II) modification of SV40 DNA occurs preferentially in (G+C) rich regions: Implication into the mechanism of action. Biochem Biophys Res Commun 108:16-23, 1982.

104. Zwelling LA, Kohn KW: Effects of cisplatin on DNA and the possible Relationships to Cytotoxicity and mutagenicity in mammalian cells. In: Prestayko AW, Crooke ST (eds), Cisplatin, pp 21-31, New York, Academic press, Inc., 1980.

105. Roberts JJ, Thomson AJ: The mechanism of action of antitumor platinum compounds. Prog Nucl Acid Res Mol Biol 22:71-133, 1979.

106. Matsumoto N, Sekimizu K, Horikoshi M, Ohtsuki M, Kidani Y, Nari S: Preferential inhibition of the activity of a stimulatory protein of eukaryotic transcription by platinum (II) Complexes. Cancer Res 43:4338-4342, 1983.

107. Macomber PB, O'Brien RL, Hahn FE: Chloroquine: Physiological basis of drug resistance in Plasmodium berghei. Science 152:1374-1375, 1966.

108. Clarke DH: The use of phosphorus 32 in studies on plasmodium gallinaceum. II. Studies on conditions affecting parasite growth in intact cells and in lysates. J Exper Med 96:451-463, 1952.

109. Schellenberg KA, Coatney GR: Influence of antimalarial drugs on nucleic acid synthesis in Plasmodium gallinaceum and P. berghei. Biochem Pharmacol 6:143-152, 1961.

110. Parker FS, Irvin JL: The interaction of chloroquine with Nucleic acids and nucleoproteins. J Biol Chem 199:897-909, 1952.

111. Cohen SN, Yielding KL: Spectrophotometric studies of the interaction of chloroquine with deoxyribonucleic acid. J Biol Chem 240:3123-3131, 1965.

112. Davidson MW, Griggs BG, Boykin DW, Wilson WD: Molecular structural effects involved in the interaction of quinolinemethanolamines with DNA. Implications for antimalarial action. J Med Chem 20:1117-1122, 1977.

113. Gutteridge WE, Trigg PI, Bayley PM: Effects of chloroquine on Plasmodium knowlesi In Vitro. Parasitol 64:37-45, 1972.

114. Warhurst DC: Chemotherapeutic agents and malaria research. In: Taylor AER, Muller R (eds),Br Soc Parasitol., Symp Vol 11: Chemotherapeutic agents in the study of parasites, pp 1-28, Blackwell Oxford, 1973.

115. Warhurst DC, Baggaley VC: Autophagic vacuole formation in P. berghei in vitro. Trans Roy Soc Trop Med and Hyg 66:5, 1972.

116. Van Jaarsveld PP, Lippoldt RE, Nandi PK, Edelhoch H: Effects of several antimalarials and phenothiazine compounds on the formation of coat structure from clathrin. Biochem pharmacol 31:793-798, 1982.

117. Nandi PK, Van Jaarsveld PP, Lippoldt RE, Edelhoch H: Effect of basic compounds on the polymerization of clathrin. Biochem 20:6706-6710, 1981.

3. Metabolism-Dependent Toxicities of Cyclophosphamide and Protection by N-Acetylcysteine and Other Thiols

H.L. GURTOO, M.J. BERRIGAN, J. LOVE, A.J. MARINELLO, J.H. HIPKENS, S.D. SHARMA, S.K. BANSAL, B. PAUL, P. KOSER, R.F. STRUCK and Z. PAVELIC

ABSTRACT

Our investigations spanning over the past six years have implicated cyclophosphamide (CP) metabolite acrolein in some specific biochemical and systemic toxicities of CP. Acrolein is implicated in the depletion of hepatic glutathione, in the depression of hepatic microsomal mixed function oxidase system (MFO), and in the induction of urotoxicity either *per se* or in conjunction with other CP metabolites. Acrolein-associated toxicities appear to arise as a consequence of the formation of covalent adducts between acrolein and critical sulfhydryl groups in protein-bound thiols. These specific toxicities of CP are blocked by exogenous thiols such as N-acetylcysteine (NAC) and mesnum (2-mercaptoethanesulfonate). However, combination of CP with the exogenous thiols does not interfere with the immunosuppressive (i.e. myelosuppressive) and carcinostatic properties of CP, which appear to be the consequence of metabolism-dependent formation of the alkylating metabolites of CP, presumably phosphoramide mustard.

INTRODUCTION

Cyclophosphamide (2-[bis(2-chloroethyl)amino]tetrahydro-2H-1,3,2-oxazaphosphorine 2-oxide) is an important anticancer drug used in the treatment of a variety of cancers in humans and in experimental animals [1, 2]. In addition, because of its immunosuppressive activity, CP has found application in the treatment of some autoimmune diseases and in the preparation of patients for tissue and organ transplantation [1, 3, 4]. Inactive *pe se,* CP is activated by the hepatic cytochrome P450-dependent mixed function oxidase system. The activated metabolites, believed to be responsible for the chemotherapeutic activity and toxic manifestations of CP, could be quanti-

F.M. Muggia (ed.), Experimental and Clinical Progress in Cancer Chemotherapy
© *1985, Martinus Nijhoff Publishers, Boston. ISBN 0-89838-679-9. Printed in the Netherlands.*

tatively reduced by the cytosolic oxidase/reductase-mediated detoxification of their precursor metabolic intermediates such as 4-hydroxy-CP [5, 6]. The major pathway of CP metabolism, illustrated in Figure 1, involves the formation of 4-hydroxy-CP which rearranges to its ring-opened isomer aldophosphamide; the latter can undergo non-enzymatic β-elimination to release acrolein and phosphoramide mustard. Alternatively, both 4-hydroxy CP and aldophosphamide can be acted upon by cytosolic reductases/oxidases and converted to essentially detoxified products 4-keto CP and carboxyphosphamide, respectively [5, 6].

Hepatic microsomal mixed function oxidase complex (MFO) – comprised of a lipid fraction, NADPH:cytochrome P450 reductase and cytochrome P450 – activates and/or detoxifies a host of chemicals including drugs, anticancer agents, pesticides, carcinogens, mutagens, teratogens and some endogenous substrates [7, 8]. Molecular oxygen and the cofactor NADPH are obligatory requirements for the catalysis of MFO-mediated reactions. MFO is an inducible enzyme complex and the diversity of the system is dependent on the multiplicity of the terminal oxidase, cytochrome P450. During recent years multiple forms of cytochrome P450 have been described, depending upon the species, strain and the inducing agent employed. Multiplicity of cytochrome P450 has been established on the basis of differences in various characteristics which include: spectral properties; substrate, inhibitor and induction specificities; immunological properties; and mobility on gel electrophoresis [9–11]. Recently, several cDNA clones and genomic clones representing different forms of cytochrome P450 have been isolated and their diversity confirmed by DNA sequence analysis [12–14].

The toxic and the carcinostatic effects of CP are believed to be a consequence of covalent interaction between the active metabolites of CP and the target tissue macromolecules. DNA cross-linking by CP metabolite phosphoramide mustard is believed to represent the ultimate cytotoxic lesion that accounts for the carcinostatic effects of CP. Various systemic toxicities of CP include hematopoietic depression, alopecia, nausea, vomiting, hemorrhagic cystitis and others [1].

During the past six years we have been involved in defining the nature of the active metabolites of CP capable of covalent interaction with tissue macromolecules and of relating these interactions to various toxic manifestations of CP. It is hoped that this approach will allow a better understanding at the molecular level of the biological effects of CP and lead to development of knowledge with clinical applicability for the intervention of at least some of the undesirable toxicities of CP, without compromising its carcinostatic and immunosuppressive properties. We hope that this report will demonstrate the fruitfulness of this approach.

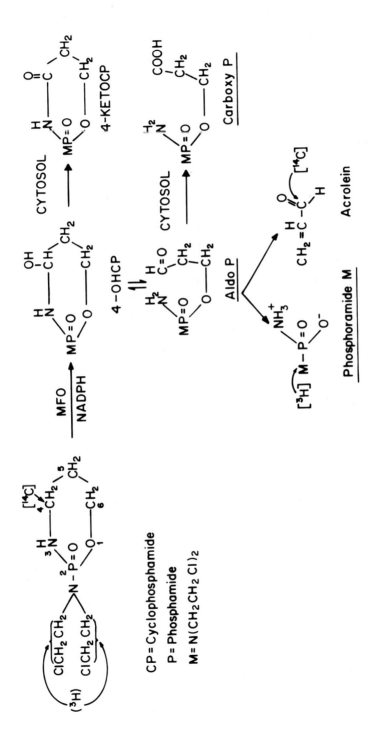

Figure 1. Metabolic fate of cyclophosphamide.
MFO, mixed-function oxidase; 4-OHCP, 4-hydroxycyclophosphamide; 4-KETO-CP, 4-ketocyclophosphamide; Aldo-P. aldophosphamide; Carboxy P, carboxyphosphamide.

METHODS

Various methodologies, analytical techniques and protocols employed in the studies reported in this article have been described in reasonable details previously [15, 16].

Text

In 1969 and early 1970's various investigators reported that several anti-cancer drugs, especially alkylating agents such as cyclophosphamide (CP), are able to depress the hepatic microsomal mixed function oxidase (MFO) system and its various enzymatic activities [17–19]. However, this depression was attributed to the ability of these agents to produce a generalized depression of protein synthesis. Our first report in 1976, in which we examined not only hepatic MFO activities but also the activities of some conjugation and hydrolytic pathways, suggested that CP produced a specific depression of hepatic MFO which probably results from the suicidal inactivation of cytochrome P450 during the metabolism of CP [15]. In other words, the data suggested that a metabolite of CP is able to destroy/denature cytochrome P450. To pursue this line of thought we set out to define the nature of various CP metabolites capable of binding covalently to macromolecules. Both *in vitro* and *in vivo* investigations were started. By this time the major pathway of the hepatic microsomal metabolism of CP, outlined in Figure 1, was well known. Since this pathway suggested that acrolein and phosphoramide mustard, derived from 4-hydroxy-CP, would retain radioactive labels in C-4 and chloroethyl groups, respectively, when CP labeled in these atoms is metabolized, we decided to investigate metabolism-mediated binding of [^{3}H-chloroethyl]CP and [^{14}C-4]CP to proteins and nucleic acids in an *in vitro* incubation system employing hepatic microsomes (or a reconstituted cytochrome P450 system), nucleic acid (calf thymus DNA or E. Coli tRNA), specifically labeled CP and various cofactors. While at that time [^{14}C-4]CP was commercially available, [^{3}H-chloroethyl]CP was procured from Amersham/Searle as a custom order preparation. The results of one of these experiments are given in Figure 2.

To our amazement we found that ^{14}C-radiolabel from [^{14}C-4]CP essentially binds exclusively to proteins in the incubation, whereas ^{3}H-label from [3H-chloroethyl]CP binds predominantly to nucleic acid. Our results demonstrated greater then 80-fold binding of the ^{14}C-label to microsomal proteins, relative to the ^{3}H-label, and binding of the ^{3}H-label to nucleic acids was favored 10–40 fold over the ^{14}C-label. By reference to Figure 1 it is evident that the binding of ^{14}C-label implicates acrolein, whereas that of the ^{3}H-label implicates phosphoramide mustard. To verify further the involvement of acrolein, chemical features of acrolein – i.e., the presence of a free aldehyde group and a reactive vinylic double bond – suggested that chemi-

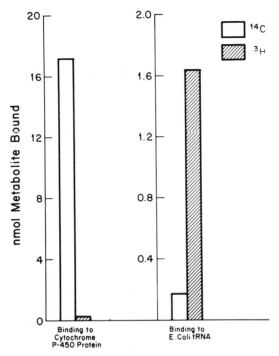

Figure 2. Metabolism-dependent binding of ^{14}[C-4]cyclophosphamide and [^{3}H-chloroethyl]cyclophosphamide to cytochrome P450 and E. coli tRNA, catalyzed by the reconstituted purified cytochrome P450 system.

A reconstituted cytochrome P450-containing system was used in these studies. The system contained in a buffered solution the following: cytochrome P450 purified from phenobarbital pretreated rats to a specific activity of 15–17 nmoles/mg protein, NADPH: cytochrome P450 reductase, dilauroyl phosphatidylcholine, ^{3}H-CP or ^{14}C-CP, E. coli tRNA, NADPH. At the end of the incubation tRNA and proteins were precipitated and treated to remove any non-covalently bound radioactivity. Background values derived from identical incubations lacking NADPH only have been subtracted.

cals with a free amino and/or a free sulfhydryl group should block binding of the ^{14}C-label to the protein in the incubation during the metabolism of ^{14}C-CP. The results of these investigations are given in Table 1. Among the chemicals containing a free amino group (e.g. semicarbazide, glycine and lysine) semicarbazide and glycine blocked the binding by 80 and 50%, respectively, whereas lysine failed to have any effect. Chemicals containing an amino and a sulfhydryl groups were most potent: glutathione inhibited the binding by 90% and cysteine by 88%. N-acetylcysteine, which contains only a sulfhydryl group, was able to block the binding by 70%. These data, while implicating acrolein, suggested that both a free amino group and/or a free thiol were effective in interacting with acrolein and thereby preventing its binding to the proteins. Since acrolein is known to form a thiazolidine type derivative with cysteine, the binding experiments suggested the possible isolation of such a metabolite. Repeated attempts to isolate this conjugate of acrolein and cysteine failed; however, its formation in the incubation was demonstrated by cochromatography of the chloroform-extracted aqueous phase of the incubations with a synthetic conjugate of acrolein and cysteine [16]. These results established that acrolein is formed during the metabolism of ^{14}C-CP and that it binds covalently to proteins, and also forms a thiazolidine type of conjugate with free cysteine added to the incubation. The observation that lysine, which is the major source of free amino groups in proteins (other than the terminal amino group), did not interact with acrolein, as indicated by its inability to block the binding of the ^{14}C-label, suggested that acrolein binds to proteins via reaction involving addition of a thiol group to the acrolein double bond and probably not via the reaction between the aldehyde group of acrolein and the free amino-group of cysteine, which is required in the formation of a thiazolidine conjugate. An earlier report from this laboratory [20] and that of Ashoor and Chu [21] had demonstrated that the binding of aflatoxin B_{2a}, which cleaves to form aldehyde-containing products, depends upon the reaction between free aldehydes of aflatoxin B_{2a} cleavage products and free protein amino groups of lysine, as this reaction was inhibited by about 70% by free lysine. We seized upon this experience and compared the effects of various chemicals, including lysine, on the binding of ^{3}H-aflatoxin B_{2a} and ^{14}C-CP to hepatic microsomes, and as expected, found that while lysine inhibits the binding of aflatoxin B_{2a} as reported [21], it does not inhibit the binding of ^{14}C-CP [16].

Table 1. Effects of amino acids and other compounds on the binding of [14][C-4] cyclophosphamide to rat hepatic microsomal proteins in in vitro incubation systems [1]

Chemical	Concentration used mM	[14]C] Cyclophosphamide bound to protein as % of control activity
None		100
Glutathione	4	10
Cysteine	4	12
N–Acetylcysteine	4	30
Semicarbazide	4	20
Glycine	4	50
Lysine	4	105

[1] Hepatic microsomes from phenobarbital-treated rats were incubated with NADPH and [14][C-4] cyclophosphamide in the presence or absence of various inhibitors of the binding of ^{14}C to hepatic microsomes. At the termination of the incubation, the microsomal protein was precipitated, treated to remove noncovalently bound radioactivity, digested and counted. Incubations lacking NADPH served to obtain a background value which has been subtracted. In various experiments, 45–55 nmol of [14][C-4] cyclophosphamide metabolite were bound to 1 mg of microsomal protein, and this value represents 100% of control activity.

Taken together these investigations led to the conclusion that acrolein is binding to hepatic microsomal proteins via interaction between the double bond in acrolein and cysteine thiol groups in proteins.

Acrolein is known to interact covalently with glutathione [22]. This report, in conjunction with our observations showing that acrolein-associated ^{14}C-label binds to microsomal proteins and that this binding is effectively blocked by glutathione and cysteine, posed the following questions: (a) what are the biological effects of this binding; (b) does acrolein, formed *in vivo* during CP metabolism, deplete glutathione; (c) can cysteine block the *in vivo* depression of hepatic MFO by CP; (d) what other toxicities of CP are due to acrolein; (e) can N-acetylcysteine or other thiols block any of these toxicities and (f) if N-acetylcysteine (or other thiols) is able to block some of the undesirable toxicities of CP, will this drug combination compromise the carcinostatic activity of CP.

DEPRESSION OF HEPATIC MFO BY CP AND ITS PROTECTION BY THIOLS

To determine specificity of binding of the ^{14}C-label with various protein components in hepatic microsomes, gel electrophoresis-autoradiography of hepatic microsomes or purified cytochrome P450 modified with ^{14}C-CP was carried out and the results were compared with those obtained in experiments in which hepatic microsomes or purified cytochrome P450 was modified with ^{14}C-acrolein in the absence of NADPH, which is required for the metabolism of ^{14}C-CP. In all experiments in which either hepatic microsomes or purified cytochrome P450 were used to metabolize ^{14}C-CP in the presence of NADPH, cytochrome P450, as determined by gel electrophoresis-autoradiography, was the major protein component to which ^{14}C-label became bound. No binding occurred in the absence of NADPH or when ^{3}H-chloroethyl CP was used (instead of [^{14}C-4]CP) either in the presence or absence of NADPH. Similarly, ^{14}C-acrolein without any metabolism (in the absence of NADPH) produced major binding to cytochrome P450 [23].

To determine the biological effects of the binding of CP metabolite(s) to microsomal proteins, effects of various CP metabolites on the spectral integrity of cytochrome P450 were examined *in vitro* in the absence of metabolism. The results of some of these studies are illustrated in Figure 3. Of the various analogs and metabolites tested (e.g. CP, ifosfamide, trofosfamide, 4-keto-CP, acrolein, phosphoramide mustard, nor-nitrogen mustard, and 4-hydroxy-CP, which undergoes spontaneous decomposition with the release of acrolein) only acrolein and 4-hydroxy-CP produced denaturation of cytochrome P450. This denaturation was associated with a decrease in absorbance at 450 nm and an increase at 420 nm in the reduced CO-com-

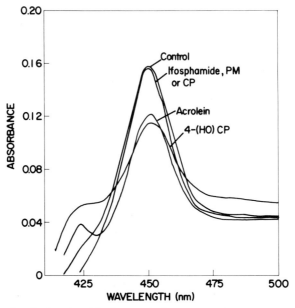

Figure 3. Effects of cyclophosphamide, its metabolites, and analogs on the spectral integrity of cytochrome P450 in rat hepatic microsomes.

Rat liver microsomes were incubated with acrolein (0.7 or 7 mM final concentration) or other cyclophosphamide metabolites or analogs (7 mM final concentration) for 30 mins at 37 °C in an initial volume of 1.2 ml. At the termination of the incubation, the volume was adjusted to 10 ml with 0.1 M phosphate buffer (pH 7.4) and the reduced CO-complexed spectrum of cytochrome P450 was recorded as described [16]. The compounds tested included: PM, phosphoramide mustard; CP, cyclophosphamide; 4-(HO)CP, 4-hydroxycyclophosphamide; 4-keto CP, 4-ketocyclophosphamide; acrolein, ifosfamide and others. Details described previously [16].

plexed difference spectrum. Nearly identical to the potential of various chemicals with a free amino and/or a free sulfhydryl group to block the binding of the ^{14}C-label from ^{14}C-CP, these chemicals, especially cysteine, glutathione and *N*-acetylcysteine, effectively blocked acrolein-induced denaturation of cytochrome P450. As expected, lysine essentially afforded no protection against acrolein. In addition to acrolein, which as suggested earlier (vide supra) appears to interact with free thiol groups in proteins, thiol reagents, such as *p*-hydroxymercuribenzoate and phenylmercuric acetate, produced an identical type of denaturation of cytochrome P450; and this denaturation also, as in the case of acrolein, was blocked by cysteine. Furthermore, at suboptimal concentrations, the effects of thiol reagents and acrolein were additive. Preincubation of hepatic microsomes with aminopyrine, a substrate of the hepatic mixed function oxidase, provided complete protection against acrolein-induced denaturation of cytochrome P450. Taken together, these observations lend strong support to the hypothesis that CP metabolite acrolein denatures hepatic cytochrome P450 by covalent interaction with sulfhydryl group(s) in or near the enzyme active site.

Inactivation (or destruction) of hepatic cytochrome P450 by various chemicals has been reported by a number of investigators. These compounds belong to different chemical types and include compounds containing double or triple bonds [24–28], sulfur-containing compounds, e.g. parathion [29, 30] and carbon disulfide [31–33], and carbon tetrachloride [24, 34]. In all these cases, cytochrome P450-mediated metabolism is an obligatory requirement.

Various mechanisms have been suggested to explain events leading to the destruction of cytochrome P450 [24]. Some of these mechanisms include: epoxide formation from double or triple bonds which culminates in the alkylation of the heme moiety of the cytochrome P450; generation of free radicals, which lead to peroxidative destruction of cytochrome P450, e.g. carbon tetrachloride; metabolic desulfuration of sulfur-containing chemicals which leads to release of elemental sulfur capable of binding covalently to sulfhydryl groups in cytochrome P450 apoprotein. In comparison to these potential mechanisms, the mechanism proposed for the metabolism dependent destruction of hepatic cytochrome P450 by CP is novel in that it implicates the formation of addition products between the acrolein double bond and free thiols in or near the enzyme active site.

Having found earlier that CP causes a specific depression of various hepatic MFO activities *in vivo* [15] and having established *in vitro* that CP metabolite acrolein binds to cytochrome P450 and causes its denaturation [16], both of which can be blocked by thiols such as N-acetylcysteine, it was of interest to ascertain whether CP-induced *in vivo* depression of MFO could be blocked by N-acetylcysteine. The effects of a single dose of CP (180–200 mg/kg) on hepatic cytochrome P450 content, NADPH: cytochrome P450 reductase, and on various MFO activities, e.g. aryl hydrocarbon hydroxylase, aminopyrine demethylase and metabolism of ^{14}C-CP, were investigated (Figure 4). In different experiments, CP produced a 25–50% depression of all these activities including the hepatic cytochrome P450 content. N-acetylcysteine and another thiol, mesnum (2-mercaptoethane sulfonate), given just before CP, almost completely reversed the effects of CP [23]. These investigations demonstrated that appropriate thiols, such as N-acetylcysteine, were effective in neutralizing the biochemical toxicologic effects of the CP metabolite acrolein. However, these investigations did not evaluate whether these beneficial effects of thiols were being achieved at the expense of the desired properties of CP, i.e. chemotherapeutic and immunosuppressive activities. This is addressed later in this article.

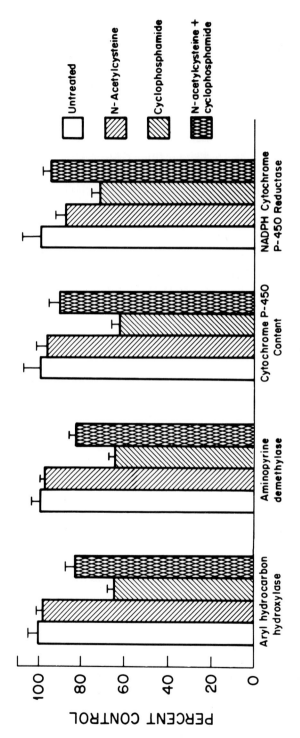

Figure 4. Protection by N-acetylcysteine against CP-induced depression of hepatic mixed function oxidase system and NADPH:cytochrome P450 reductase.

Each group was comprised of at least four rats and the experiment was repeated 2 to 4 times. (Permission to republish the data from Ref. 42 obtained from Cancer Research).

EFFECTS OF CYCLOPHOSPHAMIDE ON HEPATIC GLUTATHIONE LEVELS

Since CP metabolism in the liver generates acrolein which is known to interact with glutathione [16, 22, 35], it was of importance to evaluate the role of glutathione in the toxicity of CP and *vice versa*. Dose-response studies were carried out to determine the effects of CP and several of its metabolites on hepatic glutathione levels. The results are shown in Figure 5. CP caused a dose-dependent depletion of hepatic glutathione in mice. CP was nearly as effective as the well known glutathione depletor diethyl maleate. The effects of acrolein paralleled the effects of CP; however, phosphoramide mustard, the alkylating metabolite of CP, was an order of magnitude less active. Furthermore, when time dependence of hepatic glutathione depletion by CP was examined, maximum depletion was produced at 4-hr after CP administration, and at suboptimal doses the effects of a combination of CP and diethyl maleate were additive [35].

As shown in Figure 6 a single dose of CP (200 mg/kg) prevented normal weight gains in rats over a period of 8 days. Treatment with diethyl maleate

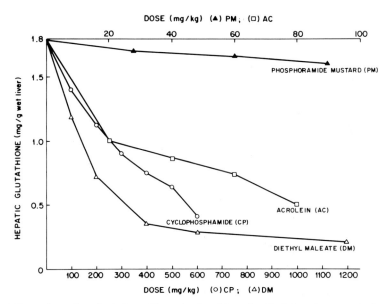

Figure 5. Dose-dependent depletion of hepatic glutathione by diethyl maleate, cyclophosphamide, phosphoramide mustard and acrolein in mice.

Six C3Hf/HeHa mice in each group were given i.P. Injections of different doses of phosphoramide mustard (PM), acrolein, diethyl maleate, or cyclophosphamide (CP). Two hr later, the mice were killed by cervical dislocation, and the livers were quickly removed, placed on ice, and immediately assayed individually for the levels of reduced glutathione. Each point is the mean of 6 animals. Individual values in each group varied less than 10% from the mean value. (Permission to reproduce the data from Reference 35 obtained from Cancer Research).

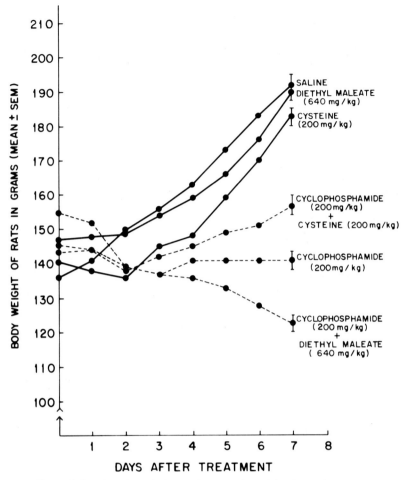

Figure 6. Effects of CP, Cysteine, diethyl maleate, and combinations of these agents on body weight gain of Sprague-Dawley rats.

Male rats (4 rats/gtoup) received 0.9% NaCl solution i.p., cycteine, diethyl maleate, or cyclo-phosphamide (CP), or combinations of CP and diethyl maleate or of CP and cysteine. Diethyl-maleate and CP were given as single doses. One-half of the 200-mg/kg dose of cysteine was given twice daily for 3 days prior to the administration of CP, whereas diethyl maleate was given in a single dose 30 min before CP. Daily weight gain over the next 7 days was recorded for each animal. Each point represents the mean of 4 animals. Bars, S.E. (Permission to reproduce the data from Reference 35 obtained from Cancer Research).

and CP produced a weight loss, whereas cysteine alone or diethyl maleate alone were unable to block the normal weight gain achieved on day 8. However, the rats, while failing to gain weight after CP, showed significant weight gain when pretreated with cysteine for up to three days prior to CP administration.

Taken together these results demonstrate that CP metabolite acrolein, which not only denatures cytochrome P450 and binds to proteins, also depletes hepatic glutathione and retards normal body weight gain; all these nocuous effects of acrolein could be blocked by appropriate thiols.

EFFECTS OF THIOLS ON THE TOXICITY AND CHEMOTHERAPEUTIC ACTIVITY OF CP

In addition to the biochemical toxicities elucidated in our laboratories over the past several years and reported here, CP is known to produce several systemic toxicities. Significant among them are urotoxicity and myelosuppression [1]. Urotoxic effects of CP can be dose-limiting [36, 37] and have proven fatal [38]. Extensive hydration of the patient may alleviate CP-induced urotoxicity but this treatment modality has been criticized for being difficult to maintain properly and also provides only partial protection against urotoxicity. Acrolein, while reported not to participate in the cytotoxicity of CP [39], has been implicated in the production of hemorrhagic cystitis following CP administration [40–42]. Since we had found that the biochemical toxic effects of acrolein *in vivo* could be neutralized by pretreatment with thiols, e.g. mesnum and N-acetylcysteine, we expected to be able to block the urotoxic effects of CP by thiols. A rat model system was developed to evaluate bladder lesions histologically. Four days following a single dose of CP (180–200 mg/kg) to rats, bladders were removed, fixed and examined for histology. While the bladders from saline treated, N-acetylcysteine-treated and mesnum-treated rats looked normal under the microscope, the bladders of rats treated with CP showed extensive pathology which included: thickened and spongy walls; hemorrhagic lesions; prominent edema in the perivesicular tissue; necrosis; bloody exudate in the lumen which contained fibrin, cellular debris and inflammatory cells; and various focal changes in the intact areas of the epithelium which included thinning, atypia and karyorrhexis. However, the bladders of rats that received a combination of CP and a thiol (N-acetylcysteine or mesnum) showed essentially no pathological changes. These results are illustrated in Figure 7. Other investigators have also achieved a diminution of the urotoxic effects of CP in man and animals with N-acetylcysteine and mesnum [42–45].

The parallelism between the deleterious effects of CP on hepatic MFO and the urinary bladder and the fact that both these lesions are reversed by thiols strongly implicate a common pathway involved in the induction of these lesions. The common pathway appears to be the production of the toxic metabolite acrolein during the hepatic MFO-mediated metabolism of CP.

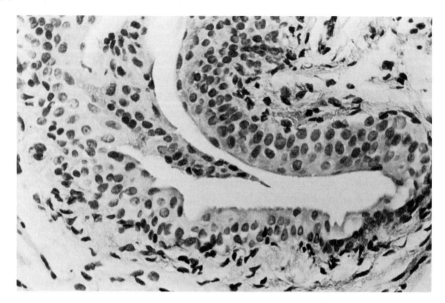

Figure 7. Histological changes in the bladders of rats treated with cyclophosphamide in the absence and the presence of treatment with *N*-acetylcysteine (NAC).

Bladders were fixed and sections stained with hematoxylin and eosin stain for examination at a magnification of 500. Other details are described elsewhere [42]. (Permission to reproduce these results from Ref. 42 obtained from Cancer Research).

A. A bladder from a control rat

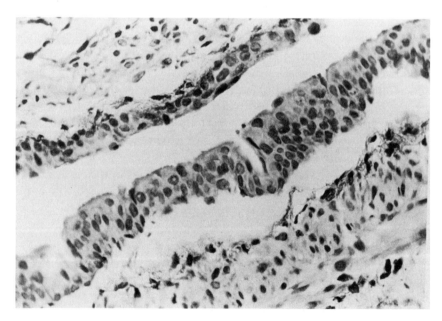

B. A bladder from NAC-treated rats

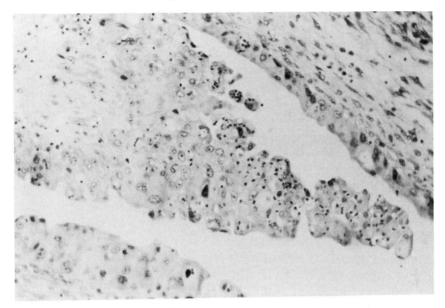

C. A bladder from cyclophosphamide-treated rats

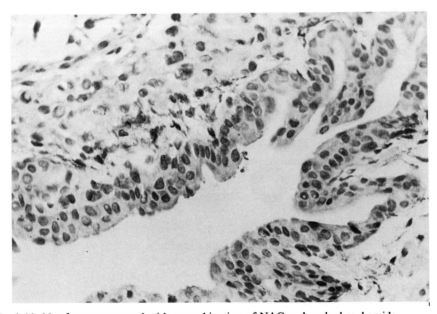

D. A bladder from rats treated with a combination of NAC and cyclophosphamide.

Immunosuppressive properties of CP have been exploited in the treatment of some chronic diseases of autoimmune etiology and in the preparation of patients for tissue and organ transplantation [1, 3, 4]. The possibility that thiols, because of their interaction with acrolein and/or possibly with other metabolites of CP, could mitigate the immunosuppressive properties of CP was examined in rats. After a single injection of CP (180 mg/kg) alone or following pretreatment with N-acetylcysteine or mesnum, rats were sacrificed on day 4 and the degree of CP-induced leucopenia was evaluated. While N-acetylcysteine had no effect on the WBC count, CP reduced the count by greater than 94% and neither N-acetylcysteine nor mesnum were able to block the effects of CP [42]. These results suggest that acrolein is not responsible for the leucopenic effects of CP and therefore implicate the involvement of other CP metabolites, possibly the alkylating metabolite phosphoramide mustard. Several reports have demonstrated that a number of alkylating agents are myelosuppressive.

It is gratifying to speculate that thiols such as N-acetylcysteine and mesnum could be combined with CP to alleviate acrolein-related toxicities. However, limitations of such interventions should not be underestimated. Since thiols entrap electrophiles, it is conceivable that the use of thiols could interfere with the chemotherapeutic activity of CP, which is believed to be due to the alkylating metabolite phosphoramide mustard [1]. However, our data comparing depletion of hepatic glutathione by acrolein and phosphoramide mustard suggest that thiols may not interfere with the chemotherapeutic activity of CP, since the affinity of phosphoramide mustard for glutathione, a major source of endogenous thiols, was found to be an order of magnitude weaker than that of acrolein [35]. This assumption is further strengthened by the observation that CP-induced myelosuppression, which is believed to be a consequence of the formation of alkylating metabolites of CP, was not affected either by N-acetylcysteine or by mesnum [42]. Based on these observations it could be predicted that combination of appropriate thiols with CP, while protecting against urotoxicity and possibly other acrolein-related toxicities, should not interfere with the chemotherapeutic activity of CP. Indeed, combinations of N-acetylcysteine (or cysteine) and CP were found not to interfere with the cytotoxic effects of CP against Walker 256 carcinosarcoma [23, 35, 42]. Also, the effects of ifosfamide against L1210 leukemia were not compromised by N-acetylcysteine [46]. Using mesnum, we have recently reported that combination of this drug with CP, while alleviating the urotoxicity, did not produce any interference with the carcinostatic activity of CP against Walker 256 carcinosarcoma [23].

ACKNOWLEDGEMENT

The authors would like to thank Miss Karen Marie Schrader for her assistance in the preparation of this manuscript.

Supported by Grants CA-23634 and CA-24538 from the National Cancer Institute, Bethesda, MD.

ABBREVIATIONS

Abbreviations used are: CP, cyclophosphamide; ^{14}C-CP, ^{14}[C-4]cyclophosphamide; ^{3}H-CP, [^{3}H-chloroethyl]cyclophosphamide; MFO, microsomal mixed function oxidase system; NAC, N-acetylcysteine.

REFERENCES

1. Friedman OM, Myles A, Colvin M: Cyclophosphamide and related phosphoramide mustards. In: Rosowsky A (Ed), Advances in Cancer Chemotherapy, pp 143–204, Marcell Dekker, Inc. New York, 1979.
2. Gershwin ME, Goetzl EJ, Steinberg AG: Cyclophosphamide: Use in practice. Ann Int Med 80:531–540, 1974.
3. Santos GW, Sensenbrenner LL, Anderson PN, Burke PJ, Klein DL, Slavin RE, Schacter B, Borgaonkar DS: HL-A- Identical marrow transplants in aplastic anemia and acute leukemia employing cyclophosphamide. Transpl Proc 8:607–610, 1976.
4. Zinke H, Woods JE: Donor pretreatment in cadaver renal transplantation. Surg Gyn and Obstet 145:183–188, 1977.
5. Cox PJ, Phillips BJ, Thomas P: The enzymatic basis of the selective action of cyclophosphamide. Cancer Res 35:3755–3761, 1975.
6. Hipkens JH, Struck RF, Gurtoo HL: Role of aldehyde dehydrogenase in the metabolism-dependent biological activity of cyclophosphamide. Cancer Res 41:3571–3583, 1981.
7. Conney AH: Pharmacological implications of microsomal enzyme induction. Pharmacol Rev 19:317–366, 1967.
8. Gelboin HV: Benzo(a)pyrene metabolism, activation and carcinogenesis: Role and regulation of mixed function oxidases and related enzymes. Physiol Rev 60:1107–1166, 1980.
9. Guengerich FP: Isolation and purification of cytochrome P450 and the existence of multiple forms. Pharmac Therap 6:99–121, 1979.
10. Guengerich FP, Dannan GA, Wright ST, Martin MV, Kaminsky LS: Purification and characterization of liver microsomal cytochrome P450: Electrophoretic, spectral, catalytic and immunochemical properties and inducibility of eight isozymes isolated from rats treated with phenobarbital or β-naphthoflavone. Biochemistry 21:6019–6030, 1982.
11. Lu AYH, West SB: Multiplicity of mammalian microsomal cytochrome P450. Pharmac Rev 31:277–295, 1980.
12. Fujii-Kuriyama Y, Mizukami Y, Kawajiri K, Sogawa K, Muramatsu M: Primary structure of a cytochrome P450: Coding nucleotide sequence of phenobarbital-inducible cytochrome P450 cDNA from rat liver. Proc Natl Acad Sci USA 79:2793–2797, 1982.
13. Mizukami Y, Fujii-Kuriyama Y, Maramatsu M: Multiplicity of deoxyribonucleic acid sequences with homology to a cloned complementary deoxyribonucleic acid coding for rat phenobarbital-inducible cytochrome P450. Biochemistry 22:1229–1233, 1983.

78

14. Mizukami Y, Sogawa K, Suwa Y, Muramatsu M, Fujii-Kuriyama Y: Gene structure of a phenobarbital-inducible cytochrome P450 in rat liver. Proc Natl Acad Sci USA 80:3958–3962, 1983.

15. Gurtoo HL, Gessner T, Culliton P: Studies of the effects of cyclophosphamide, vincristine and prednisone on some hepatic oxidations and conjugations. Cancer Treat Rep 60:1285–1293, 1976.

16. Gurtoo HL, Marinello AJ, Struck RF, Paul B, Dahms RP: Studies on the mechanism of denaturation of cytochrome P450 by cyclophosphamide and its metabolites. J Biol Chem 256:11691–11701, 1981.

17. Tardiff RG, DuBois KP: Inhibition of hepatic microsomal enzymes by alkylating agents. Arch Intl Pharmacol 177:445–456, 1969.

18. Donelli MG, Franchi G, Rosso R: The effect of cytotoxic agents on drug metabolism. Eur J Cancer 6:125–126, 1970.

19. Donelli MG, Garattimi S: Drug metabolism after repeated treatments with cytotoxic agents. Eur J Cancer 7:361–364, 1971.

20. Gurtoo HL, Campbell TC: Metabolism of aflatoxin B_1 and its metabolism-dependent and independent binding to rat hepatic microsomes. Mol Pharmacol 10:776–789, 1974.

21. Ashoor SH, Chu F-S: Interaction of aflatoxin B_{2a} with amino acids and proteins. Biochem Pharmacol 24:1799–1805, 1975.

22. Izard C, Libermann C: Acrolein. Mutation Res 47:115–138, 1978.

23. Gurtoo HL, Marinello AJ, Berrigan MJ, Bansal SK, Paul B, Pavelic ZP, Struck RF: Effect of thiols on toxicity and carcinostatic activity of cyclophosphamide. Seminars in Oncology 10:35–45, 1983.

24. DeMatteis F: Loss of liver cytochrome P450 caused by chemicals. In: DeMatteis F, Aldridge WN (eds), 'Handbook of Experimental Pharmacology' Vol. 44:95–127, Springer-Verlag, New York, 1978.

25. DeMatteis F, Gibbs AH, Unseld A: Loss of haem from cytochrome P450 caused by lipid peroxidation and 2-1lllyl-2-isopropylacetamide. Biochem J 168:417–422, 1977.

26. Ortiz-de-Montellano PR, Kunze KL: Inactivation of hepatic cytochrome P450 by allenic substrates. Biochem Biophys Res Commun 94:443–449, 1980.

27. Ortiz-de-Montellano PR, Kunze KL: Self-catalyzed inactivation of hepatic cytochrome P450 by ethynyl substrates. J Biol Chem 255:5578–5585, 1980.

28. Ortiz-de-Montellano PR, Mico BA: Destruction of cytochrome P450 by ethylene and other olefins. Mol Pharmacol 18:128–135, 1980.

29. DeMatteis F: Covalent binding of sulfar to microsomes and loss of cytochrome P450 during the oxidative desulfuration of several chemicals. Mol Pharmacol 10:849–854, 1974.

30. Poore RE, Neal RA: Evidence for extrahepatic metabolism of parathion. Toxicol Appl Pharmacol 23:759–768, 1972.

31. Bond EJ, DeMatteis F: Biochemical changes in rat liver after administration of carbon disulfide, with particular reference to microsomal changes. Biochem Pharmacol 18:2531–2549, 1969.

32. DeMatteis F, Seawright AAS: Oxidative metabolism of carbon disulfide by the rat. Effect of treatments which modify the liver toxicity of carbon disulfide. Chem-Biol Interac 7:375–388, 1973.

33. Hunter AL, Roberts RA: Inhibition of hepatic mixed-function oxidase activity *in vitro* and *in vivo* by various thiono-sulfur-containing compounds. Biochem Pharmacol 24:2199–2205, 1975.

34. Smuckler EA, Arrenius E, Hultin T: Alterations in microsomal electron transport, oxidative N-demethylation and azo-dye cleavage in carbon tetrachloride and dimethylnitrosamine-induced liver injury. Biochem J 103:55–64, 1967.

35. Gurtoo HL, Hipkens J, Sharma SD: Role of glutathione in the metabolism-dependent tox-

icity and chemotherapy of cyclophosphamide. Cancer Res 3584–3591, 1981.

36. Buckner CD, Rudolph RH, Fefer A, Clift RA, Epstein RB, Funk DD, Neiman PE, Slichter SJ, Storb R, Thomas ED: High dose cyclophosphamide therapy for malignant disease. Cancer (Phila) 29:357–365, 1972.

37. Philips FS, Sternberg SS, Cronin AP, Vidal PM: Cyclophosphamide and urinary bladder toxicity. Cancer Res 21:1577–1589, 1961.

38. Tolley DA, Castro JE: Cyclophosphamide-Induced cystitis of the urinary bladder of the rats and the treatment. Proc R Soc Med 68:169–171, 1975.

39. Wrabetz E, Peter G, Hohorst HJ: Does acrolein contribute to the cytotoxicity of cyclophosphamide. J Cancer Res Clin Oncol 98:119–126, 1980.

40. Brock N, Stekar J, Pohl J, Niemeyer V, Scheffler G: Acrolein, the causative factor of urotoxic side-effects of cyclophosphamide, ifosfamide, trofosfamide and sufosfamide. Arzneim Forsch 29:659–661, 1979.

41. Cox PJ: Cyclophosphamide cystitis-identification of acrolein as the causative agent. Biochem Pharmacol 28:2045–2049, 1979.

42. Berrigan MJ, Marinello AJ, Pavelic Z, Williams CJ, Struck RF, Gurtoo HL: Protective role of thiols in cyclophosphamide-induced urotoxicity and depression of hepatic drug metabolism. Cancer Res 42:3688–3695, 1982.

43. Morgan LR, Donley PJ, Harrison EF: The control of ifosfamide induced hematuria with N-acetylcysteine. Proc Amer Assoc Cancer Res 22, 190, 1981.

44. Scheef W, Klein HO, Brock N, Burkert H, Gunther U, Hoefer-Janker H, Schnitker J, Voigtmann R: Controlled clinical studies with an antidote against the urotoxicity of oxazaphosphorines: Preliminary results. Cancer Treat Rep 63:501–505, 1979.

45. Kedar A, Simpson CL, Williams P, Moore R, Tritsch G, Murphy GP: The Prevention of cyclophosphemide-induced bladder swelling in rat by i.v. administration of sodium -2-mercaptoethane sulfonate. Res Commun Chem Pathol Pharmacol 29:339–348, 1980.

46. Kline L, Gang M, Woodman RJ, Cysyk RL, Venditti JM: Protection with N-acetyl-L-cysteine against isophosphamide toxicity and enhancement of therapeutic effect in early murine L1210 leukemia. Cancer Chemotherapy Rep 57(part 3):299–304, 1973.

4. Cell Surface Membranes as a Chemotherapeutic Target

THOMAS R. TRITTON and JOHN A. HICKMAN

1. INTRODUCTION

DNA has held the center stage as a target for antineoplastic drugs essentially since the beginning of cancer chemotherapy. The DNA as target concept has been productive, of course, because it has led to the development of a spectrum of drugs which are useful for treating human cancer. Moreover, many of these drugs have been thought to act at the level of DNA, either by binding to the nucleic acid directly or by interference with the enzymes participating in its biosynthesis. The insistence on DNA as the receptor for anticancer drug action has also served, at least to some extent, to distract attention from other potential targets and mechanisms. However, during the last decade numerous laboratories have contributed to the idea that the cell surface or plasma membrane may represent an attractive target both for new classes of drugs and as an alternative explanation for the action of certain existing agents. The cell surface offers several advantages as the receptor for antineoplastic drug action: (a) the outer surface of a cell is the first structure encountered by a drug and thus represents the first level at which specificity could operate. In this sense the plasma membrane acts as a screen or filter to regulate further access of the cell to agents with which it comes in contact; (b) the cell surface is intimately involved in the regulation of a host of biological functions. Thus, disruption of these functions could be cytotoxic; (c) the past several years of cancer research have led to a very detailed understanding of the fact that concrete differences exist between the surfaces of cancer and normal cells, including the presence in neoplastic cell membranes of substrates for oncogene products (Amini and Kaji, 1983). Consequently, one expects that it should be possible to design drugs to specifically exploit the differences between normal and abnormal cells.

To our knowledge no one has systematically attempted to design anew any anticancer drugs which act by attacking membranes. This is probably a

F.M. Muggia (ed.), Experimental and Clinical Progress in Cancer Chemotherapy
© *1985, Martinus Nijhoff Publishers, Boston. ISBN 0-89838-679-9. Printed in the Netherlands.*

result of the fact that while DNA is a well defined target with well under-stood geometries of drug interactions, membranes are not. Thus, a lipid bilayer comprising many different types of molecules with undefined spatial relationships to each other, and conducting a baffling variety of biochemical processes, presents a formidable problem for medicinal chemists attempting to construct pharmacologic agents which carry out specific mechanisms. Because of this complexity, the approach of cancer chemotherapists inter-ested in this area has been to investigate current or existing drugs by asking whether they cause pharmacologic disruption of measurable membrane functions. The rationale of this research is that if a drug has the cell surface as part or all of its target for action, the drug must be capable of modulating the biological properties of the cell surface. The state of the art is principally

Table 1. Cancer chemotherapeutic agents for which evidence exists suggesting membrane actions. The drugs are classified according to a traditional scheme; the membrane action refer-ence refers to the particular section of this review where such work is discussed

Alkylating agents

Drug	Membrane actions
Mustards:	
Mechlorethamine (HN2)	fluidity, ion gradients, cyclic nucleotides, functional activities, covalent interaction, ultrastructure
tris(chloroethyl)amine (HN3)	ion gradients
cyclophosphamide	cyclic nucleotides
chlorambucil	fluidity, cyclic nucleotides, immobilized drugs
Aziridinyl compounds:	
Trenimon	ion gradients, cyclic nucleotides, functional activi-ties
Nitrosoureas:	
BCNU	lectin interaction, composition

Antimetabolites

Drug	Membrane actions
Folic Acid Analogs:	
Methotrexate	lectin interaction, composition
Pyrimidine Analogs:	
5-fluorouracil	composition, ion gradients
cytosine arabinoside	fusion, model membranes
Purine Analogs:	
6–thioguanine	lectin interaction, composition

a cataloging effort, that is, work which observes and reports on various membrane effects of selected anticancer drugs, with relatively little attention to the detailed mechanisms involved. A diversity of publications exists and this review attempts to gather in one place much of the established literature. Because the area is relatively new, and heretofore unreviewed we believe it is useful at this stage to follow the cataloging scheme. The information could have been categorized by drug type, but we choose instead to present the record in terms of the properties of membranes in order to consciously shift away from the more traditional classification of antineoplastic drugs. Table I summarizes the results both in terms of drug type and reported membrane actions. It will become evident for the reader that a large fraction of the published work on membrane effects concerns adriamycin and the anthracyclines. This is partly a historical accident in that adriamycin happened to be the first antineoplastic for which extensive evidence concerning membrane action was accumulated. In addition, adriamycin also possesses an amphipathic structure that leads one to expect possible membrane activities. There is considerable evidence that many of the other anticancer drugs may also possess membrane activity as well, however, and

Natural products	
Drug	Membrane actions
Adriamycin	lectin interaction, fluidity, fusion, ion gradients, functional activities, composition, receptors, ultrastructure, immobilized drugs, model membranes
VP16	fusion, model membranes
vinca alkaloids	ion gradients, functional activities, composition, model membranes
mitomycin C	ion gradients
bleomycin	lectin interaction, fluidity, functional activities, composition
actinomycin D	lectin interaction, functional activities, composition

Miscellaneous agents	
Drug	Membrane actions
cis-platinum	lectin interaction, ion gradients, cyclic nucleotides, composition, functional activities
m-AMSA	ion gradients, composition, covalent interactions
ellipticine	model membranes
neocarzinostatin	functional activities

the relative dominance of adriamycin in this area may not persist in the future.

Several areas are not reviewed here. We are concerned principally with the plasma membrane or cell surface because it is the most prominent membrane studied to date. Thus mitochondrial, nuclear, endoplasmic reticular and other intracellular membranes are not discussed here, although they may be equally valid as targets for drug action. Likewise, in order to limit the discussion, we have tended to concentrate on the relationship of anticancer or cytotoxic action to membrane effects, rather than on side effects or other toxicities associated with the antineoplastic pharmacopaeia. Also neglected are the areas of biological response modifiers, drug transport and induction of cellular differentiation, all of which are of increasing importance to new thinking in cancer chemotherapy and all of which may involve the cell surface. For reviews of these areas the interested reader is referred to De Luca and Shapiro (1981), Sirotnak *et al.* (1979), and Hozumi (1983).

2. INTERACTION OF CELL SURFACES WITH LECTINS

Lectins are plant proteins with multivalent recognition sites for the various carbohydrate groups which are present on cell surface membranes. There exists a wide variety of individual lectin types with differing specificity for individual carbohydrates. Because they bind with high affinity to cell surfaces these proteins have been widely used to probe the structural alterations which surface membranes may undergo as cells engage in processes like adhesion, differentiation and recognition (Sharon and Lis, 1972). Some of the original excitement in this area arose when it was discovered that tumor cells are more easily agglutinated or cross-linked by multivalent lectins than are non-tumor cells (e.g. Burger and Goldberg, 1967). Although the reasons for this apparent tumor cell specificity are not entirely clear, this type of work laid the foundation for sensitive assays of lectin mediated cell agglutination which were later used to determine if anticancer drugs modulated surface properties that were reflected by changes in agglutination. The original work in this area was done by Hwang and Sartorelli (1975). These investigators incubated Sarcoma 180 cells with various anticancer drugs for 1–7.5 hours and then measured changes in the agglutination rate stimulated by concanavalin A (Con A) or wheat germ agglutinin (WGA). 6-Thioguanine and bleomycin inhibited the lectin induced agglutination although the purine antimetabolite required a much longer exposure time to elicit the effect. In contrast, chromomycin A_3, adriamycin, BCNU and methotrexate all enhanced the rate of agglutination compared to untreated cells. It is significant that not all cytotoxic agents alter lectin-induced agglutination, how-ever, since 5-fluorouracil, ara-C and 5-fluorodeoxyuridine were inactive in this assay (Hwang and Sartorelli, 1975; Naiwo and Quan, 1980). Moreover, cis-platinum treatment increases the agglutination rate of splenocytes but decreases the agglutination rate of Dalton's lymphoma cells with both Con A and WGA (Prasad and Sodhi, 1981). Apparently, these lectin effects are specific for both the drug under study and the exact array of surface carbo-hydrates presented by the cells. One additional comment may be relevant: the kinetics of agglutination involve both a preliminary lag phase followed by the actual agglutination. Unless specified control experiments are done, it may be difficult to tell if the effect of drug treatment is to lengthen or shorten the lag phase or to alter the agglutination rate itself. Most, but not all, of the publications in this area address this complication.

Later work has revealed additional details of the drug-induced alteration of cell surfaces detected by lectins. Murphree *et al.* (1976, 1981) showed that a correspondence exists between the concentration of adriamycin required for cytotoxicity to Sarcoma 180 cells in culture and effects on cell aggluti-nation by Con A. Also, the agglutination changes are not due either to alterations in the number of surface carbohydrate receptors or to the rate of occupancy of the receptors by the lectin molecule. By contrast, 6-thioguan-ine, which has the opposite effect to adriamycin on the agglutination rate, also is different by virtue of the fact that the binding of lectin to the receptor is altered by the drug because of a reduction in the number of surface receptors. This may account for the observation that the effects on 6-thio-guanine on lectin-induced agglutination require several hours of drug expo-sure, whereas adriamycin causes the effect rapidly.

Incubation of human red blood cells with adriamycin over the concentra-tion range 10^{-7} to 10^{-5} M has no effects on morphology of the discocytes but, like wheat germ agglutinin (Anderson and Lovrien, 1981), the drug can prevent the dramatic morphological transformation to the echinocyte form (Mikkelson *et al.*, 1977). This transformation is brought about by ATP depletion or by increasing intracellular calcium concentration. A number of hypotheses exist as to how this change in shape is controlled within the membrane, although the most prominent explanation is that the lectin bind-ing protein glycophorin modulates these changes. It has been found that adriamycin at a concentration of 10^{-7} molar not only resembles the lectin in preventing the morphological transformation, but that N-acetylglucosam-ine, known to reverse the effect of the lectin (Anderson and Lovrien, 1981), can also reverse that of adriamycin (Chahwala and Hickman, in prepara-tion). This observation may allow an in-depth dissection of the effects of adriamycin not only upon lectin interactions but also on events within the cytoskeleton, which are well-understood in the red cell. Adriamycin binding to spectrin is also of probable significance to these events, and such an interaction was reported by Mikkelson *et al.* (1977).

It is possible that the actions of the anticancer drugs on lectin mediated processes are not closely associated with the mechanisms leading to cytotoxicity. To address this question Siegfried and Tritton (1979) studied both adriamycin resistant S180 sublines and inactive anthracycline analogs in the agglutination assay. These workers found that a) adriamycin enhances the agglutination of sensitive but not 10-fold resistant cells; and b) the cytotoxically inactive aglycone moiety of adriamycin was also inactive in the lectin-agglutination tests. These results lend further credence to the idea that membrane processes revealed by lectin probes may indeed be related to membrane events which mediate the anticancer action of the drug. Additionally, Fico *et al.* (1977) and Cannellakis and Chen (1979) have shown that the *in vivo* antitumor activity of a series of diacridine compounds had a highly significant inverse correlation with the ability of the compounds to enhance the agglutination rate of P388 cells by Con A or wheat germ agglutinin. Moreover, no correlation of antitumor activity with drug effects on DNA or RNA synthesis or on cellular uptake of the diacridine could be demonstrated. Consequently these workers have proposed that this class of compounds have a site of action at the cell surface.

Cell agglutination involves not only static cross-linking by multivalent lectins, but also dynamic mobility of lectin receptors (Horowitz *et al.*, 1974). This receptor mobility has important functional consequences. Wang and Edelman (1978) have shown that there is a direct correlation between concanavalin A receptor mobility and the ability of the lectin to stimualte DNA synthesis in lymphocytes. Thus, components of the cell surface which control receptor mobility may be involved in the regulation of cell proliferation. Since the anticancer agents influence cellular replication by exerting cytotoxicity, as well as promote changes in lectin interaction at the surface, a potential mechanism of cytotoxic action could involve modulation of surface receptors involved in normal growth control.

3. MEMBRANE FLUIDITY

The concept of fluidity dominates much of the current thinking about biological membranes. This notion is so central because it embodies the idea that membranes are dynamic, that is, a fluid environment allows the rotations and translations that membrane molecules need to undergo in order to function. Knowing the importance of membrane fluidity and its regulation, it is not surprising that many types of pharmacologic agents act by modulating fluidity (e.g. local anesthetics and polyene antibiotics; Pang *et al.*,

1979; Archer, 1975). Several of the more important anticancer drugs have also been shown to alter membrane fluidity. However, since many nonspecific small molecules are capable of stimulating fluidity changes simply by virtue of binding to membranes, it becomes important to attempt to link any observed fluidity alterations with biological functions of the drug. Each of the studies discussed here attempts to do this.

A short discussion of methodology is in order. There are numerous techniques for measuring membrane fluidity. Most of the commonly used approaches are spectroscopic and rely on the fact that the spectral properties of a given probe molecule depend on the amount of motion the probe undergoes. Since a highly fluid membrane allows a high degree of motion and a more solid membrane allows less motion, it is clear that a spectral property which depends on motion can report on membrane fluidity. Two different techniques are used in the studies to be described below. One approach is fluorescence depolarization measurements. If a fluorescent molecule is excited with polarized light, the emitted light will have a lower degree of polarization if the molecule rotates before emission. The amount of rotation is governed by how fluid the environment of the probe is; hence high polarization is associated with low fluidity and vice versa. The most common fluorescence probe is diphenylhexatriene (DPH) which, due to its lipid solubility, partitions into membrane when incubated with cells. The measured polarization can be used to calculate a 'microviscosity' of the membrane, but this extrapolation has been criticised (e.g. Lakowicz et al., 1979) so most workers simply report relative polarization values in control and treated cells, which provides information on relative membrane fluidity changes. The other commonly employed fluidity probe is a nitroxide free radical attached to a fatty acid. This probe gives an electron paramagnetic resonance spectrum whose characteristics depend on the amplitude of motion allowed by a given membrane environment. The results are usually expressed as an order parameter with values from 0 for no order (high fluidity) to 1 for complete order (rigid). Both the fluorescence and spin label spectra are principally sensitive to rotational motion and thus treatments which change the fluidity of membranes alter the rotational motion of the probe molecule.

Grunicke et al. (1982) showed that the alkylating agent nitrogen mustard increased the fluorescence polarization of DPH in Ehrlich ascites cells. Their interpretation was that alkylation of the cell surface is accompanied by a decrease in membrane fluidity. Furthermore, the cytotoxic action of the drug on cell multiplication was directly proportional to the change in polarization as well as to changes in the activity of cell surface Na^+/K^+ ATPase. Similar results are seen with chlorambucil and it seems reasonable to infer that alkylating agents do indeed alter membrane fluidity (and other membrane properties as well) and that such alterations may be associated with inhibition of tumor cell growth.

Although the principal antitumor mechanism of bleomycin is thought to be scission of DNA, Lazo *et al.* (1983) have provided evidence that the plasma membrane of endothelial cells may be the target for the notorious pulmonary toxicity of this drug. They observed, using spin labeling, that treatment of cultured bovine pulmonary artery endothelial cells with bleomycin caused an immediate increase in plasma membrane fluidity that persisted for at least 24 hours. In association with this fluidity change was a decrease in the activity of the cell surface enzyme, angiotensin converting enzyme (ACE). An important control experiment in this work was that desamido bleomycin A_2 (a bleomycin metabolite which is not a pulmonary toxin) did not increase fluidity or decrease ACE activity. Apparently, it will be important to determine if bleomycin also alters the fluidity characteristics of tumor cells, but at present it appears that alteration of endothelial cell fluidity may be important in the pathogenesis of drug induced pulmonary fibrosis.

The most comprehensive studies of membrane fluidity effects of an antineoplastic agent have been with adriamycin (Murphree *et al.*, 1981, 1982; Wheeler *et al.*, 1982; Siegfried *et al.*, 1983). It was originally shown that adriamycin induces a decrease in membrane fluidity of exposed cells and that the effect is dose-dependent and rapid. It is possible that this fluidity response may be a primary event in the initiation of cytotoxicity by adriamycin. However, since many compounds can modulate membrane fluidity (Jain *et al.*, 1975) and most of them are not effective antineoplastic agents, one is left with a dilemma of interpretation in determining whether or not the effect of a drug on membrane fluidity is a primary event in its biological mechanism of action, or is simply a result of the fact that many substances will alter fluidity nonspecifically in the course of interaction with cellular membranes. To attempt to address this problem, conditions which influence the cytotoxic action of adriamycin were analyzed for their ability to influence in parallel ESR detected changes in the fluidity of S180 cell membranes.

Sarcoma 180 cells made hypoxic by exposure to 95% N_2/5% CO_2 and thereby more sensitive to the cytotoxic action of adriamycin (Kennedy *et al.*, 1983) exhibit an increase in membrane fluidity. The enhanced inhibition of cell survival exhibited by adriamycin against the hypoxic cells was completely reversible upon reoxygenation and this reversal of the enhanced cytotoxicity followed the same time course of reoxygenation as the reversal of the order parameter changes. These findings indicate that (a) a change in membrane fluidity in the region of the paramagnetic molecule is caused by exposure of Sarcoma 180 cells to an atmosphere of low oxygen tension, and

(b) this change in the property of the membrane appears to be coupled to the enhanced cytotoxicity of the anthracycline in hypoxic cells.

Further evidence that the physical state of the membrane may be a determinant of the cytotoxicity of the anthracylines was found in studies comparing the order parameter of anthracycline sensitive and resistant Sarcoma 180 sublines. A progressive increase in membrane fluidity was found as cells developed increasing resistance to this antibiotic (Siegfried et al., 1983). Likewise, Wheeler et al. (1982) showed that progressively increasing resistance to adriamycin in MDAY-K2 cells was associated with decreased polarization of DPH i.e. increased fluidity. Complicating the issue, Glaubiger et al. (1983) recently reported that P388 cells resistant to adriamycin were more rigid than sensitive cells. Apparently, the direction of the change in membrane fluidity with progressive insensitivity to the drug depends on the cell line under study, but these changes in the fluidity properties of membranes appear to be coupled to the expression of anthracycline resistance.

Since it is clear that the fluidity of membranes plays an important role in regulating biological function (Melchior and Steim, 1976), the correlations found between fluidity, hypoxia and sensitivity to adriamycin are suggestive of a direct relationship between these phenomena. Moreover, the magnitude of the fluidity changes observed, although representing a change of only a few percent in the spectral order parameter, are of a size known to result in the modulation of pharmacologic processes. For example, Pang et al. (1979) have shown that small changes in fluidity caused by exposure to anesthetics are coupled to large changes in membrane permeability. Likewise, tolerance to ethanol is closely associated with a small change in membrane fluidity measured in membranes obtained from whole mouse brain using 5-doxyl stearic acid as the spin probe (Chin and Goldstein, 1977). Specific membrane enzymes can also be regulated by changes in fluidity. Illustrating this point, changes in the cholesterol content of membranes caused the activity of Na^+, K^+-ATPase to decrease by 200 to 300 percent when the order parameter decreased by only 2% (Sinensky et al., 1979). In addition, the cell surface enzymes adenylate cyclase, 5'-nucleotidase and cAMP phosphodiesterase are all modulated by small changes in fluidity induced by the local anesthetic benzyl alcohol (Gordon et al., 1980). Of course, it is possible that fluidity changes can be selective in effecting changes in membrane functions, with large effects on one function and little or no modulation of others. Data discussed elsewhere suggest that this is indeed the case with some anticancer drugs.

The problem at hand is to determine whether the general effect of a perturbation in lipid fluidity is related to the cytotoxic action of a drug, in particular adriamycin. It has been shown that the drug can be actively cytotoxic under conditions where it only interacts with the cell surface (Tritton and Yee, 1982). Thus, it is logical to hypothesize that membrane properties would be involved in the action of the drug. The existing data do not allow the development of a simple model because cells rendered more sensitive to adriamycin by hypoxia and cells selected for decreased sensitivity to this antibiotic both show an increase in membrane fluidity compared to appropriate controls. Since the probe measures bulk fluidity (Bales and Leon, 1978; Campisi and Scandella, 1980) it is clear that the overall fluidity of the membrane may control specific responses in different ways. Separated neighborhoods or domains within the membrane regulate different biologic processes, and each domain may respond to different stresses or conditions to preserve the functioning of the cell in an optimal manner. In fact, the results offer positive experimental support for the concept of segregated domains within a cell surface membrane. As each membrane neighborhood changes, one may observe similar effects on a general property such as fluidity but vastly different responses by the cell to the drug. The important findings of the fluidity work, however, are that the adaptive response to hypoxia and the emergence of drug resistance, both of which result in changes in adriamycin cytotoxicity, also lead to a change in membrane fludiity and that the drug itself causes a dose dependent increase in membrane fluidity. Taken together all the results suggest that fluidity effects at the cell surface may be important in the mechanisms of action of the anthracyclines which have previously been thought to act primarily at intracellular sites.

4. MEMBRANE FUSION

The fusion of one membrane with another is a phenomenon which occurs constantly in biological systems. Processes ranging from viral infection to exocytosis require a membrane fusion event to proceed (Poste and Nicolson, 1978) and thus it is not surprising to find that pharmacologic disruption of fusion has profound consequences on cellular function (Tritton et al., 1977). The exact mechanisms governing membrane fusion are under intensive study in many laboratories and, although a comprehensive picture is not in hand, one expects many of the more salient details to be understood in the next few years.

Evidence exists showing that cytosine arabinoside, VP-16, and adriamycin are all capable of modulating membrane fusion. Koehler et al. (1983) have discussed the fact that although the principal mechanism of action of ara-C is thought to involve DNA synthesis and repair, other mechanisms may also be present at high doses of the drug. They discovered several membrane lesions by high dose ara-C including an inhibition of phospholipid vesicle fusion. VP-16, on the other hand, is a potent inducer of fusion in this system. The ability to alter lipid vesicle (liposome) fusion has been even more thoroughly studied with adriamycin using proton NMR to follow the fusion reaction (Murphee *et al.*, 1982). The basic concept in this approach is that fusion of smaller vesicles to form larger ones slows the molecular motion of the lipids. This, in turn, causes the proton resonances to broaden such that, as larger liposomes are formed, the motion becomes slower, and finally in the limit of very large fused vesicles, no resonance is observed. That is, the signal intensity decreases with time as fusion occurs. In pure phosphatidyl choline vesicles, fusion proceeds very slowly if at all, and addition of adriamycin does not cause any change. If, however, the bilayer contains small amounts (0.1–10%) of cardiolipin adriamycin markedly enhances the rate of liposome fusion. The ability of adriamycin to greatly stimulate the fusion rate of cardiolipin-containing liposomes is unique, both because Ca^{2+} (a known fusogen) does not have this ability and because the effect is limited only to cardiolipin and not to acidic phospholipids as a class. Thus, adriamycin interacts in a specific manner with cardiolipin containing vesicles to alter their fusion characteristics.

Liposomal vesicles are a useful model system for studying physicochemical aspects of drug-membrane interactions, but this system does not necessarily predict events which will occur in real biological membranes. Necco and Ferraguti (1979) have performed experiments to test possible membrane fusion effects of adriamycin in cultured skeletal muscle cells. Such myoblasts can fuse in culture to form myotubes and, indeed, adriamycin can inhibit this fusion process. It is interesting that the effect of the drug is to *inhibit* fusion, since the work with liposomes showed a *stimulation* of fusion. The authors of the myoblast study argue that the effect of adriamycin is to block a Ca^{2+} dependent fusion mechanism which may involve proteins associated with the cell surface; this would be an inoperable mechanism in liposomes. It is clear, however, that adriamycin (as well as the other antineoplastics mentioned above) can alter the interactions that are involved in membrane fusion with potential consequences on biological function.

5. OF IONS, GRADIENTS AND POTENTIALS

The transport of ions across the cell membrane is important for maintenance of internal ion homeostasis, the coupled mechanisms of ion and nutrient transport, and the transmission of messages *via* excitation response coupling. Interest in the role that ions may play in the control of normal cell proliferation and in neoplasia has been increasing and is the subject of two recent and excellent volumes (Boynton *et al.*, 1982; Leffert, 1980). Much of the work shows that there are differences in internal ion concentration found in normal and neoplastic cells and in ion dependency for cell growth. Thus, for the chemotherapist these studies provide some interesting observations which are potentially exploitable for the design of novel chemotherapeutic agents and may also relate to the mode of action of some present drugs, reviewed below.

Sodium ion content is increased in a variety of rapidly dividing tumour cells when compared with either rapidly dividing normal cells or preneoplastic cells (Cameron et al., 1980; Smith et al., 1981; Zs-Nagy et al., 1981). The reason for this is not clearly established but presumably relates to a difference in function of either membrane permeability to sodium or to altered ion-exchange processes modulated by membrane proteins, or possibly to the fact that the high glycolytic rate of neoplastic cells results in the necessity for elevated sodium-proton exchange. A recent study has shown that the diuretic drug amiloride, which blocks the sodium-proton antiport (Cragoe, 1979), has antineoplastic effects both in vitro and in vivo (Sparks et al., 1983). Treatment of murine tumors in vivo with an intensive but non-toxic schedule of amiloride resulted in tumor regression and a parallel loss of their intracellular sodium, more particularly of nuclear sodium. Amiloride has a number of non-specific effects, for example inhibition of protein synthesis (Leffert, 1980), and it remains to be determined whether the antineoplastic effects are really causally related to changes in sodium ion concentration. Notwithstanding such cautions the result represents activity of a new class of compound and a totally novel and exciting approach to chemotherapy which should be eagerly followed up.

Neoplastic cells, derived from a wide variety of sources, show a marked decrease in their requirement for external calcium in order to support growth in vitro when compared to their normal counterparts (Balk, 1971; Boynton & Whitfield, 1976; Parsons et al., 1983). In avian sarcoma virus transformed rat NRK cells this fall in calcium requirement is coincident with the expression of the membrane-bound viral oncogene product pp60[src] (Durkin et al., 1981). Again, the basis for this profound change is obscure. It may be that calcium homeostasis is altered in neoplasia in terms of the content of free and bound calcium in cellular compartments, or that transformation bypasses a normally calcium-dependent step of cell growth, or that such a step is more sensitive to low concentrations of the ion.

The coupling of ion fluxes, one to another, is an extremely complex process mediated by the plasma membrane, and perturbation of such fluxes by membrane active drugs may have tremendous consequences on the control of cell proliferation. Such perturbations may also influence electrochemical gradients which result in the cell membrane potential (Em). Changes in Em also play a role in the control of proliferation (Boonstra, 1982; Kieter,

1980), although a direct causal role may be unlikely (Deutsch & Price, 1982). Once again, differences between normal and neoplastic cells exist with regard to this membrane-mediated property (Mikkelson & Koch, 1981) which may be exploitable by the chemotherapist.

Although it is attractive to speculate that interference with the intricacies of ion-modulated control of proliferation may constitute a facet of the mode of action of membrane-active antitumour drugs, less elegant ways of explaining cytotoxicity may also exist at this level. For example, the collapse of the one thousand fold gradient of calcium across the cell membrane (from extracellular fluid to cytoplasm) may constitute a final common pathway of cell death (Schanne et al., 1979; Farber, 1981). The release of the major calcium store in mitochondria to the cytoplasm, where free calcium is normally in the micro- to nanomolar concentration range, by a variety of toxins also has a profound effect on membrane structure and cell function (Jewell et al., 1982).

Alteration of ionic homeostasis by subjecting cells to hypotonic shock results in the degradation of DNA (Williams et al., 1974), presumably through strand breakage, and it is possible that DNA damage and membrane damage may not be mutually exclusive events when the multimodal effects of the antineoplastic drugs are considered. For example, in a study of the mode of action of the acridine methanesulphonic acid m-AMSA a possible relationship between ionic changes and DNA damage was speculated on by Ralph (1980). Incubation of PY815 cell nuclei in a hypotonic salt solution in the absence of m-AMSA produced strand breaks in DNA which resembled those produced in intact cells by m-AMSA, and the author suggested that the drug may affect the compartmentalization of divalent cations in the nucleus, changing specific endonuclear activity. While it may be the case that drug treatment and hypotonicity both change DNA conformation by quite different mechanisms, which results in the nicking of the strained double helix, it would be interesting to study in some depth what effects changes in ion flux and concentration have on DNA integrity and function. For example, the potassium ion ionophore valinomycin is cytotoxic and a morphological examination of the nuclei of treated cells suggested parallels between its effects and those of radiation (Whitfield and Perris, 1968).

Even some of the very early studies of the prototypical alkylating agents, the mustards, had suggested that their vesicant effect was exerted by reaction with the cell surface (Peters, 1947). More recent studies with nitrogen mustard (HN2) have shown that at cytotoxic concentrations (10^{-5} to 10^{-6} M) the cellular uptake of ^{86}rubidium, a potassium congener, is profoundly inhibited in both mouse PC6A plasmacytoma cells (Baxter et al., 1982) and Ehrlich ascites cells (Grunicke et al., 1982). Baxter et al. (1982) suggested that this inhibition might be the result of the covalent cross-linking of the membrane-bound, sulfhydryl containing enzyme Na$^+$ K$^+$-AT-Pase, an enzyme known to be sensitive to other cross-linking agents (Freedman, 1979; Sweadner, 1977). A monofunctional analogue of nitrogen mustard which is devoid of antineoplastic activity and cannot cross-link biological macromolecules was shown not to affect ^{86}Rb transport, suggesting that indeed the target, whatever its nature, has to be cross-linked (Baxter et al., 1982). This work with HN2 has not yeat progressed to the level which unequivocally proves Na$^+$ K$^+$-ATPase to be the target for this alkylating agent. Grunicke et al. (1982) provide no evidence other than the fact that ^{86}Rb transport was inhibited while Baxter et al. (1982) used indirect evidence by showing that nitrogen mustard inhibits sodium-dependent amino acid transport, by the so-called ASC system, but not sodium-independent amino acid transport by the L system. This implies some specificity to the mustards' action on the membrane and suggests that the sodium gradient appeared to be dissipated. It is possible that the inhibition of the rubidium transport is indirect, exerted through nitrogen mustard-induced changes in membrane fluidity; for example, Grunicke et al. (1982) showed that 10^{-6} M HN2 increased Ehrlich ascites cell membrane viscosity from 1.62 poise to 2.1 poise, as estimated by diphenylhexatriene fluorescence polarization. Most interestingly, a cell line resistant to HN2 showed comparatively little change under similar conditions. As mentioned above, changes in the fluidity of a membrane may exert profound effects on protein function, and this may contribute to the observed inhibition of ion transport (Pang et al., 1979). Studies of the effects of nitrogen mustard on sodium dependent aminoacid transport of a-aminoisobutyric acid into rat L5178Y cells are somewhat at variance with these studies. Ankel et al. (1982) reported that after 1 hour treatment at 10^{-3} M, uptake was inhibited by 60%, yet was increased at lower concentrations. Trenimon also had variable effects according to concentration and neither agent was claimed to affect the electrophoretic mobility of membrane proteins.

Certainly nitrogen mustards react with cytoskeletal components of the membrane and studies on alkylating agent interaction with the cytoskeleton of erythrocytes, where the components are well defined, have provided specific evidence regarding the interaction. Levi (1965) used nucleated chicken erythrocytes and membrane ghosts to study the effects of nitrogen mustard on reaction with both nucleoprotein and the membrane. Fixation of the ghost membranes by low concentrations of HN2 (10^{-6} M), as measured by inhibition of swelling under hypertonic conditions, was considered to be due to interaction with 'stroma' material of the membrane. Later studies, utilizing HN3 [tris(chloroethyl)amine], the trifunctional analogue of HN2, identified more precisely that in human erythrocytes spectrin was cross-linked (Wildenauer & Weger, 1979; Wildenauer et al., 1980). Interestingly, in the former study a comparison of the distribution of ^{14}C-HN3 between membrane and cytoplasmic protein showed that it reacted preferentially with the membrane. These are enucleate cells and therefore no comparison could be made to levels of chromatin binding. A 'fixation' of the membrane, as judged by prevention of the morphologically dramatic discocyte-echinocyte transformations, was produced by HN3 and was attributed directly to the cross-linking of spectrin rather than to changes in its phosphorylation state which may have been induced by HN3.

Another possible explanation of the observed inhibition of ion transport by nitrogen mustard is that it occurs as the result of changes in cyclic nucleotide concentrations. It appears that in certain tissues Na$^+$ K$^+$-ATPase activity may be modulated *via* the action of an elevation in the intracellular concentration of cyclic adenosine monophosphate (cAMP) (Luly *et al.*, 1972). As reviewed in more detail in the next section, alkylating agents elevate cAMP levels in tumour cells apparently through inactivation of the membrane bound, low Km form of cAMP phosphodiesterase (Tisdale & Phillips, 1975a, b, c). In a study of the inhibition of ^{86}Rb$^+$ transport into Ehrlich ascites cells by the alkylating aziridinyl benzoquinone Trenimon, Ihlenfield *et al.* (1981) showed that cAMP levels were elevated without a concomitant alteration in activity of either adenylcyclase or phosphodiesterase. No explanation for this was given, but it is possible that adenylcyclase and Na$^+$ K$^+$-ATPase may be 'linked' enzymes in the membrane, the one modulating the effect of the other, and sharing a common pool of ATP as substrate (Hadden *et al.*, 1972; Lelievre, 1977).

A number of reports of the action of Trenimon on cell membrane function, and particularly ion transport in Ehrlich ascites cells, have appeared from Grunicke's laboratory (Ihlenfield *et al.*, 1981; Grunicke *et al.*, 1980; Grunicke *et al.*, 1979). Unlike nitrogen mustard, Trenimon's effects on amino acid transport were not restricted to those dependent upon a sodium gradient (Baxter *et al.*, 1982), which may suggest that it is less specific in its action on the membrane (Ihlenfield *et al.*, 1981). The authors suggest that Na$^+$K$^+$-ATPase is the target for the drug, but no direct evidence is presented to support this supposition, other than the observations of its effects on ^{86}Rb transport.

In the two review papers Grunicke provocatively reports that the question of whether alkylating agent-mediated effects are important to cytotoxicity has been tested by utilizing polyethylenimine polymer-bound chlorambucil, which is said to interact only with the cell surface. As discussed more fully below, this preparation was found to be cytotoxic to Ehrlich ascites cells. Details of the study will apparently appear in the near future.

Strangely perhaps, the alkylating agent cyclophosphamide, labeled in both the chloroethyl groups (^{3}H) and the ring (^{14}C), failed to significantly alkylate red cell membranes when metabolically activated by rabbit liver microsomes. Most of the reaction with membrane components was found to be associated with acrolein, generated from the breakdown of the ring (Wildenauer and Oehlmann, 1982). The fate of the alkylating moeity was not pursued and it is possible that it reacted with the protein of the activating system. A provocative report that phosphoramide mustard, which is released from the spontaneous breakdown of metabolically generated 4-hydroxycyclophosphamide, does not enter the cell (Lenssen & Mohorst, 1979) may also be relevant.

In a strangely oriented study of the toxic effects of the akylating agent mitomycin-C, cell membrane potentials of hepatocytes were measured and a fall in both potassium activity and membrane potential was observed (Okada *et al.*, 1980). This was circumvented in part by administration of coenzyme Q_{10} and the authors presume that the toxicity of mitomycin-C, and 5-fluorouracil used in the same study, relate to their undefined effects on cellular energetics. Restoration of ATP levels by administration of CoQ_{10} was claimed to reactivate Na^+K^+-ATPase activity and thus to reestablish the potassium equilibrium potential.

More specific studies on interaction between membranes and the platinum compounds, especially *cis*-dichlorodiaminoplatinum (cisplatin) provide another twist to the idea of membrane mediated cytotoxicity (Scanlon *et al.*, 1983). The hydrated derivative of cisplatin, monoaquoplatin, was found to inhibit sodium-dependent amino acid uptake into murine L1210 cells. This included the uptake of methionine for which these cells are auxotrophic, an auxotrophy common to many neoplastic cells. Scanlon *et al.* (1983) argue that this inhibition of methionine uptake will ultimately inhibit cell growth and may be an important facet of cisplatin's cytotoxic action. In L1210 cells with a 180-fold resistance to cisplatin, the degree of methionine auxotrophy was found to be reduced in that the cells were less sensitive to methionine deprivation, and a relationship between this change and their sensitivity to cisplatin was implied (Gross *et al.*, 1983). In these studies no attempt was made to define or determine the mechanism of inhibition of the sodium-dependent transport system. It may be that, like HN2, inhibition could be *via* the sodium pump. Unpublished studies, from the laboratory of one of the present authors, have shown that cisplatin inhibited ^{86}Rb uptake into mouse plasmacytoma cells, possibly by cross-linking sodium potassium ATPase while the *trans* isomer, which has no antineoplastic activity, did not (Hickman & Spurgin, unpublished). On the other hand, the ASC system of amino acid transport is itself composed of a sulfhydryl containing protein (Kwock, 1981) and it is also possible that direct inhibition of this system may occur. A paper by Van den Berg *et al.* (1981) on cisplatin toxicity is of relevance here. Frog skin epithelial ion fluxes were studied as a model for those events in the kidney which lead to cisplatin-induced nephrotoxicity. Permeability to sodium was increased in this model by a high concentration of cisplatin (10^{-3} M), the effects of which were, however, studied immediately after its addition at 22°. Of particular interest was the finding that *trans*-platin, platinum chloride or sulphate had no effects on the same concentration, implying both that heavy metal toxicity *per se* was not responsible for the changes in ion flux and that the *cis* geometry of the coordinate was important for membrane changes. These authors raise the question of selective toxicity, relevant to all of the antitumor studies reported here, in that they wished to address the striking absence of cisplatin-induced hepatotoxicity, despite its high accumulation in this tissue, whilst transporting epithelia showed special vulnerability. Such questions may provide clues as to how inhibition of a ubiquitous enzyme such as Na^+K^+-ATPase may yet produce selective tumor cell cytotoxicity, when changes in ion flux are a process associated not only with transporting tissue but also proliferating cells. This question is addressed further below.

Many studies of the effects of adriamycin on membrane structure and certain aspects of function have been reviewed here. The changes in fluidity of the plasma membrane of S180 sarcoma cells observed by Murphree *et al.* (1981) altered the plasma membrane order parameter to a degree which suggested that the function of integral membrane proteins such as Na^+K^+-ATPase may be affected. These changes in order parameter were seen at concentrations of adriamycin in the range of 10^{-7} to 10^{-4} M, and occurred within 30 minutes of exposure to the drug. Most published studies on the *in vitro* cytotoxicity of adriamycin show that a five log cell kill can be achieved by exposure to less than 10 μM for 1 hour, so that Murphree *et al.* were observing effects well within the cytotoxic concentration range of the drug. It might be hypothesized, as indeed implied by Murphree *et al.* (1982), that such profound and rapidly induced changes may affect the permeability of the plasma membrane to ions. The effects of adriamycin on ion flux have been the subject of a number of studies. The majority of these have used relatively high concentrations of the drug (10 μM and above) for the reason that the objectives of the studies have been related to the mechanism of the cumulative cardiotoxicity induced by the drug (Olsen *et al.*, 1974; Necco *et al.*, 1976; Solie & Yuncker, 1978; Revis & Marasic, 1979; Gosalvez *et al.*, 1979; Villani *et al.*, 1980; Caroni *et al.*, 1981; Azuma *et al.*, 1981) rather than to its mechanism of cytotoxicity to tumour cells. It is possible, although not proven, that these are related. At concentrations greater than 10 μM the effects of adriamycin on ion flux are complex. Villani and coworkers (Villani, 1978; Caroni *et al.*, 1981) suggest that the fast exchangeable pool of calcium is decreased by adriamycin treatment of the intact heart or heart muscle preparations. This fast exchangeable fraction is often considered not to involve transmembrane flux but instead to be that associated with exchange within the glycocalyx (Borle, 1975). However, some evidence was provided that sodium-calcium exchange across the sarcoplasmic reticulum membrane may be inhibited, a result which would be compatible with the increase in calcium concentration observed in the hearts of rabbits (Jaenke, 1976; Olson, 1974) or rats (Arena et al., 1975) chronically treated with adriamycin. In studies of the effects of adriamycin on ion flux in other cell types the picture is even less clear, but generally does not support the hypothesis that the drug alters either the permeability to ions or protein associated transport of ions at concentrations within the range of standard cytotoxicity tests. Landolph et al. asked the question whether or not the so-called ouabain-like effects of adriamycin (Olsen et al., 1974) mimicked the effects of the cardiac glycoside on mouse fibroblasts. At concentrations which were cytotoxic to C3H/10T1/2 cells in the range 10^{-8} to 10^{-6} M no alteration in rubidium transport was observed, unlike the effects of ouabain, and inhibition was observed only at supralethal concentrations which were 10^4 fold greater than those for cytotoxicity (IC_{50} for Rb^+ uptake of 2×10^{-3} M). This raises doubts regarding the report of Gosalvez et al. (1979) that adriamycin was a potent inhibitor of $Na^+ K^+$-ATPase activity with an IC_{50} on rabbit heart microsomes of 10^{-13} M, and indeed two other reports have failed to substantiate these claims (Kim et al., 1980; Solomonson & Halabrin, 1981).

Dasdia et al. (1979) studied the effects of 10^{-7} M adriamycin on both calcium flux and the sodium and potassium content of HeLa cells. Although the authors discuss the implications of their results to the cytotoxic action of adriamycin, they surprisingly chose a concentration which they claim to be nontoxic to HeLa cells. Analysis of ^{45}Ca flux data suggests that the fast exchangeable pool was influenced by adriamycin, but the change was not statistically significant. Efflux kinetics were also unchanged. Despite this, the authors claim that a mobilisable pool of intracellular calcium is increased and they relate this to the now doubtful claim of Gosalvez et al. (1979) that adriamycin inhibits $Na^+ K^+$-ATPase. A fall in the K/Na ratio of HeLa cells after 10^{-7} M adriamycin is reported, although the precise mechanism whereby this would induce a rise in intracellular calcium is not stated.

Anghileri (1977) has reported that adriamycin, at an unstated concentration, inhibits calcium uptake into Ehrlich ascites cell mitochondria. The study attempts to relate this inhibition to an interaction of adriamycin with mitochondrial membrane phospholipids. This is contrary to the findings that cardiac mitochondria accumulate calcium during an adriamycin induced toxicity, but the result may relate to whatever concentration was used in the study.

We have recently measured both ^{45}Ca flux and intracellular calcium pools in L1210 cells treated with concentrations of adriamycin which produce a 3 log cell kill (2 to 5 µM) and find no difference in the treated cells after 4 hours of exposure to adriamycin (Hickman *et al.*, in preparation). Continuous exposure to 10 µM of adriamycin, with regular assessment of intracellular calcium pools by the use of arsenazo III (Bellomo *et al.*, 1982) showed a moderate increase in both cytoplasmic and mitochondrial calcium concentration but only after 4 hours of treatment. Our findings raise some questions not only regarding the functional changes that adriamycin induces in membranes, but also with respect to hypotheses that adriamycin-associated free radical formation may contribute to cell death. Free radical formation from the quinone menadione reduces hepatocyte mitochondrial calcium (Jewell *et al.*, 1982). We find adriamycin to produce no reduction in L1210 cell mitochondrial calcium pools (Hickman *et al.*, in preparation). Further evidence which suggests that adriamycin, at least in the cytotoxic concentration range, does not alter ion permeability or transport, comes from studies of the effect of the drug on the cell membrane potential (Em) of both human red blood cells and L1210 leukemia cells. Changes in Em may reflect complex coupled changes in transmembrane ion concentration, and such changes have also been suggested to be involved in the control of cell proliferation (Boonstra, 1983; Kiefer, 1980). In human red blood cells 10^{-7} M adriamycin has profound effects on the cytoskeleton, as assessed by inhibition of the morphological changes from discocyte to echinocyte forms (Mikkelson *et al.*, 1977), but had no effect on Em as measured by the accumulation of the radiolabeled lipophilic cation triphenylmethylphosphonium (TPM$^+$) (Chahwala *et al.*, 1982). At 10^{-4} M adriamycin a hyperpolarization was observed which was not due to calcium influx and stimulation of potassium efflux (Chahwala *et al.*, in preparation). This hyperpolarization is somewhat difficult to explain. Harper *et al.* (1979) showed that 20 µM and above of adriamycin inhibited calcium activated efflux of potassium which normallly leads to hyperpolarization, so that changes involving other than calcium and sodium levels may be involved, possibly protein conformational rearrangements.

With respect to adriamycin-induced changes in the permeability of ions, the picture is at present incomplete and it would be difficult at present to support any hypothesis that adriamycin actions at the cell surface may interfere with either the control of proliferation mediated by ion flux or with ionic homeostasis, for example, by inducing a dramatic change in intracellular calcium which would be potentially lethal. The work discussed here lays a useful foundation however, because it demonstrates that there are indeed drug effects on cell surface mediated ion permeability. The task for future efforts is to sort the disparate observations into a cohesive explanation and to exploit this property of the cell surface for pharmacologic manipulation.

6. CYCLIC NUCLEOTIDES

The role of cyclic nucleotides in the control of cell proliferation and differentiation is clearly a complex one, and evidence is accumulating to suggest that temporal changes in their intracellular concentrations are more important than absolute concentrations (Whitfield *et al.*, 1980). It was earlier considered that transformation was related to low intracellular concentrations of cAMP (cyclic-3′,5′-adenosine monophosphate) (Otten *et al.*, 1971) and a number of studies, related below, used this as their basis in order to investigate whether cytotoxic agents could be effective in altering the course of cell growth through changes in cAMP concentrations *via* action at cell membranes.

A fascinating series of papers from Tisdale (1974) and Tisdale and Phillips (1975a, b, 1976a-c) strongly implicate the inactivation of the low Km form of cAMP phosphodiesterase, which is considered to be membrane bound (Russell and Pastan, 1973), in the mechanism of action of the 2-chloroethylamine alkylating agents and *cis*-platin. Tisdale (1974) first demonstrated that the bifunctional alkylating agent chlorambucil, but not a monofunctional analogue incapable of performing crosslinking reactions, inactivated the low Km form of beef heart phosphodiesterase. Chlorambucil inactivated this form with a velocity constant which was three times that of the soluble high Km form. Treatment of rat Walker carcinoma cells *in vitro* with 2×10^{-5} M chlorambucil brought about a doubling of their intracellular cAMP concentration within one hour (Tisdale and Phillips, 1975c), and a similar change was obtained with the phosphodiesterase inhibitor aminophylline at a concentration producing a similar amount of toxicity as chlorambucil. That the changes in cAMP concentrations were not a reflection of cell death alone was suggested by the lack of effect of cytotoxic concentrations of the antifolate drug methotrexate (Tisdale and Phillips 1975b). In the treated Walker cells the low Km form of phosphodiesterase was inhibited by chlorambucil, but direct proof of its alkylation and presumably its crosslinking (since monofunctional analogues were inactive) is still lacking.

The alkylating agent-induced elevation of cAMP concentration activated cAMP protein kinase activity in Walker cells; this was mimicked *in vitro* by addition of dibutyryl cAMP. When dbcAMP activated the kinase to the same degree as chlorambucil it was almost equally toxic, strongly supporting the hypothesis that cell death is related to the change in cAMP levels. Unfortunately, the targets for phosphorylation were not identified (Tisdale and Phillips, 1976b). Perhaps the most convincing data for the relationship between drug-induced elevation of cAMP and cytoxoxicty came from the finding that as Walker cells were made progressively more resistant to chlorambucil, parallel falls in the amount of the low Km form of membrane-bound phosphodiesterase were observed (Tisdale and Phillips, 1976a). When a 20-fold resistance had been induced the apparent V_{max} of this low Km form fell from 40% to 15% of the total phosphodiesterase activity and this continued to fall as further resistance was induced.

Elevation of intracellular cAMP levels was shown after treatment of Walker cells with nitrogen mustard, merophan, 4-ethoxy cyclophosphamide (an activated form of cyclophosphamide) and cis platin. Interestingly, the nitrosourea BCNU did not elevate cAMP concentrations in Walker carcinoma cells. This may be a reflection of the different geometry of the crosslinking reactions which the β-chloroethylamine alkylating agents, such as the mustards, can perform via a five atom bridge versus a two atom bridge formed after nitrosourea decomposition to a chloroethyldiazo species.

As mentioned elsewhere, the aziridinylbenzoquine Trenimon elevated cAMP levels in Ehrlich ascites cells which had been treated in vivo with a tumor-curative dose, but this change was brought about by an indirect mechanism, not involving phosphodiesterase inhibition or activation of adenyl cyclase (Ihlenfield et al., 1981).

Howard et al. (1980) reported that vinca alkaloids alter cAMP metabolism in L1210 cells by a mechanism which may involve the microtubular system of the cytoskeleton acting as a regulator of plasma membrane enzyme activity. Both the synthesis of cAMP by adenylcyclase and its breakdown by phosphodiesterase appear to be regulated at the level of the cytoskeleton (Margolis and Wilson, 1979). It was shown that vinca alkaloids prolonged the elevation of cAMP concentration induced by hormonal stimuli, which may be caused by either a failure of the mechanism of coupling between the hormone receptor and adenylcyclase in such a way as to prevent auto-regulation, or to increase the efficiency of such coupling. Clearly such effects may unbalance the cells' response to hormonal factors regulating proliferation.

Several workers have noted changes in the concentration of cGMP levels both in vivo and in vitro in response to anthracyclines (e.g. Lehotay et al., 1982). Although cGMP levels have been implicated in the control of proliferation and as such could be a target for drug action, the work performed with the anthracyclines is not directed at understanding the mechanisms of anticancer activity, but with the side effect of cardiac toxicity, so we will not discuss it further here.

7. ALTERATION OF INTRINSIC MEMBRANE FUNCTIONAL ACTIVITIES

In addition to carrying out the permeability, fusion and fluidity tasks discussed above, biological membranes also perform a wide variety of catalytic and receptor mediated functions. It is reasonable to suppose that certain of these functions would be vital to cellular replication and that inhibition by toxic agents would prevent cell growth. There is ample evidence that certain anticancer agents, particularly adriamycin, do in fact alter essential cell membrane functional activities. Since there is no systematic way to classify these kinds of membrane activities, we present a representative list below:

(1) Zuckier and Tritton (1983) have shown that adriamycin can stimulate an up regulation or increase in the number of cell surface receptors for epidermal growth factor (EGF). Their results show that this anticancer agent has the property of altering the normally active regulatory mechanisms that the cell surface has over growth control. Thus, a potential cell surface mediated mechanism of action of this agent is that alterations in membrane receptor levels by the drug lead to altered cellular responses to physiological regulators.

(2) Many kinds of cell surface receptors undergo capping and patching phenomena, both spontaneous and ligand-induced, and these processes may be important steps in transducing the biological effects of certain receptors (Pastan and Willingham, 1981). Gosalvez et al. (1978) showed that adriamycin inhibits the capping of lymphocyte surface immunoglobulins at the extremely low concentration of 10^{-15} M. Likewise, Yahara et al. (1979) showed that neocarzinostatin, but not bleomycin, mitomycin C or Ara-C, inhibited ligand-independent cap formation of lymphocytes. Both groups speculate that the drug effects may be due to modification of cytoskeletal components like microtubules and microfilaments, but other explanations, including alteration of membrane fluidity, are possible. Since the surface dyanamics of various receptors are intimately involved in biological function, however, alterations by pharmacologic agents may be a significant effect and we expect further research in this area may be enlightening.

(3) Transglutaminase is an enzyme involved in the regulation of receptor endocytosis and hormone induced cell surface down-regulation. Several important amine containing antineoplastic agents are substrates for transglutaminase including actinomycin D, adriamycin, mithramycin and bleomycin (Russell and Womble, 1982). Although the exact mechanism is unclear, transglutaminase may function by mediating the coupling of receptor occupancy to biological function through conjugation of endogenous polyamines to regulatory sites in the cell. In this scheme, then, the role of cytotoxic anticancer drugs may be to compete as substrates for transglutam-

inase and thus alter the ability of the cell to correctly regulate membrane processes.

(4) One of the principal functions of the plasma membrane is to act as a permeability barrier and to transport important molecules to the cell interior. If pharmacologic agents were to interfere with the cells' usual ability to concentrate required nutrients, this could upset growth patterns and lead to cytotoxicity. In another section we discuss the evidence that this may indeed be the case for ions like K^+ and Ca^{2+}. It has also been shown that transport of molecules like uridine and 2-deoxyglucose are inhibited by adriamycin (Choudhury et al., 1982). Alkylating agents produce more complex effects on transport: tris (2-chloroethyl)amine inhibits aminoisobutyric acid uptake but Trenimon can either inhibit or increase the uptake of this amino acid, depending on the length of drug exposure (Anhel et al., 1982). These kinds of studies are still in their early stages, but it is clear that cellular toxicity of these classes of anticancer agents may result, at least in part, from alteration of transport properties of the plasma membrane.

(5) Crane et al. (1980) have demonstrated that adriamycin affects several enzymes in liver plasma membrane that oxidize NADH, xanthine, NADPH and ascorbic acid. These authors have discussed the idea that since these redox functions are implicated in the ability of the cells to respond to cyclic nucleotide mediated growth control, then alteration by adriamycin could be involved in either the therapeutic or toxic side effects of drug administration.

(6) Tökes et al. (1981) found that adriamycin treatment of mouse Sarcoma 180 cells, human BT-20 adeocarcinoma cells and primary cultures of mouse heart muscle cells caused an elevation in the expression of cell surface proteases. The meaning of these observations will not be clear until further work is done, but it is provocative to note that the pattern distribution of surface proteases has been implicated in normal growth control as well as its loss in neoplasia (Reich et al., 1975).

(7) Membranes play an important role in electrophysiological events. Rabkin and Bose (1981) showed that adriamycin prolongs the action potential duration and refractory period without altering resting membrane potential in canine Purkinje fibers. This effect was not reversed when the drug was washed out and thus may contribute to the cardiac electrophysiological malfunctions which occur during adriamycin treatment. In a different experimental system, vincristine and vinblastin altered spontaneous end plate potential in synaptic membranes (Hort-Legrand and Metral, 1976). The latter drug has a much more pronounced effect which may be related to its greater ability to disrupt bilayer structure, as demonstrated by the differential scanning calorimetric results of Ter-Minassian-Saraga et al. (1981).

(8) Although it is a cytoplasmic enzyme, the calcium phospholipid de-

pendent protein kinase (or c-kinase), can be induced both to phosphorylate membrane proteins and to bind to cell membranes by phorbol tumor promoters. Furthermore, the enzyme is regulated by a variety of agents including the anticancer drugs adriamycin (Katoh *et al.*, 1981) and alkyl lysophospholipid (Helfman *et al.*, 1983). By contrast, the cyclic nucleotide dependent protein phosphorylation systems do not seem to be sites of action of these drugs. The exact roles played by c-kinase are unclear, but the enzyme is involved in controlling cell growth and differentiation and is activated by membrane active compounds. Thus the cytotoxicity of some anticancer drugs may be related to disrupting the normal phosphorylation pattern of this enzyme. To establish this, one would have to identify phosphorylated substrates which play a role in growth control and demonstrate linkage of disrupted phosphorylation with drug action. To date, this has not been accomplished.

(9) Aggarwal and Niroomand-Rad (1983) showed that cisplatinum inhibited three plasma membrane enzymes (Ca^{2+}-ATPase, Na^+K^+-ATPase and 5′-nucleotidase) both *in vitro* and *in vivo* using a Sarcoma 180 cell line. The mechanism of inactivation has not been elucidated, but the authors speculate that inhibition of plasma membrane enzymes may be responsible, at least in some part, for cell death.

8. MEMBRANE COMPOSITION

It is clear that the protein and lipid composition of cellular membranes will determine their ability to function normally. A great deal of effort has been expended in showing that the composition varies among many individual membrane species when comparing normal versus tumor cells (Wallach, 1975). These differences, especially at the cell surface membrane, raise the intriguing possibility that antineoplastic drugs can be selective for tumor cells by virtue of the fact that the cancer cell presents a different surface to the drug than does its normal counterpart. This selectivity could be manifested regardless of the ultimate target for drug action, whether it be on the cell surface or at some intracellular site such as DNA. Unfortunately, little progress has been made in exploiting membrane differences for the design or use of anticancer drugs but this remains a promising area for future research efforts. There is published information, however, on the change induced in surface composition by anticancer drug action and on the changes in cell surfaces accompanying the acquisition of drug resistance. These two topics will be taken up now.

a. *Effects of drugs on surface proteins and glycoproteins*

It is not unreasonable to expect that treatment of susceptible cells with a cytotoxic agent would alter the spectrum of proteins expressed by the translation process. Furthermore, if one could identify specific changes induced by drug action, this might offer clues on the mechanism of drug induced cell kill. Surprisingly, however, little work has been done in this area. In one study, Adler and Tritton (1984) using a double labeling technique and one dimensional gel electrophoresis, found that adriamycin treatment of Sarcoma 180 cells caused no detectable changes in the pattern of overall cellular protein synthesis. The level of detectable resolution in these experiments was about 0.5 % so the authors concluded that drug treatment did not alter the overall phenotypic expression of protein synthesis but that subtle changes would not be detected by their technique. It is likely that sensitive two dimensional gel electrophoresis techniques could uncover the changes in protein synthesis patterns elicited by antineoplastic drugs, so this seems the most suitable approach for future work in this largely unexplored area.

In a different approach using mastocytoma P815 cells labeled on the cell surface with a protein specific paramagnetic spin label, Sinha and Chignel (1979) showed that treatment with adriamycin, acridines and diacridines, actinomycin D, AMSA and cis-platinum all induced subtle changes in membrane protein conformation as detected by EPR spectra. These workers concluded that such changes in protein structure alter significant membrane functions such as glucose or ion transport which could be important in controlling the action of the drugs on cell proliferation.

Rather than looking at total cellular or membrane proteins, several groups have studied drug induced changes in glycoprotein expression. Since most glycoproteins are ultimately found on the cell surface, this approach is relatively specific for this target site in the cells under study. Kessel (1979) for example found that adriamycin markedly enhanced the incorporation of radioactive fucose into membrane glycoproteins of P388 cells without affecting the overall uptake of leucine into the protein fraction. The consequence of the so altered glycoprotein was an overall increase in the net negative charge of the cell surface. These changes were not observed in similarly treated adriamycin resistant cells. 5-Fluorouracil has somewhat different effects on glycoprotein expression since, unlike adriamycin, this drug alters somewhat the incorporation of leucine into glycoproteins, while simultaneously decreasing the uptake of fucose (Kessel, 1980). Glucosamine incorporation, on the other hand, was increased by 5-FU.

Other studies in this area also have been published. For example Marks *et al.* (1983) showed that N,N-dimethyl formamide altered glycoprotein biosynthesis in colon carcinoma cells. Lazo *et al.* (1979) found that 6-thioguanine reduced the incorporation of mannose into surface glycoproteins, and that this in turn reduced the ability of S180 cells to specifically interact with ConA by reducing the number of available glycoprotein receptors for the lectin. The changes in mannose incorporation were also associated with an alteration of cellular ultrastructure. It is clear from these various studies that many of the existing anticancer agents can modulate the pattern of glycoprotein expression. In general though, the mechanisms whereby these alterations in glycoprotein composition occur are not known. Nonetheless, a great deal of effort has been expended in the design and testing of sugar analogs which could be selectively cytotoxic by virtue of incorporation into glycoproteins or modulation of glycoprotein synthesis. The rationale in this work is two-fold: (1) cancer cells contain membrane glycoprotein changes which may be in part responsible for loss of growth control so it may be therapeutically useful to alter or inhibit the biosynthesis of variant tumor cell surfaces and (2) by analogy with existing antineoplastics, new agents which alter glycoproteins may also be useful anticancer agents. A detailed review of this type of work is beyond the scope of this paper so the interested reader is referred to Bernacki *et al.* (1979).

b. *Effects of drugs on cell surface lipid composition*
Although the technology for doing so exists, the effect of drugs on phospholipid composition of cell surface membranes has not been comprehensively researched. The reasons for this are probably two: (1) because there are literally hundreds of identifiably different lipid components in the membranes of mammalian cells, identifying the complex interrelationships between the levels of the various components is a formidably tedious task and (2) it has not been clear that such knowledge would aid in the design or use of anticancer agents. Recent work has been published, however, showing that antineoplastics do indeed alter the lipid composition of the plasma membrane of exposed cells and that these alterations may be linked to the pharmacologic action of the drugs. Thus, we believe that this newly developing area holds some promise for uncovering new leads in cancer therapy.

Schroeder *et al.* (1981) showed that the spindle inhibitors colchicine and vinblastine altered the plasma membrane content of phospatidyl serine and phosphatidyl glycerol in mouse LM fibroblasts, but did not change the assymetry or distribution of phosphatidyl ethanolamine. The authors discuss the evidence for the likelihood that small alterations in lipid composition can considerably alter the activity of membrane bound proteins and suggest this as a potential contribution to the mechanism of action of these drugs. Interferon, too, alters the phospholipid composition of S180 cells by modulating the fatty-acyl chains (Chandrabose and Cuatrecasas 1981). It has also been shown that adriamycin (Schlager and Ohanian, 1979, 1980) enhances the sensitivity of hepatoma cells to antibody-complement killing and that the effect is correlated with drug-induced changes in cellular lipid and fatty acid composition. Adriamycin also stimulates MDCK cells to deacylate cellular lipids and produce prostaglandins (Ohuchi and Levine, 1978). Taken together these types of studies suggest that (1) the cytotoxic action of certain antineoplastic agents is associated with changes in lipid composition; (2) modifications of cellular lipid composition by drugs can affect the outcome of humoral immune attack at the cell surface and (3) drug treatment can induce the surface cyclooxygenase pathways which lead to prostaglandin mobilization.

The possibility has been widely discussed that membrane lipid peroxidation is involved in the mechanism of cardiac toxicity invoked by adriamycin (Mimnaugh et al., 1981, 1982; Kharasch et al., 1982; Patterson et al., 1983; Jensen, 1983). Since the drug molecule contains a quinone functionality, it can be enzymatically reduced to a semiquinone which can in turn activate molecular oxygen. This process stimulates lipid peroxidation, particularly in mitochondrial and microsomal preparations. We are not aware of any published reports demonstrating lipid peroxidation at the cell surface so, although it is a postulated mechanism for a deleterious side effect of adriamycin action, lipid peroxidation has not yet been implicated as directly involved in the therapeutic anticancer action of this agent.

c. *Membrane protein changes associated with anticancer drug resistance*
Several cell lines have been shown to have acquired altered surface glycoproteins when selected for resistance to antiproliferative agents (reviewed in Ling, 1983). The best characterized of these are CHO cells, originally selected for resistance to colchicine, but shown to be cross-resistant to many drugs including actinomycin D, adriamycin and melphalan. Examination of the plasma membrane of these cell lines by surface-labeling techniques has revealed the presence of a 170,000 dalton glycoprotein which is apparently unique to the resistant mutants. The protein has been isolated and characterized (Riordan and Ling, 1979) and termed the 'P-glycoprotein' because of its presumed functional role in regulating membrane permeability to the drugs. Beck et al. (1979) have characterized a very similar protein in human leukemic lymphoblasts (CCRF-CEM). More recently, Peterson et al. (1983) observed a similar glycoprotein in vincristine/daunomycin resistant Chinese hamster lung cells (DC-3F), which proved to be a family of glycoproteins when resolved by two dimensional gels. The relationship between the various subtypes of modified glycoproteins and the patterns of drug resistance and cross-resistance are not established. It is also not firmly established that permeability is the controlling factor in drug resistance, so it is not yet clear

what mechanistic role the P-glycoprotein plays. Because the protein is closely associated with resistance however, two interesting possibilities emerge: (1) since the cell surface seems to have some involvement in the acquisition of resistance, it may be possible to alter the cell surface to overcome resistance, and (2) if surface glycoproteins are a general marker for multiple drug resistance, this fact could serve as the basis for a clinically useful assay of potential sensitivity of a patient to a drug treatment regimen.

Other workers have shown that drug resistant cells have an altered ability to incorporate sugars into surface glycoproteins (as opposed to increased content of an existing glycoprotein as described in the previously discussed work). Wheeler *et al.* (1982) found that adriamycin resistant MDAY-K2 cells had increased content of cell surface sialic acid and Garman and Center (1982) showed that resistant Chinese hamster lung cells had increased glucosamine incorporation, as well as a 100,000 dalton surface membrane protein altered in its ability to be iodinated. Salles *et al.* (1982) have reported that Chinese hamster lung cells resistant to ellipticine have altered surface morphology; this probably results from altered composition. It is too early to be certain whether these types of observations will enhance our understanding of drug resistance, but it is evident from the available work that changes in the cell surface proteins may play an important role in the resistant phenotype.

d. *Membrane lipid changes associated with anticancer drug resistance*
Since the lipid milieu of a membrane controls the ability to carry out functional processes, it would not be surprising to find altered lipid composition in drug resistant cells if the membranes were indeed involved in the resistance mechanism. Ling (1975) found little difference in the phospholipid/cholesterol ratio between his sensitive and resistant CHO cell lines suggesting that this parameter was not an important one. In a more comprehensive study, however, Adler and Tritton (1984) investigated the composition of 10 lipid species in 5 sublines of S180 of progressively increasing resistance to adriamycin. There are dramatic differences among the various lipid classes in the resistant lines but none of the changes vary systematically with the degree of resistance. Glaubiger *et al.* (1983) also have results showing phospholipid changes in adriamycin resistant P388 cells. Thus, although single lipid types do not correlate directly with drug sensitivity, the results from several laboratories suggest that the overall pattern of lipid content may regulate the ability of a cell to react to the presence of a cytotoxic anticancer drug.

9. MODIFICATION OF MEMBRANE COMPOSITION OR STRUCTURE TO AFFECT
   DRUG ACTION

It has been implicit throughout this review that the structure and composition of a membrane dictate the functional interactions which are possible for that given membrane. In turn, alteration of membrane structure or composition could lead to altered biological activity, so it should be feasible to modulate access or mechanism of action of any drug which passes through or acts on a biological membrane, by lipid substitution. The viability of this idea has been demonstrated recently. For example, Schiffman and Klein (1979) showed that amphotericin B sensitivity could be induced in cells in culture by fusing the growing cells with ergosterol-containing liposomes. Amphotericin B is an antifungal agent whose mechanism of action is thought to involve disruption of cell membranes containing certain sterols (like ergosterol). Moreover, insertion of amphotericin B into tumor cell membranes can augment the antitumor activity of mainline agents including adriamycin, BCNU, actinomycin D and melphalan (Medoff *et al.*, 1981; Ozols *et al.*, 1983). In attempting to modify the fluidity of L1210 cells, Burns *et al.* (1979) found that fatty acid supplementation of the growth medium resulted in cell surface membranes that were altered both in their fluidity characteristics and the ability to transport methotrexate. For adriamycin, which unlike methotrexate may act directly on the cell surface rather than requiring transport, two groups have shown that cytotoxicity of the drug can be enhanced by altering the fatty acid, phospholipid or cholesterol composition of L1210 cell membranes (Spiegel *et al.*, 1983; Tritton, 1983). Other workers have shown that membrane active local anesthetics (dibucaine, tetracaine, butacaine, lidocaine and procaine) can potentiate the cytotoxic activity of both bleomycin (Mizuno and Ishida, 1982) and adriamycin (Chlebowski *et al.*, 1982). The mechanism of this effect has not been elucidated but it seems reasonable that it is a result of the ability of the local anaesthetics to disrupt the fluidity of the lipid bilayer. It has also been demonstrated that alteration of surface proteins by trypsin treatment of cells changes drug sensitivity (Barranco *et al.*, 1980). Viewed as a whole, these kinds of approaches to membrane modification are only now in their infancy, but it is evident from the results obtained to date that alteration of cell surface composition, with associated changes in the structure and activity of the membrane, can have profound consequences on drug action.

10. COVALENT INTERACTION OF ANTICANCER DRUGS WITH MEMBRANES

The inhibition of cell growth by alkylating agents is usually attributed to alkylation of DNA (Ludlum, 1975). It is also possible that quinone containing molecules like the anthracyclines can, via reduction, form reactive alkylating species and there is evidence for covalent DNA modification (Moore, 1977; Sinha and Gregory, 1981). There is, however, no direct proof that DNA alkylation leads to cytotoxicity and it is not unreasonable to propose that chemically reactive drug species could also covalently modify the components of membranes, and that this mechanism could be the primary one leading to pharmacologic action. Some evidence supporting this idea exists. Ihlenfeldt *et al.* (1981) Baxter *et al.* (1982) and Grunicke *et al.* (1979, 1982) have published a series of papers showing that the alkylating agents modify the plasma membrane of cells in culture, presumably by covalent interaction. Moreover, these effects are correlated with inhibition of the membrane transport of thymidine, amino acids and glucose, as well as with the inhibition of cell surface Na^+K^+-ATPase and with decreases in membrane fluidity. The authors conclude that alkylation of membrane targets are responsible for this alteration in cellular function, and suggest that, since the plasma membrane plays such an important role in the regulation of cell division, that alkylating agents bring about their primary cytotoxic lesion by alkylation of the plasma membrane. This idea is by no means proven, but is attractive and under intense study in these laboratories. Further discussion of this topic appears elsewhere in this review.

There have been findings reported that certain other antineoplastics may covalently cross-link to membrane proteins. The purported DNA intercalator m-AMSA, for example, rapidly reacts with membrane proteins of red blood cell ghosts by covalently attaching to exposed sulfhydryl groups (Wong *et al.*, 1983). Adriamycin can be activated by microsomes and NADPH to form a semiquinone species which covalently labels microsomal membrane proteins (Ghezzi *et al.*, 1981). Again, these reactions have not been linked in any way to the biological function of the drugs, but they are observations which must be contended with when considering possible mechanisms of pharmacologic action.

11. MEMBRANE RECEPTORS FOR ANTICANCER AGENTS

The idea that there may exist formal membrane receptors for anticancer drugs is relatively unexplored for two reasons: (1) most of the existing drugs have been thought to have well-defined intracellular receptors such as enzymes (e.g. ribonucleotide reductase for hydroxyurea) or DNA (e.g. for actionomycin D); and (2) it has been considered unlikely that cells would synthesize a receptor whose sole purpose is to mediate cell death. Elsewhere in this paper we have discussed the evidence that anticancer drugs alter pre-existing receptors with defined functions, but there is only one major publication suggesting the existence of a drug-binding receptor whose major function is to mediate anticancer drug action (Taylor *et al.*, 1981). These workers identified and isolated two distinct macromolecular lipid complexes from L1210 tumors either sensitive or resistant to an anticancer terephthalanilide. This drug, as well as Cain quinoliniums, a carbanilide, anthraquinones and adriamycin, all bind to one of the macromolecular lipids. Equilibrium binding studies showed a correlation with drug efficacy, in that specific site concentration and orientation appear to be required in order for a particular drug to have *in vivo* activity. A number of questions remain unanswered about this system, including the cellular distribution of the lipids, the exact chemical makeup and possible subunit structure, and the mechanism whereby binding of a macromolecular lipid with a drug participates in pharmacologic activity. Nonetheless this is an intriguing lead because it suggests the existence of a primary drug-binding site, consisting of membrane components and possibly membrane associated, which must be occupied in order for drug action to occur.

There is some indirect evidence *against* the idea of a formal drug receptor for anthracyclines on the cell surface. Yee *et al.* (1983) have shown that daunomycin can be photochemically incorporated into the plasma membrane of S180 cells in culture. If a formal drug receptor existed on the surface, its occupation by drug should lead to the eventual endpoint of duanomycin action, namely cell death. This was not found to be the case since up to 200,000 daunomycin molecules could be photochemically incorporated into the S180 cell surface without affecting cell viability. Thus, either a receptor exists which has only very low affinity for the drug, or there is not a major class of receptors on the cell surface whose occupancy by photoincorporated drug is directly coupled to cell death.

Wingard *et al.* (1983) have also obtained circumstantial evidence against a formal anthracycline membrane receptor using immobilized drugs (see additional discussion below). On the other hand, preliminary results from Hickman's laboratory (unpublished) showing that N-acetyl glucosamine can apparently prevent adriamycin from freezing discocyte human red cells in that morphology may contradict this (see action on lectins).

12. ALTERATION OF CELL SURFACE ULTRASTRUCTURE

Observation, usually by electron microscopy, of the morphology of cell surfaces can give indication of whether drug treatment has altered the gross structure and organization of the plasma membrane. Several antineoplastic agents have been documented to cause such changes. Erythrocytes in particular are a favorite cell type for morphologic investigation, and adriamycin,

112

daunomycin and tris (2-chloroethyl)-amine all alter red blood cell morphology and increase susceptibility to lysis (Schioppocassi and Schwartz, 1977; Mikkelson *et al.*, 1977; Wildenauer *et al.*, 1980). It has been suggested that these changes are due to specific binding of the drugs to the cell surface protein spectrin, which is known to be involved in maintaining red cell surface morphology, but this proposition has not been rigorously tested. Myers *et al.* (1982) showed that an adriamycin-iron complex caused destruction of erythrocyte ghost membranes. These workers have proposed a model in which the drug-iron complex acts by first binding to the membrane, followed by generation of high local concentrations of reactive oxygen species which catalyze destruction of membrane structure. Adriamycin also induces changes in the surface structure of liver cells (Rogers *et al.*, 1983), CHO cells (Walling and Ord, 1982) and neuroblastoma cells (Schengrund and Sheffler, 1982). One is tempted to speculate that the severe drug-induced changes in surface ultrastructure that can be observed by electron microscopy must be linked to disruption of cellular function, but there are no investigations which sort out the complex cause and effect relationships which may exist.

13. THE USE OF IMMOBILIZED DRUGS TO SEPARATE CELL SURFACE FROM INTRACELLULAR MECHANISMS

Almost all of the work described in this review is of the cataloging variety, that is, experiments which show that various anticancer drugs have effects on measurable functions of membranes. These kinds of experiments can not be offered as proof that the pharmacologic mechanism of the drug in question is related to the effect being measured. Perhaps the most direct experimental way to separate cell surface from intracellular effects of a pharmacologic agent is by attachment to insoluble supports. One can then ask the question, Does the drug have biological activity under conditions where its access to the interior of the cell is prevented? This approach is conceptually straightforward and, at least on paper, simple because the drug can be permanently attached to a support larger than cells and thus cannot penetrate past the cell surface by diffusion, transport, or endocytosis. This approach, of course, is based on the assumption that drug activity is not lost because of coupling to another material. The validity of this assumption will vary with the drug and the specific functional groups of the drug molecule used for the coupling; however, the fact that immobilized drugs can retain their activity has been substantiated and summarized elsewhere (Venter, 1982). This approach has been taken by previous investigators to elucidate the mechanism of certain agents. For example, Laporte *et al.* (1977) showed that agarose-immobilized polymyxin B was as effective at inhibiting bacterial growth as free drug. These workers used careful controls to demonstrate that the bound drug was not released from the complex and made a convincing argument that the effects of polymyxin B on gram-negative bacteria were due to a specific outer membrane lesion.

In studies with immobilized drugs it is especially pertinent to demonstrate rigorously that sufficient drug is not being released to account for the results attributed to the immobilized material. This problem is especially noticeable with drugs bound to agarose preparations, where for certain linkages the leakage rate may be as high as 1% of the bound drug per hour (Vaugelin *et al.*, 1975). Thus, each study must be carried out with suitable controls to document the absence of appreciable leakage rates.

Many anticancer drugs have been attached to high molecular weight supports in attempts to increase the specificity of the drug for a specific target (e.g. immobilization to antibodies), or to create sustained release drug preparations, or for use in affinity chromatography (see Venter (1982), for a review of these areas) but most of these kinds of studies have not been designed to separate cell surface from intracellular effects, since most kinds of drug-carrier molecules can be internalized by cells. However, two antineoplastics (chlorambucil and adriamycin) have been immobilized for this latter purpose and these studies will be discussed now.

Chlorambucil is a classical alkylating agent which is presumed to act by covalent interaction with DNA. Grunicke *et al.* (1979) have attached chlorambucil to polyethyleneimines of various chain lengths by chemistry which has not been disclosed. They showed that pure polyethyleneimine polymers did not affect the multiplication of Ehrlich ascites cells in culture, but that chlorambucil-polyethyleneimine conjugates were cytotoxic. Unfortunately, no studies were undertaken to show if either (1) the free drugs leaked off the polymer, or (2) the polymer (MW $\sim 30,000$ daltons) was taken into the cell interior by endocytosis. Thus, although these results are intriguing and offer some indication that cell surface alkylation may be important in chlorambucil action, further work is necessary before one can feel confident about this interpretation.

Better evidence for a cell surface mediated cytotoxicity exists for adriamycin, since two independent research groups have done extensive work on immobilizing this drug and its congeneric relatives, although the exact approach taken has been different in each laboratory. Tritton's group (Tritton and Yee, 1982; Tritton *et al.*, 1983; Wingard and Tritton, 1983) have approached the problem by attaching anthracycline molecules to cross-linked polymers which are very much larger in diameter (50–200 μ) than cells (~10 μ). These investigators have attached both adriamycin and carminomycin by several chemistries involving different orientations of the drug molecule and different key linkages (see refs. cited above for details). Results have been obtained by measuring cytotoxicity by both cloning and growth inhibition and by assay for free drug inside cells by HPLC. The principal findings may be summarized as follows:

(1) Immobilized adriamycin and carminomycin can kill cells under conditions where no demonstrable free drug has been accumulated in the cells. The limit of detectable drug inside the cells (both L1210 and S180) is lower than that which can be measured at non-cytotoxic concentrations of free, native anthracycline. Thus, these drugs can be actively cytotoxic without entering the cells.

(2) The cytotoxic action does not depend on a specific type of support since agarose, beaded dextran and polyvinyl alcohol are all effective.

(3) Adriamycin can be attached to the polymer by either alkylation or acylation reactions of the amino sugar moiety of the molecule and either preparation is cytotoxically active.

(4) The reverse orientation of the anthracycline on the polymer, *i.e.* through the aglycone ring, also yields an active species. These results (3) and (4) suggest that a precise orientation of the drug on the cell surface is not required for biological activity, but rather the mere presence of the drug is sufficient to cause derangement of growth. The implication of this conclusion is that a formal drug receptor for anthracyclines, which could ordinarily require the ligand to bind in a specific geometry, is not present on the cell surface.

(5) Fluorescence microscopy of the adriamycin-agarose beads showed a uniform distribution of drug fluorescence. Thus the surface, and hence cell-available, concentration of drug can be calculated. When this is done it is found that immobilized adriamycin is 2 to 3 orders of magnitude more potent than free adriamycin when comparing the total available concentration.

(6) Because the amount of cytotoxicity that can be achieved by immobilized preparations is limited to one or two logs of cell kill (albeit with a very low concentration of drug), and because increasing the time of exposure of cells to bead/drug conjugates does not greatly increase the cytotoxicity, it appears that the ability to kill cells by surface attack undergoes a type of down regulation. Put differently, the presence of immobilized adriamycin stimulated cells to reduce their susceptibility to further membrane-mediated kill by removing the structures which mediate this type of toxicity.

The Tökes' group approach to this problem has differed in three regards: (1) the attachment matrix is polyglutaraldehyde; (2) the linkage of drug to polymer is a Schiff base; and (3) the microspheres formed are many diameters smaller than typical cultured cells (about 0.4 m compared to 10–20 μ cell size). These workers find, however, that adriamycin attached covalently to polyglutaraldehyde microspheres is cytotoxically active (Tökes *et al.*, 1982; Rogers *et al.*, 1983). Using scanning electron microscopy these workers observed interaction of the drug-polymer conjugates with the cell surface and striking alterations in membrane morphology similar to those produced by toxins like menadione which act through intracellular mechanisms (Jewell *et al.*, 1982). However, the Tökes group claims to find little polymer or free drug inside the cells (L1210 and rat liver cells). Consequently, it is concluded that adriamycin retains its cytocidal activity and ability to alter surface ultrastructure even when it is restricted to interaction solely at the cell surface. Tökes *et al.* (1982) and Rogers *et al.* (1983) also report that polyglutaraldehyde coupled adriamycin is capable of overcoming drug resistance, possibly due to 'multiple interactions' at the cell surface, i.e. the continued presence of the drug at the plasma membrane at high concentration may overcome the resistance mechanism.

These kinds of studies using immobilized preparations of anticancer drugs to force action at the cell surface are extremely provocative, although in a sense more questions are raised than answered. For example, what is the mechanism by which cell surface interaction leads to cell death? Possibly, one or more of the many membrane activities of anticancer drugs discussed in this review is the primary lesion. This remains an open question. Another problem is how to apply the knowledge obtained about membrane mechanisms of antineoplastics to practical clinical application. It seems unlikely that large polymers will prove generally useful as therapeutic agents, although certain types of tumors could be susceptible. Rather, we think that it will be necessary to design a new generation of non-penetrating low molecular weight drugs which take advantage of surface mediated cytotoxicity but which do not enter cells. Such drugs would offer several advantages:

(1) They would not undergo intracellular degradation, sequestration or distribution.

(2) They might be used at low concentrations, since the results obtained to date suggest that surface attack is much more potent than attack at intracellular targets. The ability to use smaller doses might obviate some of the obnoxious side effects of treatment using cytotoxic agents.

(3) The undesirable toxicities of anticancer drugs (e.g. cardiotoxicity with adriamycin) are probably mediated at intracellular sites and thus non-penetrating congeners could avoid such deleterious side effects.

It is evident that the concept of membrane mediated cancer cell kill is new and rather underdeveloped. However, it is also evident that great potential exists for improving the therapeutic usefulness of pharmacological agents by exploring this approach, and we believe that research efforts in this direction will provide fruitful results over the next several years.

14. INTERACTION OF ANTICANCER DRUGS WITH MODEL MEMBRANES

There are at least two major reasons for studying the interaction of drugs with model membranes: (1) One of the criteria for establishing a membrane target for an agent is that the drug must have the ability to interact with membrane components; and (2) once a membrane target is established as a binding site, the model membrane can be used to establish the chemical details of drug-membrane interaction. The most widely employed model membrane system for studying drug interactions is the phospholipid vesicle, or liposome (Tritton *et al.*, 1977).

The liposome system has several advantages over natural cell membranes for defining the physicochemistry of drug action. Liposomes are exceedingly simple; sonicated dispersions of phospholipids produce small vesicles of fairly uniform size (on the order of 300 Å), consisting of a single bilayer surrounding an aqueous space (Huang, 1969). The membrane composition both in terms of the polar head group and the fatty acid side chains is accurately known, since pure phospholipids can be employed as starting materials. In this way, both the surface charge density and interior hydrocarbon fluidity can be controlled. Furthermore, membranes of practically any lipid composition can be prepared, and purified proteins or other molecules can be incorporated into either the aqueous or hydrocarbon phases. Such vesicles can be prepared on the large scale necessary for certain types of physical measurements without the complex manipulations required to purify cellular membranes. Most importantly, liposomes would appear to be relevant models of biological membranes, as they have the basic phospholipid bilayer structural element of the membrane.

Several anticancer drugs have been shown to interact with and modify the properties of model membranes. Koehler *et al.* (1983) used calorimetric techniques to show that cytosine arabinoside increased the solid $\Leftrightarrow$ fluid transition temperature of phospholipid vesicles, and suggested that the results indicated an effect of the drug on the relative populations of cooperatively melting phases in a mixed lipid system. The more lipid soluble VP-16 had the effect of broadening the transition curve and decreasing the enthalpy of the phase transition, i.e. the solid $\Leftrightarrow$ fluid transition was forced to become less cooperative in the presence of the drug. Likewise, Ter-Minassian-Saraga *et al.* (1981) found that vincristine and vinblastine lowered the T_m of dipalmityl phosphatidylcholine liposomes, but these drugs had the unusual property of increasing the transition enthalpy, possibly because they cause formation of coexisting drug-contaminated domains within the membrane which melt with high enthalpy. The amphipathic molecule, ellipticine, also has strong interactions with model membranes. Terce *et al.* (1982) and El Mashak and Tocanne (1980) have used monolayers of acidic phospholipids to characterize this drug's interaction with membranes. Using surface pressure and surface potential measurements, these investigators found that ellipiticine interacts strongly with phospholipids, regardless of the membrane surface pressure or the nature and physical state of the lipid acyl chains. The interaction is stabilized by both electrostatic and hydrophobic forces and caused a large film expansion and modification of the phase properties of the membrane in a manner similar to cholesterol. It is apparent that ellipticine inserts between the lipid molecules to cause these rather large alterations in membrane structure. Although DNA has been considered as a target for ellipticine binding and action, it is evident from these results that biological membranes, because they can be extensively modulated by the drug, could also be a potential target for the pharmacologic action.

Adriamycin has been studied more comprehensively than any other anticancer drug with respect to its ability to interact with model membranes and membrane lipid components. The overall aim of this work has been to learn both about the drug molecule and how it interacts with membranes, and also to draw inferences about membrane structure and organization in general. Through such experiments, the various investigators involved have derived some important clues about how the structure of the anthracyclines, as well as of the membrane components, contribute to the specificity of interaction. This work will be summarized next.

One of the original questions asked was – Does adriamycin alter liposome membrane fluidity? Using light scattering as a means of detection, Tritton et al. (1978) found that adriamycin decreases the solid ⇔ fluid transition temperature (T_m) of membranes of varying composition. Thus the drug in general increases membrane fluidity. However, when a low level of cardiolipin (0.1–10%) is inserted into a lecithin membrane matrix, drug interaction causes the opposite effect on the thermal transition, i.e. adriamycin makes these membranes *less* fluid. This differential effect of adriamycin on the fluidity of membranes containing cardiolipin is quite remarkable and could provide an explanation for the specificity of the cytotoxic action of the drug on tumors, because evidence exists (Wallach, 1975; Bergelson et al., 1970, 1974) indicating that certain neoplastic cells, unlike their normal counterparts, contain cardiolipin in their plasma membranes, and thus present a different surface to the drug than non-malignant cells. Moreover, this concept may explain, at least in part, the notorious cardiac toxicity of this agent, in that heart muscle, which is rich in respiring mitochondria, might be a sensitive target because membranes of mitochondria are the major repository for cardiolipin in normal cells. Thus it is suggested that the phospholipid composition and distribution in cellular membranes may play an important role in determining the susceptibility of neoplastic cells to the anthracycline antibiotics, as well as the toxic side effects of these agents on heart tissue.

Other investigators have shown that in organic solvents, cardiolipin and adriamycin molecules form a specific complex of reasonably high affinity (Duarte-Karim *et al.*, 1976; Schwartz and Kanter, 1979). This complex is stabilized by ionic interactions between the negatively charged phospholipid and the positively charged aminosugar of the anthracyclines, as well as π electron overlap. The next question thus becomes, does the interaction between drug and isolated cardiolipin molecules also pertain when the cardiolipin is an integral part of a phospholipid bilayer? Goormaghtigh *et al.* (1980a, b; 1982) have studied this problem thoroughly using both lipid monolayers and sonicated liposomes as model membranes. By using a combination of surface potential and equilibrium binding techniques as well as absorption spectroscopy and ^{31}P NMR spectroscopy, these workers showed that adriamycin forms a specific complex with cardiolipin membranes but not with neutral phospholipids. The association constant is as high as for DNA ($\sim 2 \times 10^6$ M^{-1}) and the limiting stoichiometry is 2 adriamycin moles per mole of cardiolipin. An important property of cardiolipin containing bilayers is the ability of this phospholipid to provoke structural polymorphism (Goormaghtigh *et al.*, 1982). Normal bilayer structure predominates in pure cardiolipin membranes in the absence of divalent cations, but addition of Ca^{2+}, for example, causes formation of intrabilayer inverted micelles and hexagonal phases which may be functionally important in biological membranes containing cardiolipin. Mitochondria in particular are the principal cellular location of cardiolipin and correctly structured mitochondrial membranes are undoubtedly required in respiration. Goormaghtigh *et al.* (1982) showed by elegant microscopic and ^{31}P NMR work that adriamycin inhibited the formation of non-bilayer structures in model membrane systems and proposed that this may provide a structural explanation for the damage caused by adriamycin to cardiac muscle, *i.e.* direct mitochondrial alteration. Recent work from this laboratory has provided additional verification of these concepts by demonstrating that adriamycin can transfer electrons from NADH to cytochrome C and coenzyme Q in cardiac mitochondrial membranes (Goormaghtigh *et al.*, 1983). The authors proposed, although no direct proof is shown, that a specific adriamycin-cardiolipin complex is an intermediary in this redox process.

Further understanding of the structural basis for this cardiolipin effect has come from studies taking advantage of the intrinsic fluorescence emission of adriamycin (Karczmar and Tritton, 1979). In these studies only small mole fractions (0.01–0.03) of cardiolipin are present in a phosphatidyl choline matrix to more closely approximate the surface of a tumor cell. Fluorescence titration studies of equilibrium binding showed that the differences in the interactions of adriamycin with cardiolipin containing membranes, as compared to those of other phospholipid compositions, are not due to an increased binding but rather to an altered membrane structure when this lipid is present. Thus, unlike the pure cardiolipin membranes, low amounts of this phospholipid in a bilayer do not create a unique binding site for adriamycin. It was also demonstrated that I^- ions, which quench adriamycin fluorescence by collision with the excited state, can serve as a molecular dipstick on the location of the drug within the bilayer. These quenching studies show that adriamycin is partially, but not completely, buried in the liposomal membrane. Goldman et al. (1978) also concluded that daunomycin and adriamycin are localized at the polar/apolar interface in phospholipid bilayers, based on measurements of the rotational rate from fluorescence depolarization data. Karczmar and Tritton (1979) further demonstrated that, both in the presence and absence of cardiolipin, the bulk of adriamycin is more accessible below the T_m then above it; that is, a solid membrane tends to exclude the drug from deep penetration. Above the T_m, where the membrane is in the fluid state, the presence of cardiolipin alters the nature of the liposome-adriamycin interaction. In this case, the fluorescence quenching data suggests that the presence of small amounts of cardiolipin (3%) in a lecithin matrix creates two types of binding environments for the drug, one relatively exposed and the other more deeply buried in the membrane. The temperature dependence of the adriamycin fluorescence and the liposome light scattering reveal that cardiolipin also alters the thermal properties of the bilayer, as well as its interaction with adriamycin. At low ionic strength lateral phase separations occur with liposomes of both pure phosphatidyl choline and phosphatidyl choline containing 3% cardiolipin; under these conditions the bound adriamycin exists in two kinds of environment. It is notable that only adriamycin fluorescence reveals this phenomenon; the bulk property of liposome light scattering reports only on the overall membrane phase change. These data suggest that under certain conditions the drug binding sites in the membrane are decoupled from the bulk of the lipid bilayer.

Murphree et al. (1982) obtained further evidence that cardiolipin stimulates a membrane to interact uniquely with adriamycin by studying liposome fusion. Using ^{1}H-NMR spectroscopy these workers studied the fusion rates of phosphatidyl choline vesicles both with and without small amounts of various other lipid classes. The most pertinent result of this work is that, although adriamycin can stimulate membrane fusion under certain conditions, the effect is most pronounced only when cardiolipin is present in the membranes. Thus, it is again clear that adriamycin induced effects on a membrane process (in this case fusion) are dependent on the phospholipid composition, and are particularly sensitive to the presence of cardiolipin.

Two other kinds of magnetic resonance experiments add to our understanding of this cardiolipin effect. Since one of the central functions of a membrane is to serve as a permeability barrier, Murphree *et al.* (1982) used both NMR and EPR spectroscopy to determine if adriamycin altered permeability. Using the spectral splitting caused in the proton NMR spectrum by paramagnetic Pr^{3+} ions, they showed that pure phosphatidyl choline liposomes are unaffected in their ionic permeability by drug treatment. However, when cardiolipin (0.25%) is present in the liposomal membranes, then adriamycin stimulates permeation of Pr^{3+} cations across the bilayer. ESR studies were employed to see if adriamycin is capable of altering *anion* (ascorbate) permeability. In these experiments advantage was taken of the ability of ascorbate to reduce the paramagnetic signal of spinlabeled liposomes (labeled with 5 doxyl stearic acid) at a rate which is determined by the ability of ascorbate to penetrate into the membrane. Murphree *et al.* (1982) found that adriamycin decreased ascorbate permeation into pure phosphatidyl choline liposomes, but, conversely, when cardiolipin was present (1%) adriamycin stimulated the rate of ascorbate permeation. Thus, adriamycin can alter the permeability rate of both anions and cations across the lipid bilayer depending on the lipid composition. Perhaps the most striking aspect of this work is that binding of a single adriamycin molecule to a liposome (~ 2500 lipid molecules) affects the structure of the entire liposome (Murphree *et al.*, 1982). Thus, adriamycin can cause propagation of long-range effects on membrane structure and organization; this observation may provide some explanation for the extraordinary range of cell membrane actions of this agent.

In addition to these studies on the role of membrane composition, Burke *et al.* (1983) have reported the use of fluorescence spectroscopy to investigate the effect of drug structure on the membrane interaction. They studied the liposomal interaction of a series of anthracyclines and their respective aglycones by fluorescence quenching and fluorescence polarization. The agents examined include adriamycin, daunomycin, carminomycin, AD-32, pyrromycin, marcellomycin, aclacinomycin and N,N-dimethyl adriamycin. The most intriguing result from this work is that both the binding affinity and the location within the membrane are similar for any parent/aglycone pair, but vary drastically for different chromophore structures. Thus the presence of the sugar portion of the molecule does not appear to be an important factor in determining the nature of the drug-membrane interaction, at least in an equilibrium thermodynamic sense. We expect that further studies of this type will lead to a detailed understanding of the structural facets of the anthracycline molecule which lead to effective membrane interaction.

15. CONCLUSION

Most membrane specialists and pharmacologists will not find it surprising that anticancer drugs produce a rich variety of effects on the structure and function of biological membranes. This is because membranes are inherently responsive to the action of external ligands and because many established classes of drugs are known to bring about their pharmacologic response by interaction with membranes. Classical cancer chemotherapists, however, may be somewhat startled to discover that practically every major type of antineoplastic agent, no matter what its accepted principal mechanism, has been surveyed for membrane action and found operative (Table 1). It is clear that there now exists a rather large mass of facts and observations showing that even for drugs having well-established intracellular targets, for example methotrexate and 5-fluorouracil, there is evidence for cell surface activity as well. We believe that there is little to be gained from simply collecting more observations and extending the list of membrane actions of anticancer drugs. It should be considered established that antineoplastics can be membrane active agents. The more important, and more difficult, question remaining for future work is – are these membrane effects functionally linked to pharmacologic action?

The cell surface membrane conducts a wide variety of cellular business and a variety of types of control and regulatory mechanisms have been identified. These mechanisms include receptor coupled synthesis of cyclic nucleotides, protein phosphorylation, lipid methylation, phosphatidyl inositol turnover, regulation of permeability and membrane potential and control of membrane fluidity. Disruption of these mechanisms by drugs can irreversibly alter the ability of a cell to control metabolism and proliferation, and in turn provide attractive possibilities for explaining the cytotoxic actions of antineoplastic agents. Indeed, this review shows that many of these mechanisms can be modulated by one or more anticancer drugs; the future awaits demonstration of how the membrane events are coupled to the ability of the drugs to be clinically effective. The major advantage of surface attack is that it offers the possibility of specificity of drug action since tumor cells are known to have altered plasma membranes and deranged abilities to carry out the aforementioned kinds of control mechanisms, when compared to their normal counterparts. Thus one hopes that drugs could be targeted to recognize and exploit such differences. Additionally, the use of drugs to alter specific membrane control mechanisms may represent a more sophisticated mode of cellular disruption than attempting to kill the cell by non-specific annihilation of DNA synthesis. The result of such drug action will be more selectivity for tumor cells and fewer toxic repercussions on normal cells, a result of clear significance to the advancement of cancer chemotherapy.

ACKNOWLEDGEMENTS

We thank Gerald Zuckier and Marc Adler for helpful comments on the manuscript and Ann Lovejoy for her usual editorial brilliance.

Work in the authors' laboratories was supported by the National Institutes of Health (CA 28852), the American Cancer Society (CH 212), and the Cancer Research Campaign. JAH was supported by a CRC-UICC Travel Fellowship while writing this review. TRT is the recipient of a Research Career Development Award (CA 00684).

REFERENCES

Adler M, Tritton TR: Protein and lipid composition of Adriamycin resistant S180 variants. To be submitted, 1984.

Aggarwal SK, Niroomand-Rad I: Effect of cisplatin on the plasma membrane phosphatase activities in ascites sarcoma 180 cells: A cytochemical study. J Histochem Cytochem 31:307–317, 1983.

Amini S, Kaji A: Association of pp36, a phosphorylated form of the presumed target protein for the SRC transformed by rous sarcoma virus. Proc Nat Acad Sci 80:960–964, 1983.

Anderson RA, Lovrien RE: Erythrocyte membrane sidedness in lectin control of the Ca^{2+}-A23187-mediated diskocyte $\rightleftarrows$ echinocyte conversion. Nature 292:158–161, 1981.

Anghileri LJ: Ca^{2+} transport inhibition by the antitumour agents adriamycin and daunomycin. Arzneim Forsch 27:1177–1180, 1977.

Ankel E, Ring B, Holcenberg J: Effects of alkylating agents on cell membranes of mouse leukemic cells and human erythrocytes. Fed Proc 41:1477, 1982.

Archer DB: The use of a fluorescent sterol to investigate the mode of action of amphotericin methyl ester, a polyene antibiotic. Biochem Biophys Res Comm 66:195–201, 1975.

Arena E, Arico M, Biondo F, D'Alessancro N, Dusonchet L, Gebbia N, Gerbasi F, Sangnedolce R, Rausa L: Analysis of some probable factors responsible for adriamycin induced cardiotoxicity. IInd international symposium on adriamycin, pp 160–172, European Press Medikon Belgium, 1975.

Azuma J, Sperelakis N, Hasegowa H, Tanimoto T, Vogel S, Ogura K, Awata N, Sawamura A, Harada H, Ishiyama T, Morita Y, Yamamura Y: Adriamycin cardiotoxicity: possible pathogenic mechanisms. J Molec Cell Cardiol 13:381–397, 1981.

Bales BL, Leon V: Magnetic Resonance Studies of eukaryotic cells. III. Spin labeled fatty acids in the plasma membrane. Biochim Biophys Acta 509:90–99, 1978.

Balk SD: Calcium as a regulator of the proliferation of normal but not of transformed, chick fibroblasts in a plasma-containing medium. Proc Natl Acad Sci USA 68:271–275, 1971.

Barranco SL, Bolton WE, Novak JK: Time dependent changes in drug sensitivity expressed by mammalian cells after exposure to trypsin. J Nat Can Inst 64:913–916, 1980.

Baxter MA, Chahwala SB, Hickman JA, Spurgin GE: The effects of nitrogen mustard (HN2) on activities of the plasma membrane of PC6A mouse plasmacytoma cells. Biochem Pharmacol 31:1773–1778, 1982.

Beck WT, Mueller TJ, Tanzer LR: Altered surface membrane glycoproteins in vinca alkaloid-resistant human leukemic lymphoblasts. Cancer Res 39:2070–2076, 1979.

Bellomo G, Jewell SA, Thor H, Orrenius S: Regulation of intracellular calcium compartmentation: Studies with isolated lepatocytes and t-butyl hydroperoxide. Proc Natl Acad Sci USA 79:6842–6866, 1982.

Bergelson LD, Dyatlovitskaya EV, Torkhovskaya TJ, Sorokina IB, Gorkova NP: Phospholipid composition of membranes in the tumor cell. Biochim Biophys Acta 210:287–298, 1970.

Bergelson LD, Dyatlovitskaya EV, Sorokina IB, Gorkova WB: Phospholipid composition of mitochondria and microsomes from regenerating rat liver and hepatomas of different growth rate. Biochim Biophys Acta 360:361–365, 1974.

Bernacki R, Porter C, Korytnyk W, Michich E: Plasma membrane as a site for chemotherapeutic intervention. Adr Enz Res 16:217–237, 1978.

Boonstra J, Mummery CL, van Zoelen EJJ, van der Saag PT, de Laat SW: Monovalent cation transport during the cell cycle. Anticancer Res 2:265–274, 1982.

Borle AB: Methods of assessing hormone effects on calcium fluxes in $vitro$. Methods in enzymology, XXXIX, 513–573, 1975.

Boynton AL, McKeehan WL, Whitfield JF (ed) (1982): 'Ions, cell proliferation and cancer.' Academic Press, N.Y.

Boynton AL, Whitfield JF: Different calcium requirements for proliferation of conditionally and unconditionally tumorigenic mouse cells. Proc Natl Acad Sci 73(5):1651–1654, 1976.

Burger MM, Goldberg AR: Identification of a tumor specific determinant on neoplastic cell surfaces. Proc Nat Acad Sci 57:359–366, 1967.

Burke TG, Morin MJ, Forder J, Sartorelli AC, Tritton TR: A fluorescence study of the interaction of anthracyclines with model membranes. Fed Proc 42:2169, 1983.

Burns CP, Luttenegger DG, Dudley DT, Buettner GR, Spector AA: Effect of modification of plasma membrane fatty acid composition on fluidity and methotrexate transport in L1210 Murine leukemic cells. Cancer Res 39:1726–1732, 1979.

Cameron IL, Smith NKR, Pool TB, Sparks RL: Intracellular concentration of sodium and other elements as related to mitogenesis and oncogenesis in $vitro$. Cancer Res 40:1493–1500, 1980.

Campisi J, Scandella CJ: Bulk membrane fluidity increases after fertilization or partial activation of Sea Urchin Eggs. J Biol Chem 255:5411–5419, 1980.

Canellakis ES, Chen T-K: Relationship of biochemical drug effects to their antitumor activity. I. Diacridines and the cell membrane. Biochem Pharm 28:1971–1976, 1979.

Caroni P, Villani F, Carafoli E: The cardiotoxic antibiotic doxorubicin inhibits the Na^+/Ca^{2+} exhange of dog heart sarcolemmal vesicles. FEBS Letts 130:186–186, 1981.

Chahwala SB, Hickman JA, Grundy RG: Effects of adriamycin on membrane potential of human erythrocytes. Brit J Cancer 46:501, 1982.

Chandrabose K, Cuatrecases P: Changes in fatty acyl chains of phospholipids induced by interferon in mouse sarcoma S-180 cells. Biochem Biophys Res Comm 98:661–668, 1981.

Chin JH, Goldstein DB: Drug tolerance in biomembranes: A spin label study of the effects of ethanol. Science 196:684–685, 1977.

Chlebowski RT, Block JB, Cundiff D, Dietrich F: Doxorubicin cytotoxicity enhanced by local anesthetics in a human melanoma cell line. Cancer Treat Rep 66:121–125, 1982.

Choudhury SR, Deb JK, Choudhury K, Neogy RK: Inhibition of uridine transport through sarcoma 180 cell membrane by anthracycline antibiotics. Biochem Pharm 31:1811–1814, 1982.

Cragoe EJ Jr: In: Cuthbert AW, Fanelli GM, Jr, Seriabine A (ed), Amiloride and epithelial sodium transport. pp 1–20, 1979. Urban and Schwarzenberg, Baltimore-Munich.

Crane FL, MacKellar WC, Morre DJ, Ramasarma T, Goldenberg H, Grebing C Löw H: Adriamycin affects plasma membrane redox functions. Biochem Biophys Res Comm 93:746–754, 1980.

Dasdia T, DiMarco A, Goffredi M, Minghetti A, Necco A: Ion level and Calcium Fluxes in HeLa cells after adriamycin treatment. Pharmacol Res Commun 11:9–29, 1979.

De Luca LM, Shapir SS: Modulation of cellular interactions by vitamins A and derivatives (Retinoids). Ann NY Acad Sci Vol 359, 1981.

Deutsch C, Price M: Role of Extracellular Na and K in lymphocyte Activation. J Cell Physiol 113:73–79, 1982.

Duarte-Karim M, Ruysschaert JM, Hidebrand J: Affinity of adriamycin to phospholipids: A possible explanation for cardiac mitochondrial lesions. Biochem Biophys Res Comm 71û–663, 1976.

Durkin JP, Boynton AL, Whitfield JF: The src gene product (pp60^{src}) of Arian sarcoma virus rapidly induces DNA synthesis and proliferation of calcium-deprived rat cells. Biochem biophys Res Commun 103:233–239, 1981.

El Mashak E-S M, Tocanne J-F: Interactions between ellipticine and phospholipids. Effect of ellipticine and 9-Methoxyellipticine on the phase behavior of phosphatidylglycerols. Eur J Biochem 105:593–609, 1980.

Farber JL: The role of calcium in cell death. Life Sciences 29:1289–1295, 1981.

Fico RM, Chen TK, Canellakis ES: Bifunctional intercalators: Relationship of antitumor activity of diacridines to the cell membrane. Science 198:53–56, 1977.

Freedman RB: Crossêlinking reagents and membrane organization. Trends in Biochem Sci 4:193–197, 1979.

Garman D, Center MS: Alterations in cell surface membranes in chinese hamster lung cells resistant to adriamycin. Biochem biophys Res Comm 105:157–163, 1982.

Ghezzi P, Donelli MG, Pantarotto C, Facchineti T, Garattini S: Evidence for covalent binding of adriamycin to rat liver microsomal protproteins. Biochem Pharm 30:175–177, 1981.

Glaubinger D, Ramu A, Weintraub H, Magrath I, Brereton H, Joshi A: Differences in lipid composition and structural order between anthracycline sensitive and resistant P388 murine leukemia cells. Proc Amer Assoc Cancer Res 284:284, 1983.

Goldman R, Facchinetti T, Bach D, Raz A, Shinitzky M: A differential interaction of daunomycin adriamycin and their derivatives with human erythrocytes and phospholipid bilayer. Biochim Biophys Acts 512:254–269, 1978.

Goormaghtigh E, Chatelain P, Caspers J Ruysschaert JM: Evidence of specific complex between adriamycin and negatively charged phospholipids. Biochim Biophys Acta 597:1–14, 1980a.

Goormaghtigh E, Chatelain P, Caspers J, Ruysschaert JM: Evidence for a complex between adriamycin derivatives and cardiolipin: Possible Role in cardiotoxicity. Biochem Pharm 29:3003–3010, 1980b.

Goormaghtigh E, Vandenbranden M, Ruysschaert JM, DeKruijff B: Adriamycin Inhibits the formation of non-bilayer lipid structures in cardiolipin-containing model membranes. Biochim Biophys Acta 685:137–143, 1982.

Goormaghtigh E, Pollakis G, Ruysschaert JM: Mitochondrial Membrane modifications induced by adriamycin-mediated electron transport. Biochem Pharm 32:889–893, 1983.

Gordon LM, Sauerheber RD, Esgate JA, Dipple I, Marchmont RJ, Houslay MD: The Increase in bilayer fluidity of rat liver plasma membranes achieved by the local anesthetic benzyl alcohol affects the activity of intrinsic membrane enzymes. J Biol Chem 255:4519–4527, 1980.

Gosalvez M, Pezzi L, Vivero C: Inhibition of capping of surface immunoglobuline at femtomolar concentrations of adriamycin, compound ICR5–159 and tetrodotoxin. Biochem Soc Trans 6:659–661, 1978.

Gosalvez M, van Rossum GDV, Blanco MF: Inhibition of sodium-potassium-activated adenosine 5′-triphosphatase and ion transport by adriamycin. Cancer Res 39:257–261, 1979.

Gross RB, Scanlon KJ, Kisthard H, Waxman S: Altered membrane transport properties of L1210 cells resistant to cis platin. Proc Amer Assoc cancer Res 42:281, 1983.

Grunicke H, Gantner G, Ihlenfeldt M, Harrer M, Puschendorf B: A new concept on the mode of action of alkylating agents: Interaction with the plasma membrane. Excerpta Medica International Congress Series 484:296–305, 1980.

Grunicke H, Gantner G, Holzweber F, Ihlenfeldt M, Puschendorf B: New Concepts on the

Interference of Alkylating Antitumor agents with the regulation of cell division. Adv Enzy Reg 17:291–303, 1979.

Grunicke H, Putzer H, Scheidl F, Wolf-Schreiner E, Grünewald K: Inhibition of tumor growth by alkylation of the plasma membrane. Bioscience Rep 2:601–604, 1982.

Harper JR, Jr, Orringer EP, Parker JC: Adriamycin inhibits Ca permeability and Ca-dependent K movements in red blood cells. Res Commun Chem Path Pharmac 26:277–284, 1979.

Helfman DM, Barnes KK, Kinkade JM, Vogler WR, Shoji M, Kuo JF: Phospholipid-sensitive Ca^{2+}-dependent protein phosphorylation system in various types of leukemic cells from human patients and human leukemic cell lines HL60 and K562, and its inhibition by alkyl-lysophospholipid. Cancer Res 43:2955–2961.

Hort-Legrand C, Metral S: Modifications sous l'effet de la vincristine de l'apparition des potentiels miniatures à la jonction neuromusculaire de la grenouille. CR Acad Sci (Paris) 282 Serie D:933–936, 1976.

Howard SMH, Theologides A, Sheppard JR: Comparitive effects of vindesine, vinblastine, and vincristine on mitotic arrest and hormonal response in L1210 Leukemia cells. Cancer Res 40:2695–2700, 1980.

Hozumi M: Fundamentals of chemotherapy of myeloid leukemia by induction of leukemia cell differentiation. Adv Cancer Res 38:121–169, 1983.

Huang C-H: Studies on phosphatidylcholine vesicles. Formation and physical characteristics. Biochemistry 8:344–351, 1969.

Hwang KM, Sartorelli AC: Use of plant lectin induced agglutination to detect alterations in surface architecture of sarcoma 180 caused by antineoplastic agents. Biochem Pharm 24:1149–1152, 1975.

Ihlenfield M, Gantner G, Harrer M, Puschendorf B, Putzer H, Grunicke H: Interaction of the alkylating antitumor agents 2,3,5-Tris(ethyleneimino)-benzoquinone with the plasma membrane of erhlich ascites tumor cells. Cancer Res 41:289–293, 1981.

Jaenke RS: Delayed and progressive myocardial Lesions after adriamycin administration in the rabbit. Cancer Res 36:2958–2966, 1976.

Jain MK, Wu NYM, Wray LV: Drug induced phase change in bilayer as possible mode of action of membrane-expanding drugs. Nature 255:495, 1975.

Jensen RA: Cardiotoxicity of 5-iminodaunorubicin and doxorubicin in the rat. Proc Amer Assoc Cancer Res 24:354, 1983.

Jewell SA, Bellomo G, Thor H, Orrenius S, Smith MT: Bleb formation in hepatocytes during drug metabolism is caused by disturbances in thiol and calcium ion homeostasis. Science 217:1257–1259, 1982.

Karczmar GS, Tritton TR: The interaction of adriamycin with small unilamellar liposomes: A fluorescence study. Biochim Biophys. Acta 557:306–319, 1979.

Katoh H, Wise BC, Wrenn RW, Kuo JF: Inhibition by adriamycin of calmodulin-sensitive and phospholipid-ensitive calcium-dependent phosphorylation of endogenous proteins from the heart. Biochem J 198:199–205, 1981.

Kennedy KA, Siegfried JA, Sartorelli AC, Tritton TR: Effects of anthracyclines on oxygenated and hypoxic tumor cells. Cancer Res 43:54–59, 1983.

Kessel D: Enhanced glycosylation by Adriamycin. Mol Phrm 16:306–312, 1979.

Kessel D: Cell surface alterations associated with exposure of L1210 Cells to fluorouracil. Cancer Res 40:722–324, 1980.

Kharasch ED, Novak RF: Inhibition of adriamycin stimulated microsomal lipid peroxidation by mitoxantrone and ametantrone. Biochem Biophys Res Comm 108:1346–1352, 1982.

Kiefer H, Blume AJ, Kaback HR: Membrane potential changes during mitogenic stimulation of mouse Spleen lymphocytes. Proc Natl Acad Sci USA 77:2200–2204, 1980.

Kim D-H, Akera T, Brody TM: Inotropic actions of doxorubicin in isolated guinea-pig Atria; Evidence for lack of involvement of Na+-K+-adenosine triphosphatase. J Pharm Exp Ther

214:368–374, 1980

Koechler KA, Hines JD, Mansour EG, Rustum YM, Jain MK: Evidence suggesting that high dose cytosine arabinoside effects are associated with drug-membrane interaction. Proc Amer Assoc Cancer Res 24:290, 1983.

Kwock L: Sulfhydryl group involvement in the modulation of neutral amino acid transport in thymocyte membrane vesicles. J Cell Physiol 106:279–282, 1981.

Lakowicz JR, Prendergast FG, Hogan I: Differential phase fluorimetric investigation of diphenylhexatriene in lipid bilayers. Quantitation of hindered depolarizing rotation. Biochemistry 18:508–519, 1979.

Landolph JR, Bhatt RS, Telfer N, Heidelberger C: Comparison of adriamycin- and ouabain-induced cytotoxicity and inhibition of ^{86}Rubidium transport in wildtype and ouabain-resistant C3H/10 T1/2 mouse fibroblasts. Cancer Res 40:4581–4588, 1980.

Laporte DC, Rosentahl KS, Storm DR: Inhibition of Escherichia coli growth and respiration by polymyxin B covalently attached to agarose beads. Biochemistry 16:1642–1648, 1977.

Lazo JS, Lynch TJ, Tritton TR: Bleomycin disruption of pulmonary endothelial plasma membranes. Submitted, 1983.

Lazo JS, Shansky LW, Sartorelli AC: Reduction in cell surface con A binding and mannose incorporation into glycoproteins of sarcoma 180 by 6-thioguanine. Biochem Pharm 28:583–588, 1979.

Leffert HL(editor): Growth regulation by ion fluxes. Ann NY Acad Sci Vol 339, 1980.

Lehotay DC, Levey BA, Rogersen BJ, Levey GS: Inhibition of cardiac guanylate cyclase by doxorubicin and some of its analogs: Possible relationship to cardiotoxicity. Cancer Treat Res 66:311–318, 1982.

Levi M: The effect of mustard gases upon a property of nucleated erythrocytes and their ghosts. Cancer Res 25:752–759, 1965.

Ling V: Drug resistance and membrane alteration in mutants of mammalian cells. Canad J Genet Cytol 17:503–515, 1975.

Ling V: Genetic basis of drug resistance in mammalian cells in drug and hormone resistance in neoplasia. CRC Press, in press, 1983.

Ludlum DB: Molecular biology of alkylation: An overview. In: Sartorelli AC, Johns DG (eds), Antineoplastic and Immunosuppressive Agents. Part 2, pp 6–17, 1975, Springer-Verlag.

Luly P, Barnabei O, Tria E: Hormonal control in vitro of plasma membrane bound (Na+-K+)-ATPase of rat liver. B.B.A. 282:447–452, 1972.

Margolis RL, Wilson L: Regulation of microtubule steady state in vitro by ATP. Cell 18:673–679, 1979.

Marks ME, Ziober B, Brattain DE, Syna D: Effects of N,N-dimethylformamide on plasma membrane proteins from human colonic carcinoma cells grown in vitro. Proc Amer Assoc Cancer Res 24:44, 1983.

Medoff G, Valeriote FA, Dieckman J: Potentiation of anticancer agents by amphotericin B. J Nat Cancer Inst 67:131–135, 1981.

Melchior DL, Steim JM: Thermotropic transitions in biomembranes. Ann Rev Biophys Bioeng 5:205–238, 1976.

Mikkelson RB, Koch B: Thermosensitivity of the membrane potential of normal and simian virus 40-transformed hamster lymphocytes. Cancer Res 41:209–215, 1981.

Mikkelson RB, Lin P-S, Wallach DFH: Interaction of adriamycin with human red blood cells: A biochemical and morphological study. J Molec Med 2:33–40, 1977.

Minnaugh EG, Trush MA, Gram TE: Stimulation by adriamycin of rat heart and liver microsomal NADPH-dependent lipid peroxidation. Biochem Pharm 30:2797–2804, 2804, 1981.

Minnaugh EG, Trush MA, Ginsburg E, Gran TE: Differential effects of anthracycline drugs on rat heart and liver microsomal reduced nicotinamide adenine dinucleotide phosphate-dependent lipid peroxidation. Cancer Res 42:3574–3582, 1982.

Mizuno S, Ishida A: Selective enhancement of bleomycin cytotoxicity by local anesthetics. Biochem Biophys Res Comm 105:425–431, 1982.

Moore HW: Bioactivation as a model for drug design bioreductive alkylation. Science 197:527–532, 1977.

Murphree SA, Cunningham LS, Hwang KM, Sartorelli AC: Effects of adriamycin on surface properties of sarcoma 180 ascites cells. Biochem pharm 25:1227–1231, 1976.

Murphree SA, Murphy D, Sartorelli AC, Tritton TR: Adriamycin-Liposome Interactions: A magnetic resonance study of the differential effects of cardiolipin on drug-induced fusion and permeability. Biochim Biophys Acta 691:97–105, 1982.

Murphree SA, Tritton TR, Smith PL, Sartorelli AC: Adriamycin induced changes in the surface membrane of sarcoma 180 ascites cells. Biochim Biophys Acta 649:317–324, 1981.

Myers CE, Gianni L, Simone CB, Klecker R, Greene R: Oxidative destruction of erythrocyte ghost membranes catalyzed by the doxorubicin-iron complex. Biochemistry 21:1707–1713, 1982.

Naiwu F, Guan L: Effect of Dan-shen and anticancer drugs on the cancer cell surface agglutination induced by phytohemagglutinin Zhonghua Zhongliu Zazhi 2:24–28, 1980.

Necco A, Dasdia T, DiFrancesco D, Ferroni A: Action of ouabain, oligomycin and glucagon on cultured heart cells treated with adriamycin. Pharmacol Res Commun 8:105–109, 1976.

Necco A, Ferraguti M: Influence of doxorubicin on myogenic cell fusion. Exp Molec Path 31:353–360, 1979.

Ohuchi K, Levine L: Adriamycin stimulated cancine kidney (MDCK) cells to deacylate cellular lipids and to produce prostaglandins. Prostaglandins and medicine 1:433–439, 1978.

Okada K, Yamada S, Kawashima Y, Kitade F, Okajima K, Fujimoto M: Cell injury by antineoplastic agents and influence of coenzyme Q_{10} on cellular potassiuim acticity and potential difference across the membrane in rat liver cells. Cancer Res 40:1663–1667, 1980.

Olson HM, Young DM, Prieur DJ, LeRoy AF, Reagan RL: Electrolyte and morphological alterations of myocardium in adriamycin-treated rabbits. Am J Pathol 77:439–454, 1974.

Otten J, Johnson GS, Pastan I: Cyclic AMP levels in fibroblasts, relationship to growth rate and contact inhibition of growth. Biochem Biophys Res Commun 44:1192–1198, 1971.

Ozols LF, Hogan WM, Grotzinger KR, McCoy W, Young RC: Effects of amphotericin B on adriamycin and melphalan cytotoxicity in human and murine ovarian carcinoma and L1210 leukemia Cancer Res 43:959–964, 1983.

Pang K-Y, Chang T-L, Miller KW: On the coupling between anesthetic induced membrane fluidization and cation permeability in lipid vesicles. Mol Pharm 15:729–738, 1979.

Parsons PG, Musk P, Goss PD, Leah J: Effects of calcium depletion on human cells in vitro and the anomolous behaviour of the human melanoma cell line. Cancer Res 43:2081–2087, 1983.

Pastan I, Willingham MC: Journey to the center of the cell: Role of the receptosome. Science 214:504–509, 1981.

Patterson LH, Gandecha BM, Brown JR: 1,4-Bis [2-(2-hydroxyethyl)aminolethylaminol-9,10-anthracenedione an anthraquinone antitumor agent that does not cause lipid peroxidation in vivo; Comparison with daunorubicin. Biochem Biophys Res Comm 110:399–405, 1983.

Peters RW: Biochemical research at Oxford upon mustard gas. Nature 159:149–151, 1947.

Peterson RHF, Meyers MB, Spengler BA, Biedler JL: Alteration of plasma membrane glycopeptides and gangliosides of chinese hamster cells accompanying development of resistance to daunorubicin and vincristine. Cancer Res 43:222–229, 1983.

Poste G, Nicholson GL (eds): Membrane fusion. North Holland Publishing Company, Amsterdam, 1978.

Prasad SB, Sodhi A: Effect of Cis-dichlorodiamine Platinum (II) on the agglutinability of tumor and normal cells with concanavalin A and wheat germ agglutinin. Chem Biol Int

36:355–367, 1981.

Rabkin SW, Bose D: Adriamycin induced alterations vs canine purkinje fiber action potential. Res Comm Chem Path Pharm 34:55–68, 1981.

Ralph RK: On the mechanism of action of 4′[(9-acridinyl)-aminol-Methanesulphon-M-anisidine. Europ J Cancer 16:595–600, 1980.

Reich E, Rifkin DB, Shaw E: Proteases and Biological Control, 1975. Cold Spring Harbor Press, Cold Spring Harbor, N.Y.

Revis NW, Marusic N: Effects of doxorubicin and its aglycone metabolite on calcium sequestration by rabbit heart, liver and kidney mitochondria. Life Sci 25:1055–1064, 1979.

Riordan JR, Ling V: Purification of P-glycoprotein from plasma membrane vesicles of chinese hamster ovary cell mutants with reduced colchicine permeability. J Biol Chem 254:12701–12705, 1979.

Rogers KE, Carr BI, Tökes ZA: Cell Surface-mediated cytotoxicity of polymer-bound adriamycin against drug-resistant hepatocytes. Cancer Res 43:2741–2748, 1983.

Russell T, Pastan I: Plasma membrane cyclic adenosine 3′:5′-Monophosphate phosphodiesterase of cultured cells and its modification after trypsin treatment of intact cells. J Biol Chem 248:5835–5840, 1973.

Russell DH, Womble JR: Transglutaminase may mediate certain physiological effects of endogenous amines and amine containing therapeutic agents. Life Sci 30:1499–1508, 1982.

Salles B, Charcosset JY, Jacquemin-Sablon A: Isolation and properties of chinese hamster lung cells resistant to ellipticine derivatives. Cancer Treat Rep 66:327–338, 1982.

Scanlon KJ, Safirstein RL, Thies H, Gross RB, Waxman S, Gutterplan JB: Inhibition of amino acid transport by cisplatin and its derivatives in L1210 murine leukemia cells. Cancer Res 1983, in press.

Schanne FAX, Kane AB, Young EE, Farber JL: Calcium dependence of toxic cell death: A final common pathway. Science 206:700–702, 1979.

Schengrund C-L, Sheffler BA: Biochemical and morphological study of adriamycin induced changes in murine neuroblastoma cells. Oncology 39:185–190, 1982.

Schiffman FJ, Klein I: Rapid induction of amphotericin B sensitivity in L1210 leukaemia cells by liposomes containing ergosterol. Nature 269:65–66, 1977.

Schioppocassi G, Schwartz HS: Membrane actions of daunorubicin in mammalian erythocytes. Res Comm Chem Path Pharm 18:519–531, 1977.

Schlager SI, Ohanian SH: Plasma membrane and Intracellular lipid synthesis in tumor cells rendered sensitive to humoral immune killing after treatment with metabolic inhibitors. J Nat Can Inst 63:1475–1483, 1979.

Schlager SI, Ohanian SH: Tumor cell lipid composition and sensitivity to humoral immune killing. J Immunol 125:508–517, 1980.

Schroeder F, Fontaine RW, Feller DJ, Weston KG: Drug induced surface membrane phospholipid composition in murine fibroblasts. Biochim biophys. Acta 643:76–88, 1981.

Schwartz HS, Kanter PM: Chemical interactions of cardiolipin with daunorubicin and other intercalating agents. Europ J Cancer 15:923–928, 1979

Sharon N, Lis H: Lectins: Cell-agglutinating and sugar-specific proteins. Science 177:949–959, 1972.

Siegfried JA, Kennedy KA, Sartorelli AC, Tritton TR: The role of membranes in the mechanism of action of adriamycin: Spin labeling studies with chronically hypoxic and drug resistant tumor cells. J Biol Chem 258:339–343, 1983.

Siegfried JA, Tritton TR: Adriamycin enhances the agglutination rate of sensitive, but not resistant S180 cells. Annual New England pharmacologists 8:18, 1979.

Sinensky M, Pinkerton F, Sutherland E, Simon FR: Rate limitation of $(Na^+ + K^+)$-stimulated and adenosinetriphosphatase by membrane acyl chain ordering. Proc Nat Acad Sci 76:4893–4897, 1979.

Sinha BK, Gregory JL: Role of One-electron and two-electron reduction products of adriamycin and daunomycin in DNA binding. Biochem Pharm 30:2626–2629, 1981.

Sinha B, Chignell CF: Interaction of antitumor drugs with human erythrocyte host membranes and mastocytoma P815: A spin label study. Biochem Biophys Res Comm 86:1051–1057, 1979.

Sirotnak FM, Chello PL, Brockman RW: Potential for Exploitation of Transport systems in anticancer drug design. Methods Cancer Res XVI, 381–445, 1979.

Smith NKR, Stabler SB, Cameron IL, Medina D: X-ray microanalkysis of electrolyte content of normal, preneoplastic and neoplastic mouse mammary tissue. Cancer res 41·3877–3880, 1981.

Solie TN, Yuncker C: Adriamycin induced changes in translocation of sodium ions in transpoeting epithelial cells. Life Sci 22:1907–1920, 1978.

Solomonson LP, Halabrin PR: Cardiac sodium, potassium-adenosine triphosphatase as a possible site of Adriamycin-induced cardiotoxicity. Cancer Res 41:570–572, 1981.

Sparks RL, Pool TB, Smith NKR, Cameron IL: Effects of amiloride on tumour growth and intra-cellular element content of tumour cells in vivo. Cancer Res 43:73–77, 1983.

Spiegel RJ, Nodar R, Levin M: Enhanced adriamycin cytotoxicity in L1210 cells following lipid modulation. Proc Amer Assoc Cancer Res 24:256, 1983.

Sweadner KJ: Cross Linking and modifications of Na,K-ATPase by ethyl acetimidate. Biochem Biophys Res Commun 78:962–969, 1977.

Taylor RG, Teague LA, Yesair DW: Drug-binding macromolecular lipids from L1210 leukemia tumors. Cancer Res41:4316–4323, 1981.

Terce F, Tocanne J-P, Laneele G: Interactions of elipticine with model or natural membranes. A Spectrophotometric study. Europ J Biochem 125:203–207, 1982.

Ter-Minassian-Saraga L, Madelmont G, Hort-Legrand C, Metral D: Vinblastine and Vincristine action on gel-fluid transition of hydrated DPPC. Biochem Pharm 30:411–415, 1981.

Tisdale, MJ: The reaction of alkylating agents with cyclic 3′,5′-nucleotide phosphodiesterase. Chem-Biol Interac 9:145–153, 1974.

Tisdale MJ, Phillips BJ: Adenosine 3′,5′-monophosphate phosphodiesterase activity in experimental tumours which are either sensitive or resistant to bifunctional alkylating agents. Biochem. Pharmac 24:205–210, 1975a.

Tisdale MJ, Phillips BJ: Inhibition of 3′,5′-Nuleotide Phosphodiesterase – a possible mechanism of action of bifunctional alkylating agents. Biochem. Pharmac 24:211–217, 1975b.

Tisdale MJ, Phillips BJ: Comparative effects of alkylating agents and other antitumour agents on the intracellular level of adenosine-3′,5′-monophosphate in walker carcinoma. Biochem Pharmac 24:1271–1276, 1975c.

Tisdale MJ, Phillips BJ: The effect of alkylating agents on adenosine 3′,5′-monophosphate metabolism in walker carcinoma. Biochem Pharmas 25:1793–1797, 1976a.

Tisdale MJ, Phillips BJ: The effect of alkylating agents on the activity of adenosine 3′,5′-monophosphate-dependent protein kinase in walker carcinoma cells. Biochem Pharmac 25û5–2370, 1976b.

Tisdale MJ, Phillips BJ: Alterations in adenosine 3′,5′-monophosphate-binding protein in walker carcinoma cells sensitive or resistant to alkylating agents. Biochem Pharmac 25:1831–1836, 1976c.

Tökes ZA, Csipke CP, Siegfried JM, Tritton TR: Adriamycin induced elevation of proteolytic activity measured at the cell surface. Proc Amer Assoc Cancer Res 22:28, 1981.

Tökes ZA, Rogers KE, Rembaum A: Synthesis of Adriamycin Coupled POlyglutaraldehyde microspheres and the evaluation of their cytostatic activity. Proc Nat Acad Sci 79:2026–2030, 1982.

Tritton TR, Murphree SA, Sartotelli AC: Adriamycin: A proposal on the specificity of drug action. biochem Biophys Res Comm 84:802–808, 1978.

Tritton TR, Yee G: The anticancer drug adriamycin can Be actively cytotoxic without entering cells. Science 217:248-250, 1982.

Tritton TR, Murphree SA, Sartorelli AC: Characterization of Drug-membrane interactions using the liposome system. Biochem Pharm 26:2319-2323, 1977.

Tritton TR, Wingard LB, Yee G: Immobilized adriamycin: A tool for separating cell surface from intracellular drug mechanisms. Fed Proc 42:284-287, 1983.

Tritton TR: 1983, Unpublished Results.

Van den Berg EK, Brazy PC, Huang AT, Dennis VW: Cisplatin-induced changes in sodium, chloride and urea transport by the frog skin. Kidney Int 19:8-14, 1981.

Vauquelin G, Lacombe ML, Hanoune J, Strosberg AD: Stability of isoproterenol bound to cyanogen bromide activated agarose. Biochem Biophys Res CComm 64:1076-1082, 1975.

Venter JC: Immobilized and insolubilized drugs, hormones and neurotransmitters: Properties, mechanisms of action and application. Pharm Rev 34:153-187, 1982.

Villani F, Faralli L, Piccinini F: Relationship between the effects on calcium turnover and early cardiotoxicity of doxorubicin and 4'-epi-doxorubicin in guinea pig heart muscle. Tumori 66:689-697, 1980.

Villani F, Piccinini F, Merelli P, Faralli L: Influence of adriamycin on calcium exchangeability in Cardiac muscle and its modification by ouabain. Biochem Pharma 27:985-987, 1978.

Wallach DFH: Membrane Molecules Biology of Neoplastic Cells, 1975, Elsecier, New York.

Walling JM, Ord MJ: Importance of cytoplasm/cell membrane induced by adriamycin. Brt Assoc Cancer Res Mar 29-31, 1982.

Wang JL, Edelman GM: Binding and functional properties of concanavalin A and its derivatives. J Biol Chem 253:3000-3007, 1978.

Wheeler C, Rader R, Kessel D: Membrane alterations associated with progressive adriamycin resistance. Biochem Pharm 31:2691-2697, 1982.

Whetton AD, Margison GP, Dodd NJF, Needham L, Houslay MD: (Submitted) dimethylnitrosamine modulates the activity of glucagan-stimulated adenylate cyclase for rat liver plasma membranes by altering plasma membrane fluidity.

Whitfield JF, Boynton AL, MacManus JP, Rixon RH, Sikorska M, Tsang B, Walker PR: The roles of calcium and cyclic AMP in cell proliferation. Ann NY Acad Sci 339:216-240, 1980.

Whitfield JF, Perris AD: The radiomimetic action of valinomycin on the nuclear structure of rat thymocytes. Expl Cell Res 51:451-461, 1968.

Wildenauer DB, Oehlmann CE: Interaction of cyclophosphanide metabolites with membrane proteins: an in vitro study with rabbit liver microsomes and human red blood cells. Effect of thiols. Biochem Pharmac 31:3535-3541, 1982.

Wildenauer DB, Reuther H, Remien J: Reactions of the alkylating agent tris(2-chloroethyl)-amine with the Erythrocyte membrane: Effects on shape changes of Human erythocytes and ghosts. Biochim Biophys Acta 603:101-116, 1980.

Wildenauer D, Weger N: Reactions of the trifunctional nitrogen mustard tris(2-chloroethyl)-amine (HN3) with human erythrocyte membranes in vitro. Biochem Pharmac 28:2761-2769, 1979.

Williams JR, Little JB, Shipley WV: Association of mammalian cell death with a specific endonucleolytic degradation of DNA. Nature 252:754-755, 1974.

Wingard LB: Immobilized drugs and enzymes in biochemical pharmacology: Perspectives and critique. Biochem Pharm 32:2647-2652, 1983.

Wingard L, Tritton TR: Immobilized adriamycin and carminomycin: Coupling chemistry and effects on survival of L1210 and S180 clones. In: Chaiken IM, Wilchele M, Parikh (eds) Affinity chromatography and biological recognition, 1984, Academic Press, N.Y., p 583-585.

Wong S-K, Huang C-H, Prestayko AW, Crooke ST: Fluorescent adducts produced from interactions of M-AMSA with Human Red blood cell membrane ghosts. Proc Amer Assoc Cancer Res 24:44, 1983.

Yahara I, Iwashita S, Evina T, Satake M, Ishida W: Inhibition of lipid-independent cap formation of mouse lymphocytes and raji cells by neocarzinostatin. Cancer res 39:4687, 1979.

Yee C, Carey M, Tritton TR: Photoaffinity labeling of daunomycin binding sites on the surface of S180 cells. Cancer Res 44:1898–1903, 1984.

Zs-Nagy I, Lustyik G, Zarardi B, Bertoni-Freddari C: Intracellular $Na^+:K^+$ Ratios in Human cancer cells as reveled by energy dispersive X-ray microanalysis. J Cell Biol 90:769–777, 1981.

Zuckier G, Tritton TR: Adriamycin Causes up regulation of epidermal growth factor receptors in actively growing cells. Exp Cell Res 148:155–161, 1983.

5. Development of Fluoropyrimidines: Japanese Experience

MAKOTO OGAWA, M.D.

Introduction

Eight fluoropyrimidines including 6 analogs of 5-fluorouracil (5FU) and 2 analogs of 2'-deoxy-5-fluorouridine (FUDR) have been tested clinically in Japan since 1970. Characteristically, all drugs are masked compounds of either 5FU or FUDR and the administrative method used for clinical trials has been by the oral route. This trend has been influenced by the success of oral ftotafur at a commercial level and also by the fact that oral administration is a convenient method for an outpatient clinic. In order to enter clinical trials, several experimental evidences have been required for a new compound.

Firstly, superior antitumor activity over 5FU and/or ftorafur in various animal tumors and secondly, less toxicity than either drug has been judged to be essential.

More recently, higher concentration and longer retention of 5FU in both blood and tumor tissue were judged to be a favorable factor to predict an enhanced antitumor activity in human tumors. Among 8 compounds entered in clinical trials, further clinical investigations of 1,3-Bis (tetrahydro-2-furanyl)-5-fluoro-2,4-pyrimidinedione [1] (FD1) and ethyl($\pm$)-t-6-butoxyl-5-fluorohexahydro-2,4-dioxypyrimidine-γ-5-carboxylate [2] (TAC-278) were discontinued due to central nervous toxicity and inferior activity to 5FU and ftorafur. 5'-Deoxy-5-fluorouridine [3] (5'-DFUR), a masked compound of 5FU, has almost completed phase II study by oral administration.

Two masked compounds of FUdR; 2'-deoxy-3', 5'-di-o-acetyl-5-fluoro-3-(3-methyl henzoyl)uridine [4] (FF-705) and 5-fluoro-3-(3,4-methylene-dioxybenzoyl)-2'-deoxy-β-uridine [5](TK-117) are in phase I-II studies. Thus, this review describes three compounds: ftorafur, HCFU and UFT which are commercially available at present time.

F.M. Muggia (ed.), Experimental and Clinical Progress in Cancer Chemotherapy
© *1985, Martinus Nijhoff Publishers, Boston. ISBN 0-89838-679-9. Printed in the Netherlands.*

1 *Ftorafur*

Ftorafur was synthesized by Hiller, *et al.* [6] in 1966 and the first clinical result was published by Blokhina *et al.* [7], Considerable clinical efficacy was reported in gastric, colorectal, and breast cancer with less toxicity than 5FU. The clinical study of ftorafur in Japan was initiated by intravenous administration in 1970 but it was discontinued because of intolerable central nervous toxicities including dizziness, hypotension, vomiting and others occurring in the majority of patients.

Thereafter, Kimura, Fujita *et al.* [8] at National Cancer Center found that upon oral administration ftorafur was absorbed promptly and concentrations of 5FU in the human plasma were sustained longer compared to intravenous administration. Thus clinical study of ftorafur was restarted by the oral route in 1972.

A. *Clinical Efficacy*

Doses used in Phase II study ranged from 600 mg to 1,200 mg by daily chronic administration and clinical efficacies seen in various tumors are summarized in Table 1. Furue *et al.* [9], reported a 22.2% response rate in 163 patients with advanced gastric cancer but the responses included Karnofsky's [10] 1-A response because at that time most investigators used these criteria.

Summarizing three papers [11–13], an overall response rate of 33% was obtained in 76 patients with advanced breast cancer. In colorectal cancer, Konda [12] reported 2 responders (13%) out of 16 patients and Watanabe [11] reported one responder (7%) out of 14 patients. Bedikian *et al.* [14], conducted a randomized trial comparing oral ftorafur and intravenous 5FU in advanced colorectal cancer. There were 6 partial responses (19%) in 32 patients in 5FU arm, while 7 partial responses (20%) in 35 patients in ftorafur arm. They concluded that oral ftorafur is equally effective against colorectal cancer with minimal hematologic toxicity.

B. *Toxicity*

Non-hematologic toxicities observed at a dose of 800 mg daily in Japanese study [11] are summarized comparing with those seen at a dose of 1 g/m^2 daily in the USA study [14] (Table 2). Gastrointestinal toxicities appear to be dose-related because significantly higher incidence was observed at a dose of 1 g/m^2. Bedikian *et al.* [15], conducted a phase I study escalating doses from 0.5 g/m^2 to 1.5 g/m^2 for 21 days repeated at 3-week intervals.

They reported that diarrhea was the dose limiting factor and central nervous toxicity which was the dose limiting toxicity by intravenous administration was minimal at the dosages administered. However, the CNS toxicity [16] appears to be associated with peak plasma levels according to the analysis of available literature on oral administration. Hematologic toxicity seen in Japanese and the US studies has been extremely mild.

2 1-Hexylcarbamoyl-5-fluorouracil (HCFU)

HCFU was synthesized by Ozaki, et al. [17] in 1977 as one of several carbamoyl derivatives of 5FU.

In various animal tumors [18], HCFU was the most active among various compounds in the same group and HCFU therefore was selected for further evaluation. HCFU is a masked compound converting to 5FU by either non-enzymatic pathway or hepatic enzymes through intermediates of 1-ω-carboxypenylcarbamoyl-5-fluorouracil (CPEFU) and 1-ω-carboxypropylcarbamoyl-5-fluorouracil (CRPFU) [19]. HCFU [18, 20] demonstrated superior antitumor activity over 5FU and ftorafur in L1210, colon 28, colon 38 and others. The distribution [21] studied in mice revealed that high concentrations were observed in liver, kidney and lung but distribution to brain was limited.

In preclinical toxicology [22, 23], HCFU demonstrated nearly identical gastrointestinal disturbances and bone marrow suppression as 5FU and ftorafur.

Phase I Study. Koyama et al. [24], conducted a phase I study with escalating doses from 1 mg/kg upto 21 mg/kg orally for 2 weeks.

The maximum tolerated dose was decided to be 20 mg/kg and optimal doses were judged to be 9-18 mg/kg in divided doses 2 to 3 times in a day. The dose limiting factor appeared to be central nervous toxicity including hot sensation, pollakiuria and sometimes urgency to defecate which occurred 15–120 minutes after oral administration, lasting for 30 minutes to several hours and subsided spontaneously.

Phase II Study. Koyama [25] summarized the results obtained in a multi-institutional cooperative study group as shown in Table 1.

Table 1. Clinical efficacy of Japanese fluoropyrimidines: percent responses (number/total)

Tumors	Oral ftorafur	HCFU	UFT	5FU**
Gastric cancer	22 (36/163)	20 (16/80)	27 (33/121)	23 (101/448)
Colorectal cancer	10 (3/30) 20 (7/35)*	43 (13/30)	27 (12/45)	21 (454/2107)
Breast cancer	33 (25/76)	33 (14/42)	32 (18/57)	26 (324/1263)

* Bedikian, A.Y., et al. CCT 6:181, 1983.
** Wasserman, T.H., et al. Cancer Treat Rep. Part 3 6(2):399, 1975.

There were 16 partial responses (20%) out of 80 patients with advanced gastric cancer and responding sites were primary tumor, metastatic lymph-node, metastatic liver and lesion in abdominal wall. Among 30 patients with advanced colorectal cancer, there were one complete and 12 partial responses with a high response rate of 43%. Complete disappearance of metastatic inguinal lymph nodes after resection of a primary tumor was evaluated as a complete response.

With HCFU the studies obtained 3 complete and 11 partial responses (33%) out of 42 patients with advanced breast cancer including responding sites in soft tissues and bone lesions. Time to response in these tumors was approximately 5 weeks and the mean duration was 11.5 weeks.

Toxicity. Non-hematologic toxicities seen at doses ranging from 900 mg to 1,500 mg per day are described in Table 2.

Gastrointestinal toxicity was much milder than with oral ftorafur; in addition, hematologic toxicity was negligible. However, central nervous toxicity was observed in about one-third of patients; furthermore, this toxicity was unpredictable even though these symptoms subsided spontaneously during the first week in 20-30% of patients.

The exact mechanism to develop this toxicity has not been clarified but the experimental result [26] in rats has suggested that HCFU itself and one of its metabolites CPEFU is responsible.

3 UFT

UFT is a unique combination consisting of uracil and ftofafur. Fujii *et al.* [27, 28], found that coadministration of uracil and ftorafur enhances antitumor activity of ftorafur on sarcoma-180 and AH-130, because uracil inhibits degradation of 5FU which has been released from ftorafur; conse-

Table 2. Toxicity of Japanese fluoropyrimidines

Toxicity	Incidence (%)			
	Oral Ftorafur		HCFU	UFT
	800 mg/d	lg/m^2/d	900–1500 mg/d	600 mg/d
Anorexia	32	43	16	29
Nausea & Vomiting	23	54 & 32	11	15
Diarrhea	16	27	7	6
Mucositis	4	26	0	3
Malaise	17	57	12	6
Dizziness	0	6	0.5	0

quently, 5FU levels in tumor tissues were much higher comparing to those measured after administration of ftorafur alone.

A molar ratio of ftorafur to uracil of 1 to 4 was determined to be optimal in accordance with balance of antitumor efficacy and toxicity.

Phase I Study. Taguchi *et al.* [29], reported the results obtained in phase I study. They escalated doses from 100 mg/body to 1,200 mg/body by a single oral administration but no serious toxicity was seen in this schedule. Thereafter, they administered the drug by daily chronic administration escalating doses up to 750 mg/day and found that dose limiting factor was gastrointestinal toxicity including nausea, vomiting and diarrhea which occurred in the majority of patients who received doses exceeding 750 mg/day. They, therefore, determined an optimal dose for daily chronic administration to be 600 mg/day.

During phase I study, several investigators [30–32] measured 5FU levels in human tumor tissues and found that UFT produced higher 5FU levels in human tumor tissues compared to normal tissues and these levels lasted for longer periods than levels achieved when ftorafur was administered alone.

Phase II Study. Among 121 patients with advanced gastric cancer summarizing from 8 studies in the literature [33–40], there were one complete and 32 partial responses for an overall response rate of 27.2% ranging from 12.5% to 44.4%. Durations of responses were reported to range from 5 to 47 weeks. There were scattered results reporting about clinical efficacy on colorectal cancer and 12 partial responders (26.7%) out of 45 patients were reported among studies of 8 investigators [33–37, 41–43]; in addition, durations of responses ranged from 6 to 42 weeks. Among 57 patients with advanced breast cancer [33–35 37, 38, 41, 44], there were 2 complete and 16 partial responses (31.6%) lasting for 4 to 16 weeks.

UFT produced 6 complete and 9 partial responses (34.9%) lasting from 4 to 24 weeks in 43 patients with head and neck tumors [45, 46]. A few objective responsers [33–38] were observed in hepatoma and pancreatic cancer but UFT does not appear to be as active against non-small cell carcinoma of the lung.

C. *Toxicity*

Watanabe *et al.* [33] compared toxicities seen in phase II study of UFT and ftorafur because they conducted the studies in the same group. The dose of ftorafur containing in UFT was 600 mg and that of ftorafur alone was 800 mg. They concluded that toxicities of UFT were milder than those of ftorafur.

Takino *et al.* [36] also compared toxicities of both drugs observed in their sequential studies. The doses they used were 600 mg of UFT and 800 to 1,200 mg of ftorafur. They reported that the overall incidence of gastrointestinal toxicity was slightly higher in patients treated by UFT.

COMMENT

Response rates for 3 major tumors obtained by 3 drugs are summarized and compared to these of 5FU reported by Wasserman *et al.* [47]. In gastric cancer, 4 drugs demonstrated nearly identical response rates, while in colorectal cancer HCFU showed a surprisingly high response rate although numbers of patients were relatively small. Thus further studies are necessary to confirm this result, because colorectal cancer is an unresponsive tumor to chemotherapy. Other 3 drugs indicate nearly identical activity. It was judged that all 4 drugs have a similar activity for breast cancer.

Concerning the toxicities, both hematologic and gastrointestinal toxicities of the 3 Japanese compounds are milder than 5FU.

The central nervous toxicity was infrequent at the relatively low dosage used in oral ftorafur and UFT; however it has been an obstacle for clinical use of HCFU. Specific advantages of any one of these in combinations awaits further study.

REFERENCES

1. Taguchi T E Overview of fluorinated pyrimidine derivatives under development in Japan. Jpn J Canc Chemother 8(6):834–839, 1981.
2. Koyama K: Phase II study of a new fluorinated pyrimidine, ethyl($\pm$)-t-6-butoxy-5-fluoro-2,4-dioxyheexahydropyrimidine-γ-5-carboxylate (TAC-287). Jpn J Canc Chemother 9(10):1821–1826. 1982.
3. Ota K, Kimura K: A phase II study of oral 5-deoxy-5-fluorouridine, in proceeding of International symposium on fluoropyrimidines, in press.
4. Saito T, Taguchi T: Phase I study of a new fluorouridine derivative, 2′-deoxy-3′,5′-di-o-acetyl-5-fluoro-3-(3-methyl henzoyl) uridine (FF-705). Jpn J Cancer Chemother, in press.
5. Koshimura S, Akimoto R, Takahashi Y *et al.*: Antitumor effect of a new potent agent TK177 on human gastric cancer xenografts. In: Proceeding of the Japanese Cancer Association the 42nd Annual Meeting, p 252, 1983.
6. Hiller SA, Zhuk RA, Yu Lidak M: Works of the Ist All-Union Conference on malignant tumors, Riga. pp 111–112, 1968.
7. Blokhina NG, Vozny ED, Garin AM: Results of treatment of malignant tumors with ftorafur. Cancer 30:390–392, 1972.
8. Fujita H, Ogawa K, Sawabe T, *et al.*: *In vivo* distribution of N_1-(2′-tetrahydrofuryl)-5-fluorouracil (FT-207). Jpn J Cancer Clin 18:911–916, 1972.
9. Furue H, Nakao I, Kanko T, *et al.*: Chemotherapy of gastric cancer. Jpn J Cancer Chemother 2(3):351–359, 1975.
10. Karnofsky DA: Meaningful clinical classification of therapeutic responses to anti-cancer drugs. Clin Pharmac Ther 2:709–712, 1961.

11. Watanabe HS, Yamamoto S, Naito T: Clinical results of oral UFT therapy under cooperative study. Jpn J Cancer Chemother 7(9)18–1596. 1980.
12. Konda C: The effects of oral, and rectal administration of N-(2-tetrahydrofuryl)-5-fluorouracil in the treatment of advanced cancer. Jpn J Cancer Clin 21(12:1044–1050, 1975.
13. Ishida T, Tamura N, Okamoto A, et al.: Clinical experience of oral ftorafur for recurrent breast cancer. Jpn J Cancer Chemother 1(6):999–1003, 1975.
14. Bedikian AY, Karlin D, Stroehlein J, et al.: A comparative study of oral tegafur and intravenous 5-fluorouracil in patients with metastatic colorectal cancer. Am J Clin Oncol (CCT) 6:181–186, 1983.
15. Bedikian AY, Bodey GP, Valdivieso M, et al.: Phase I evaluation of oral tegafur. Cancer Treat Rep 67:81–84, 1983.
16. Friedman MA, Ignoffo RJ: A review of the United States clinical experience of the fluoropyrimidine, ftorafur (NSC-148958).
17. Ozaki S, Ike Y, Mizuno H, et al.: 5-Fluorouracil derivatives. I. The synthesis of 1-carbamoyl-5-fluorouracils. Bull Chem Soc Jpn 60:2404–2412, 1977.
18. Iigo M, Hoshi A, Nakamura A, et al.: Antitumor activity of 1-alkylcarbamoyl derivatives of 5-fluorouracil in a variety of mouse tumors. Cancer Chemother Pharmacol 1:203–208, 1978.
19. Kobari T, Tan K, Kumakura M, et al.: Metabolic fate of 1-hexylcarbamoyl-5-fluorouracil in rats. Xenobiotica 8(9):547–556, 1978.
20. Hoshi A, Iigo M, Nakamura A, et al.: Antitumor activity of 1-hexylcarbamoyl-5-fluorouracil in a variety of experimental tumors. GANN 67:725–731, 1976.
21. Iigo M, Nakamura A, Kuretani K, et al.: Distribution of 1-hexylcarbamoyl-5-fluorouracil and 5-fluorouracil by oral administration in mice. J Pharm Dyn 2:5-11, 1979.
22. Ishimura K, Toizumi S, Inoue H, et al.:Toxicological study on 1-hexylcarbamoyl-5-fluorouracil (HCFU) (1) Subacute and chronic toxicity studies in rats. Pharmacometrics 17(4):575–595, 1979.
23. Ishimura K, Toizumi S, Neda K, et al.: Toxicological study on 1-hexylcarbamoyl-5-fluorouracil (HCFU)(2) Subacute and chronic toxicity studies in dogs. Pharmacometrics 17(4):597–615, 1979.
24. Koyama Y, Koyama Y and HCFU Clinical Study Group: Phase I study of a new antitumor drug, 1-hexylcarbamoyl-5-fluorouracil (HCFU) by oral administration. Cancer Treat Rep 64(8–9):861–867, 1980.
25. Koyama Y: Phase II study of a new fluorinated pyrimidine, 1-hexylcarbamoyl-5-fluorouracil (HCFU). Jpn J Cancer Chemother 7(7):1181–1190, 1980.
26. Horikomi K, Muramoto K, Araki K, et al.: Effect of 1-hexylcarbamoyl-5-fluorouracil (HCFU) and 1-ω-carboxypentylcarbamoyl-5-fluorouracil (CPEFU) on hypothalamic nervous in the rat. Rinshoyakuri 11(1):17–25, 1980.
27. Fujii S, Ikenaka K, Fukushima M, et al.: Effect of uracil and its derivatives on antitumor activity of 5-fluorouracil and 1-(2-tetrahydrofuryl)-5-fluorouracil. GANN 69(6):763–772, 1978.
28. Fujii S, Kitano K, Ikenaka T, et al.: Effect of coadministration of uracil or cytosine on the antitumor activity of clinical doses of 1-(2-tetrahydrofuryl)-5-fluorouracil and level of 5-fluorouracil in rodents. Gann 70(2):209–214, 1979.
29. Taguchi T, Furue H, Koyama Y, et al.: Phase I study of UFT (uracil plus futraful preparation). Jpn J Cancer Chemother 7(6):966–972, 1980.
30. Taguchi T, Nakano Y, Fujii S, et al.: Determination of 5-fluorouracil levels in tumors, blood and other tissues. Jpn J Cancer Chemother 5(6):69–74, 1978.
31. Kimura K, Suga S, Shimaji T, et al.: Clinical basis of chemotherapy for gastric cancer with uracil and 1-(2′-tetrahydrofuryl)-5-fluorouracil. Gastroenterogia Japonica 15(4):324–329, 1980.

32. Fukui Y, Imabayashi N, Nishi M, *et al.*: Clinical study on the enhancement of drug delivery into tumor tissue by using UFT. Jpn J Cancer Chemother 7(12):2124–2129, 1980.
33. Watanabe H, Yamamoto S, Naito T: Clinical results of oral UFT therapy under cooperative study. Jpn J Cancer Chemother 71(9):1588–1596, 1980.
34. Nakano Y, Taguchi T, Sakai K, *et al.*: Clinical phase II study of UFT by Cooperative Study Group. Jpn J Cancer Chemother 7(9):1569–1578, 1980.
35. Murakami M, Ota K: Clinical results of UFT therapy for malignant tumors under cooperative study (phase II study). Jpn J Cancer Chemother 7(9):1579–1586, 1980.
36. Takino T, Misawa S, Edagawa J, *et al.*: Clinical studies on the chemotherapy of advanced cancer with UFT (Uracil plus Futraful preparation). Jpn J Cancer Chemother 7(10):1804–1819, 1980.
37. Tamura Y, Okino M, Hongo H, *et al.*: Phase II study of UFT by collaborative study 8(2):302–307, 1981.
38. Majima H: Phase I and preliminary phase II study of co-administration of uracil and FT-207 (UFT Therapy). Jpn J Cancer Chemother 7(8):1383–1387, 1980.
39. Shirakawa S, Uehara N, Kita K, *et al.*: Clinical trial on the effect of UFT. Jpn J Cancer Chemother 8(1):101–105, 1981.
40. Yakeishi Y, Yoshida H, Yokota H, *et al.*: Clinical trial of UFT (Uracil-Futraful preparation) against malignant tumors. Jpn J Cancer Chemother 8(3):414–421, 1981.
41. Tominaga T, Kaneko T, Ito I: Clinical trial of UFT against advanced cancer. Jpn J Cancer Chemother 7(12):2119–2123, 1980.
42. Tosen T, Ando K, Ochiai M, *et al.*: Clinical trial on the effect of UFT. Jpn J Cancer Chemother 8(5):715–722, 1981.
43. Kunitomo K, Kuwashima T, Korematsu H, *et al.*: Clinical trial of UFT against recurrent or advanced carcinoma. Jpn J Cancer Chemother 9(1):72–78, 1982.
44. Kubo K, Ohshima N, Yamada H, *et al.*: Phase II study of 'UFT' in disseminated breast cancer. Jpn J Cancer Chemother 7(11):1971–1977, 1980.
45. Nakashima T, Matsumura Y, Nomura Y, *et al.*: Antitumor effect of UFT against malignant tumors of maxillary sinus – clinical and biochemical study – Jpn J Cancer Chemother 9(10):1729–1734, 1982.
46. Inuyama Y, Fujii M, Mashino S, *et al.*: Clinical effect of UFT therapy for head and neck cancer. Jpn J Cancer Chemother 10(1):90–96, 1983.
47. Wasserman TH, Comis RL, Goldsmith M, *et al.*: Tabular analysis of the clinical chemotherapy of solid tumors. Cancer Chemother. Rep Part 3 6(2):399–419, 1975.

6. DNA Modification by the Nitrosoureas: Chemical Nature and Cellular Repair

DAVID B. LUDLUM and WILLIAM P. TONG

1. INTRODUCTION

Compounds which react with DNA, and there are many, rank with our most effective antitumor agents. In fact, the use of nitrogen mustard and its derivatives introduced the era of effective cancer chemotherapy. Since that time, a wealth of information has accumulated about the interaction of antineoplastic agents with DNA, and certain basic hypotheses have been developed about their mechanism of action.

A major hypothesis relates the cytotoxicity of bifunctional alkylating agents to the formation of interstrand crosslinks in DNA. Evidence for crosslinking was obtained early in the investigation of alkylating agents and details of the crosslinking mechanism are now becoming available. It seems probable that differences in the nature of the crosslinks produced by different classes of DNA-modifying agents may underlie differences in the therapeutic activity of these compounds.

Following the discovery that methylnitronitrosoguanidine had activity against L1210 cells [1], other related compounds were synthesized and tested as antitumor agents at the Southern Research Institute [2]. It was noted that substitution of the methyl group by a haloethyl moiety greatly increases cytotoxicity and that haloethylnitrosoureas give a positive test for alkylating activity and react with DNA [3, 4].

We became interested in these reactions since it seemed likely that DNA modification by the haloethylnitrosoureas might be similar to modification by N-methyl-N-nitrosourea [5, 6] and different from modification by classical alkylating agents. It is now apparent that this supposition is correct and that, although haloethylnitrosoureas and nitrogen mustards both crosslink DNA, different mechanisms are involved.

In what follows, we will review the chemistry of DNA modification by the nitrosoureas and consider the role of cellular enzymes in either magnify-

F.M. Muggia (ed.), Experimental and Clinical Progress in Cancer Chemotherapy
© *1985, Martinus Nijhoff Publishers, Boston. ISBN 0-89838-679-9. Printed in the Netherlands.*

ing or repairing this damage. Since the presence or absence of cellular repair processes may play a role in determining the sensitivity of a particular cell line to cytotoxicity by the nitrosoureas, a deeper understanding of this process may ultimately contribute to the more effective use of this important class of compounds.

2. MODIFICATION OF DNA BY THE NITROSOUREAS

The DNA bases are readily modified by the haloethylnitrosoureas at the nucleoside, polynucleotide, and DNA level. However, the ready availability of polyribonucleotides led us to investigate the modification of these polymers first, thus identifying the most readily substituted bases. Substitution of the deoxyribonucleosides is similar, although the secondary structure of DNA and its organization into chromatin probably determine the extent of substitution at a particular base site in cellular DNA.

The first haloethylnitrosourea-modified nucleosides which were identified were 3-hydroxyethylcytidine and $3,N^4$-ethanocytidine [7]. Their structure clearly illustrates the transfer of a two-carbon fragment from BCNU to the base, and led to our suggestion that the initial step in DNA modification was substitution by a haloethyl group. This substituent could then react a second time to produce an intra- or interstrand crosslink [7, 8]. The haloethyl group would arise from the nitroso-bearing nitrogen in the haloethylnitrosourea structure so that a chloroethyl group would be transferred from BCNU (N,N'-bis[2-chloroethyl]-N-nitrosourea) and a fluoroethyl group from FCNU (N-[2-fluoroethyl]-N'-cyclohexyl-N-nitrosourea).

Most of the chloroethyl-substituted bases are evidently quite reactive and the only one which has actually been recovered from BCNU-treated DNA is 7-chloroethylguanine. The fluoroethyl derivatives are more stable and advantage of this fact has been taken to isolate and characterize several such nucleosides [9–12]. It was originally thought that hydroxyethyl nucleosides arose from the haloethyl nucleosides by simple hydrolysis, but the haloethyl nucleosides which have been isolated are relatively stable in aqueous solution. Thus, it appears that hydroxyethyl nucleosides arise from the interaction of a different reactive species with the nucleoside as described below.

As shown in Figure 1, derivatives of all the major DNA/RNA bases except thymine and uracil have been identified [13–15]. Mono-substituted bases bear haloethyl, hydroxyethyl, or aminoethyl groups, the latter arising from the chloroethylisocyanate generated from agents like BCNU which carry a chloroethyl group on their non-nitroso-bearing nitrogen [13].

Modified Bases

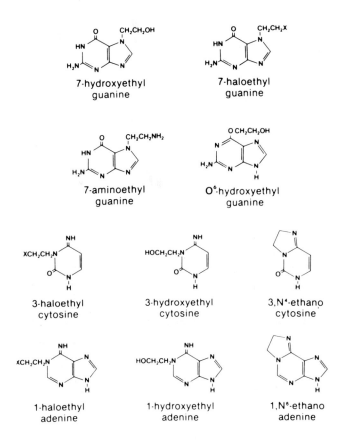

7-hydroxyethyl guanine

7-haloethyl guanine

7-aminoethyl guanine

O⁶-hydroxyethyl guanine

3-haloethyl cytosine

3-hydroxyethyl cytosine

3,N⁴-ethano cytosine

1-haloethyl adenine

1-hydroxyethyl adenine

1,N⁶-ethano adenine

Crosslinks

1-[N³-deoxycytidyl]. 2-[N¹-deoxyguanosinyl]-ethane

1,2-di-[N⁷-guanosinyl]-ethane

Figure 1. Structures of modified nucleosides and bases isolated from reactions of haloethylnitrosoureas with nucleic acids and nucleosides.

Of the modified bases shown in Figure 1, 7-hydroxyethylguanine has been found in the largest amounts. This and the other 7-substituted guanines represent modifications in the major groove of the DNA helix; the other monoadducts all represent substitution in base-pairing positions. Thus, the local structure of DNA is probably of great importance in determining the amount of DNA modification and may underlie differences in the sensitivity of cells at different stages in the cell cycle.

In line with the more extensive studies of nucleic acid modification by methylnitrosourea, it is to be anticipated that other derivatives will be identified which involve substitution at the other base nitrogens and oxygens. Furthermore, phosphate alkylation evidently occurs as shown by physical studies [16, 17] which are described in further detail below. Thus, additional studies are needed to complete the characterization of the DNA lesions produced by the nitrosoureas.

Although this review is concerned primarily with the biological significance of the nucleic acid derivatives, it is important to consider their origin since different nitrosoureas produce different distributions of products [18]. A general scheme for the generation of reactive intermediates is shown in Figure 2 [19–22]. Three chemically distinct routes labelled A, B, and C by Lown and Chauhan [19] seem to be involved. Decomposition through route B results in the formation of haloethyl nucleosides which probably cause interstrand crosslink formation [7, 8, 23, 24]. Hydroxyethyl derivatives evidently arise from decomposition via routes A and C, but both modes of decomposition could also lead to crosslink formation if the cyclic intermediates reacted in the correct sequence with neighboring nucleosides [25, 26]. As the significance of particular DNA modifications becomes more apparent, and as the distribution of lesions produced by the different nitrosoureas is elucidated, it may become possible to choose among the various nitrosoureas on this basis as well as on more classical grounds.

Most of the derivatives shown in Figure 1 are not yet available from commercial sources, but can be identified with moderate certainty in DNA hydrolysates from their chromatographic properties and ultraviolet spectra. Their structures were established originally on the basis of ultraviolet and mass spectrometry and, in most cases, by an unambiguous synthesis as described in the original papers cited above and in two previous reviews [25, 26].

Separation of the modified nucleosides and bases is readily achieved by high pressure liquid chromatography on C_{18} reverse phase columns using either acetonitrile-phosphate buffers or paired ion chromatography. The retention times of the modified nucleosides and bases actually isolated from BCNU-treated DNA are shown in Table 1. Further characterization of these derivatives is possible using the spectroscopic data contained in Table 2.

The most interesting structures isolated from BCNU-treated DNA are, of course, the crosslinked nucleosides shown at the bottom of Figure 1. We will consider the formation of the dCydCH$_2$CH$_2$dGuo crosslink (1-[N^3-deoxycytidyl],2-[N^1-deoxyguanosinyl]-ethane) in further detail below, but it is im-

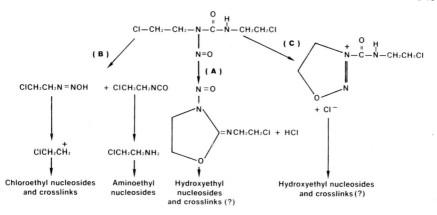

Figure 2. Proposed decomposition of BCNU and the formation of intermediates involved in the modification of nucleic acids.

portant to emphasize that it is an excellent candidate for an interstrand crosslink. It would involve the basepairing partners, cytosine and guanine, and once formed would be very difficult to repair. Thus, even if one of the altered bases were recognized and removed from a DNA strand, the other strand would still contain an altered base in the position across from it. Excision of that base would automatically result in a double-strand break.

Crosslinking cannot be the only factor involved in explaining the cytotoxicity of the nitrosoureas, however. The methylating nitrosoureas, methylnitrosourea and streptozotocin, are both effective in the treatment of certain solid tumors. The cytotoxicity of these agents is probably attributable to

Table 1. High pressure liquid chromatographic retention times for modified bases and nucleosides isolated from BCNU-treated DNA.

Compound	Retention time (min)*
7–(2–hydroxyethyl)guanine	9.1
7–(2–chloroethyl)guanine	35.7
7–(2–aminoethyl)guanine	5.9
O^6–(2–hydroxyethyl)guanine	22.3
3–(2–hydroxyethyl)deoxycytidine	7.1
3,N^4–ethanodeoxycytidine	8.3
1–(2–hydroxyethyl)deoxyadenosine	8.1
1,N^6–ethanodeoxyadenosine	12.8
1–(N^3-deoxycytidyl),2–(N^1-deoxyguanosinyl)–ethane	46.6
1,2–di(7–guanyl)ethane	29.5

* Separations on a Spherisorb ODS 5 μm (4.6 × 250 mm) column eluted isocratically with 50 mM KH_2PO_4, pH 4.5, containing 3% acetonitrile at a flow rate of 1 ml/min.

Table 2. Ultraviolet spectra of modified bases and nucleosides isolated from BCNU-treated DNA

Compound	Acid		pH 7		Base	
	max	min	max	min	max	min
7–(2–hydroxyethyl)guanine	250	228	284	260	280	257
			245	235		
7–(2–chloroethyl)guanine	250	230	284	260	280	257
			245	235		
7–(2–aminoethyl)guanine	250	230	284	260	280	257
			243	234		
O^6–(2–hydroxyethyl)guanine	288	257	282	258	284	260
			240	228		
3–(2–hydroxyethyl)deoxycytidine	280	249	274	245	266	245
3,N^4–ethanodeoxycytidine	285	243	284	250	279	254
1–(2–hydroxyethyl)deoxyadenosine	260	235	260	235	260	235
1,N^6–ethanodeoxyadenosine	261	239	267	240	267	239
1–(N^3–deoxycytidyl),2–(N^1–deoxygua-nosinyl)–ethane	278	237	275	234	259	237
	265 (s)		260 (s)			
1,2–di(7–guanyl)ethane	250	230	284	260	280	257
			245	235		

either depuration and strand scission, or to phosphate alkylation as described below.

Two extremely important features of DNA modification, crosslinking and strand scission, have been established by physical measurements on DNA exposed to the nitrosoureas. Kohn and his collaborators [23, 27–29] demonstrated that both fluoroethyl- and chloroethylnitrosoureas can produce interstrand crosslinks in DNA. Their studies utilized alkaline elution and gradient centrifugation techniques to show the existence of these crosslinks. These studies went further, however, and demonstrated that crosslink formation did indeed occur as a two-step reaction. Nucleic acids were exposed to haloethylnitrosoureas for a period of time which was presumably sufficient to allow the formation of reactive haloethyl nucleosides within one DNA strand. The DNA was then precipitated, washed free of unreacted nitrosoureas, and incubated a second time. The amount of interstrand crosslinking increased significantly over a matter of hours during the second incubation period with a half-life which seemed to be shorter for the chloroethyl- than for the fluoroethylnitrosoureas.

Lown and his co-workers [24, 30] obtained similar data with a somewhat different technique which also provided evidence for a two-step crosslinking reaction. DNA was incubated with the nitrosoureas, washed free of unreacted material, and reincubated as described above, but the amount of crosslinking was calculated from the amount of DNA renaturation which could be achieved after heat denaturation. Renaturation was determined in these experiments by measuring the fluorescence of intercalated ethidium bromide in the helical regions which reappeared in the renatured DNA.

DNA interstrand crosslink formation achieved biological significance when Kohn and his co-workers showed that the amount of interstrand crosslinking correlated with the sensitivity of a particular cell to the cytotoxic action of the nitrosoureas [31]. At the present time, it seems most likely that the interstrand crosslinks which are measured by these physical techniques are actually the dCydCH$_2$CH$_2$dGuo lesions described above.

Double-strand scission is another potentially important DNA lesion which has been demonstrated by physical methods [16, 17]. Since it is difficult to imagine a biological process which would lead to the repair of such a lesion, chain scission could also be responsible for cytotoxicity. Lown [17] has pointed out that phosphate esterification by the haloethylnitrosoureas would probably result in the formation of hydroxyethyl phosphates. These linkages would presumably constitute weak spots in the sugar phosphate backbone of DNA and could easily result in chain scission.

Of course, monoadduct formation could also be lethal. Not only do certain base modifications result in the transfer of incorrect genetic information, but many of the mono-substituted bases described above may be subject to chemical or enzymatic depurination which could lead to further genetic damage.

Thus, there are several possibilities for explaining the cytotoxicity of the nitrosoureas at a biochemical level. The problem is a challenging and fascinating one which is moving at a gratifying pace towards that goal of molecular pharmacologists – explaining the therapeutic action of a drug at a molecular level. If this goal can be reached, practical applications should follow quickly in determining and, perhaps, controlling the sensitivity of tumor cells to this group of antitumor agents.

3. CELLULAR REPAIR OF NITROSOUREA-MODIFIED DNA

The biological consequences of DNA damage depend not only on the nature of the original lesion, but also on cellular processes which repair or modify this damage further. Although it seems likely that repair would lead to resistance in most cases, error-prone repair could conceivably increase the cytotoxic action of the nitrosoureas.

Although relatively little is known about the repair of the specific lesions mentioned above, many of the mono-substituted bases are rather similar to the corresponding methyl and ethyl derivatives which have been studied in considerable detail. Accordingly, we can be guided by a knowledge of the repair of these lesions, and the reader is referred to the many excellent reviews in this area [32–39].

Table 3 lists some of the repair processes which are almost certainly involved in protecting cells from the cytotoxic action of the nitrosoureas. The first process, postreplication repair, is potentially error-prone, but can protect the cells from a wide variety of lesions by using genetic information from an undamaged stretch of DNA. Evidence for its involvement in protecting bacteria from the lethal action of the nitrosoureas is mentioned below.

Based on what is known about the repair of DNA damage induced by other chemical agents, several enzymes involved in excision repair are probably also active in the repair of nitrosourea-damaged DNA. The uvr endonuclease system apparently recognizes distortions in the DNA structure, and we have obtained some preliminary data which suggest that it provides protection against the lethal action of the nitrosoureas, perhaps by excising crosslinks [40]. DNA glycosylases have been described which remove 7-substituted guanines and the ring-opened products which can be generated from them. Such enzymes might recognize 7-hydroxyethylguanine, 7-haloethylguanine, or 7-aminoethylguanine. Similarly, glycosylases which recognize 3-methyladenine or related enzymes might release 3-hydroxyethyladenine from nitrosourea-damaged DNA.

All of these glycosylases as well as chemical depurinations would leave apurinic sites in DNA. AP endonucleases would be important in repairing these lesions, and their absence would confer special sensitivity on a cell line which failed to contain them. Finally, and of great current interest, a correlation has been established between sensitivity to the nitrosoureas and the

Table 3. Cellular repair processes for nitrosourea-induced DNA lesions

Repair process	DNA lesion recognized
Postreplication repair	Probably diverse
Excision repair	
uvr$^+$ endonucleases	Crosslinks and/or helical distortions
DNA glycosylases	7-Substituted guanines; ring-opened 7-substituted guanines; 3-substituted adenines
AP endonucleases	Depurinated sites
Transferase repair	O^6-alkylguanines

presence or absence of enzymes capable of removing methyl groups from the 6 position of guanine [41].

The relationship between cytotoxicity and repair can be studied with precision in bacterial systems because mutants are available which are deficient in specific repair processes. Tashima *et al.* [42] investigated the cytotoxicity of BCNU to four strains of *Escherichia coli* with normal or defective excision or recombination repair. Strains lacking recombination repair were particularly sensitive to the nitrosoureas while a double mutant which lacked both the uvr-A and rec-A genes seemed to be even more sensitive than the corresponding uvr-A$^+$ rec-A$^-$ strain. As mentioned above, the importance of the uvr-A gene has been confirmed by Kacinski *et al.* [40].

Just as previous work with methylnitrosourea has contributed to the understanding of the biochemistry of DNA modification by the haloethylnitrosoureas, studies of methylnitrosourea-induced mutagenesis and carcinogenesis have contributed to our knowledge of relevant repair processes. Ever since Loveless suggested that alkylation of guanine in the 6 position contributes to mutagenesis and carcinogenesis by methylnitrosourea [43], data have accumulated which support this proposal. Repair of this lesion has been described in both bacterial and eucaryotic cells [44–47]. Those cells which are capable of removing the methyl group from the O^6 position of guanine are described as MER$^+$ and are, in general, more resistant to mutation.

Possession of this trait in human tumor cell lines has been shown to correlate with resistance to the *in vitro* cytotoxicity of the haloethylnitrosoureas [29, 41]. Such MER$^+$ cells also show a decrease in DNA interstrand crosslink formation. These correlations have been attributed to the ability of a MER$^+$ strain to remove a haloethyl group from the 6 position of guanine before it could react a second time to form an interstrand crosslink [29, 41].

Although methyl- and ethylnitrosourea cause substitution in the 6 position of guanine, formation of O^6-haloethylguanine by the haloethylnitrosoureas has not been described until very recently [12] and a crosslink involving this position has not yet been detected at all. Thus, it has not been clear at a biochemical level what crosslink formation could be prevented in MER$^+$ cells. However, it has recently been shown that O^6-fluoroethylguanosine hydrolyzes to N^1-hydroxyethylguanosine [16], and this observation supports the proposal that the dCydCH$_2$CH$_2$dGuo crosslink results from an initial attack on the 6 position of guanine [15].

This route to crosslink formation is shown in Figure 3 which, at the same time, illustrates the role that O^6-alkylguanine transferase might play in preventing crosslink formation. The left-hand side of the figure shows the proposed route to BCNU crosslinking in cells which are repair-deficient, i.e.,

Proposed Crosslinking and Repair Mechanisms

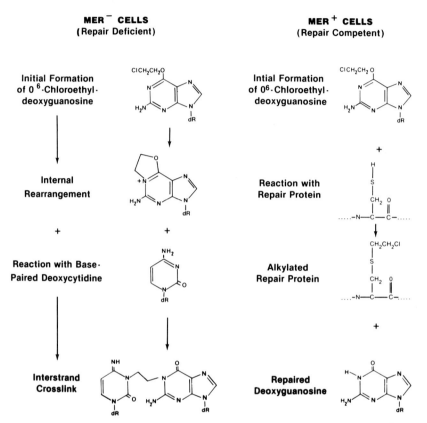

Figure 3. Proposed mechanism leading to the formation of the DNA crosslink, 1-(N³-deoxycytidyl),2-(N¹-deoxyguanosinyl)-ethane, and the role of O⁶-alkylguanine transferase in preventing crosslink formation.

lack the MER⁺ trait. Initial attack of a chloroethyl carbonium ion on the 6 position of deoxyguanosine would lead to O⁶-chloroethyldeoxyguanosine as shown in the upper left corner of this figure. An internal rearrangement would then lead to the reactive intermediate, N¹,O⁶-ethanodeoxyguanosine which would then react with its base-pairing partner, deoxycytidine, to form dCydCH₂CH₂dGuo. As mentioned above, this route to crosslink formation is supported by evidence which shows that O⁶-fluoroethylguanine is formed in DNA and that O⁶-fluoroethylguanosine rearranges and hydrolyzes to N¹-hydroxyethylguanosine [12].

This proposal would also explain the role of O⁶-alkyl transferase in preventing crosslink formation. Since the O^6-alkylguanine transferase system in MER$^+$ strains has been shown to transfer methyl [48, 49] or ethyl [50, 51] groups from DNA to a cysteine moiety, this same or a related transferase activity could probably transfer the O^6-chloroethylguanine group to the repair protein. This would lead to the formation of chloroethylcysteine and the restoration of deoxyguanosine to its original unmodified condition. Assuming that the dCydCH$_2$CH$_2$dGuo crosslink is responsible for at least some of the cytotoxic action of the haloethylnitrosoureas, this would explain the resistance of cell lines which possess the MER$^+$ trait.

4. SUMMARY

In summary, then, the haloethylnitrosoureas modify DNA extensively, attaching haloethyl, hydroxyethyl, and in the case of BCNU, aminoethyl groups to the nitrogens and oxygens of the DNA bases. Phosphate alkylation and interstrand crosslink formation have also been demonstrated by physical chemical techniques. These studies have shown that interstrand crosslink formation correlates with cytotoxicity.

Interstrand crosslink formation evidently occurs as a two-step reaction in which a haloethyl group is transferred to a base in one strand of DNA and then reacts a second time with the opposite strand of DNA. The interstrand crosslink itself probably has the structure, 1-(N^3-deoxycytidyl),2-(N^1-deoxyguanosinyl)-ethane, or dCydCH$_2$CH$_2$dGuo. This structure consists of a two-carbon bridge between the N^1 position of deoxycytidine and the N^3 position of its base-pairing partner, deoxyguanosine. Formation of this crosslink probably involves, as a first step, alkylation of the 6 position of deoxyguanosine by a haloethyl group. Removal of this group by O^6-alkylguanine transferase could then prevent the secondary reactions which lead to crosslink formation, explaining the increased resistance of cell lines which contain the MER$^+$ trait. Other repair mechanisms are probably also important in affecting the resistance of cells to the cytotoxic action of the haloethylnitrosoureas by modifying or repairing other DNA lesions.

ACKNOWLEDGEMENTS

The authors would like to acknowledge the scientific contributions of their associates, particularly Barnett S. Kramer and Charles T. Gombar. We are also indebted to Suzanne Wissel for editorial assistance and to Santas Seitz for technical assistance. This research was supported by grant CA 32171 from the National Cancer Institute, DHEW.

REFERENCES

1. Greene MO, Greenberg J: The activity of nitrosoguanidines against ascites tumors in mice. Cancer Res 20:1166–1171, 1960.

2. Montgomery JA: The development of the nitrosoureas: A study in congener synthesis. In: Prestayko AW, Crooke ST, Baker LH, Carter SK, Schein PS (eds), Nitrosoureas: Current status and new developments, New York, Academic Press, 1981, p 3–8.

3. Wheeler DG, Chumley S: Alkylating activity of 1,3-bis-(2-chloroethyl)-1-nitrosourea and related compounds. J Med Chem 10:259–261, 1967.

4. Cheng CJ, Fujimura S, Grunberger D, Weinstein IB: Interaction of 1-(2-chloroethyl)-3-cyclohexyl-1-nitrosourea (NSC 79037) with nucleic acids and proteins *in vivo* and *in vitro*. Cancer Res 32:22–27, 1972.

5. Singer B: The chemical effects of nucleic acid alkylation and their relation to mutagenesis and carcinogenesis. Prog Nucleic Acid Res Mol Biol 15:219–284, 330–332, 1975.

6. Lawley PD, Orr DJ, Jarman M: Isolation and identification of products from alkylation of nucleic acids: ethyl- and isopropyl-purines. Biochem J 145:73–84, 1975.

7. Kramer BS, Fenselau CC, Ludlum DB: Reaction of BCNU (1,3-bis[2-chloroethyl]-1-nitrosourea) with polycytidylic acid. Substitution of the cytosine ring. Biochem Biophys Res Commun 56:783–788, 1974.

8. Ludlum DB, Kramer BS, Wang J, Fenselau C: Reaction of 1,3-bis-(2-choroethyl)-1-nitrosourea with synthetic polynucleotides. Biochemistry 14:5480–5485, 1975.

9. Tong WP, Ludlum DB: Mechanism of action of the nitrosoureas I. Role of fluoroethyl cytidine in the reaction of BFNU with nucleic acids. Biochem Pharmacol 27:77–81, 1978.

10. Ludlum DB, Tong WP: Mechanism of action of the nitrosoureas II. Formation of fluoro-ethylguanosine from the reaction of BFNU and guanosine. Biochem Pharmacol 27:2391–2394, 1978.

11. Tong WP, Ludlum DB: Mechanism of action of the nitrosoureas III. Reaction of bis-chloroethyl nitrosourea and bis-fluoroethyl nitrosourea with adenosine. Biochem Pharmacol 28:1175–1179, 1979.

12. Tong WP, Kirk MC, Ludlum DB: Mechanism of action of the nitrosoureas V. The formation of O^6-(2-fluoroethyl)guanine and its probable role in the crosslinking of deoxyribonucleic acid. Biochem Pharmacol 32:2011–2015, 1983.

13. Gombar CT, Tong WP, Ludlum DB: Mechanism of action of the nitrosoureas IV. Reactions of BCNU and CCNU with DNA. Biochem Pharmacol 29:2639–2643, 1980.

14. Tong WP, Ludlum DB: Formation of the cross-linked base, diguanylethane, in DNA treated with N,N^1-bis(2-chloroethyl)-N-nitrosourea. Cancer Res 41:380–382, 1981.

15. Tong WP, Kirk MC, Ludlum DB: Formation of the crosslink, 1-[N^3-deoxycytidyl],2-[N^1-deoxyguanosinyl]-ethane, in DNA treated with N,N'-bis(2-chloroethyl)-N-nitrosourea (BCNU). Cancer Res 42:3102–3105, 1982.

16. Erickson LC, Bradley MO, Kohn KW: Strand breaks in DNA from normal and transformed human cells treated with 1,3-bis(2-chloroethyl)-1-nitrosourea. Cancer Res 37:3744–3750, 1977.

17. Lown JW, McLaughlin LW: Nitrosourea-induced DNA single-strand breaks. Biochem Pharmacol 28:1631–1638, 1979.

18. Tong WP, Kohn KW, Ludlum DB: Modifications of DNA by different haloethylnitroso-ureas. Cancer Res 42:4460–4464, 1982.

19. Lown JW, Chauhan SMS: Mechanism of action of (2-haloethyl)nitrosoureas on DNA. Isolation and reactions of postulated 2-(alkylimino)-3-nitrosooxazolidine intermediates in the decomposition of 1,3-bis(2-chloroethyl)-3-(4'-trans-methylcyclohexyl)-1-nitrosourea. J Med Chem 24:270–279, 1981.

20. Montgomery JA: The chemistry of the nitrosoureas. In: Serrou B, Schein PS, Imbach J-L (eds), Nitrosoureas in cancer treatment, Amsterdam, Elsevier, 1981, pp 13–20.
21. Colvin M, Brundrett RB, Cowens W, Jardine I, Ludlum DB: A chemical basis for the antitumor activity of chloroethylnitrosoureas. Biochem Pharmacol 25:695–699, 1976.
22. Reed DJ: Metabolism of nitrosoureas. In: Prestayko AW, Crooke ST, Baker LH, Carter SK, Schein PS (eds), Nitrosoureas: Current status and new developments, New York, Academic Press, 1981, pp 51–67.
23. Kohn KW: Interstrand cross-linking of DNA by 1,3-bis(2-chloroethyl)-1-nitrosourea and other 1-(2-haloethyl)-1-nitrosoureas. Cancer Res 37:1450–1454, 1977.
24. Lown JW, McLaughlin LW, Chang Y-M: Mechanism of action of 2-haloethylnitrosoureas on DNA and its relation to their antileukemic properties. Bioorg Chem 7:97–110, 1978.
25. Ludlum DB, Tong WP: Modification of DNA and RNA bases. In: Prestayko AW, Crooke ST, Baker LH, Carter SK, Schein PS (eds), Nitrosoureas: Current status and new developments, New York, Academic Press, 1981, pp 85–94.
26. Ludlum DB, Tong WP: Modification of DNA and RNA bases by the nitrosoureas. In: Serrou B, Schein PS, Imbach J-L (eds), Nitrosoureas in cancer treatment, Amsterdam, Elsevier, 1981, pp 21–31.
27. Ewig RAG, Kohn KW: DNA damage and repair in mouse leukemia L1210 cells treated with nitrogen mustard, 1,1-bis(2-chloroethyl)-1-nitrosourea, and other nitrosoureas. Cancer Res 37:2114–2122, 1977.
28. Kohn KW, Erickson LC, Laurent G, Ducore J, Sharkey N, Ewig RA: DNA crosslinking and the origin of sensitivity to chloroethylnitrosoureas. In: Prestayko AW, Crooke ST, Baker LH, Carter SK, Schein PS (eds), Nitrosoureas: Current status and new developments, New York, Academic Press, 1981, pp 69–83.
29. Kohn KW, Erickson LC, Laurent G: DNA alkylation, crosslinking and repair. In: Serrou B, Schein PS, Imbach J-L (eds), Nitrosoureas in cancer treatment, Amsterdam, Elsevier, 1981, pp 33–48.
30. Lown JW, McLaughlin LW: Mechanism of action of 2-haloethylnitrosoureas on deoxyribonucleic acid. Nature of the chemical reaction with deoxyribonucleic acid. Biochem Pharmacol 28:2123–2128, 1979.
31. Thomas CB, Osieka R, Kohn KW: DNA cross-linking by *in vivo* treatment with 1-(2-chloroethyl)-3-(4-methylcyclohexyl)-1-nitrosourea of sensitive and resistant human colon carcinoma xenografts in nude mice. Cancer Res 38:2448–2454, 1978.
32. Strauss BS: DNA repair mechanisms and their relation to mutation and recombination. In: Arber W, Braun W, Cramer F, Haas R, Henie W, Hofschneider PH, Jerne NK, Koldovsky P, Koprowski H, Maaloe O, Rott R, Schweiger HG, Sela M, Syrucek L, Vogt PK, Wecker E (eds), Current topics in microbiology and immunology, Vol 44, New York, Springer-Verlag, 1968, pp 1–89.
33. Roberts JJ: The repair of DNA modified by cytotoxic, mutagenic, and carcinogenic chemicals. In: Lett JT, Adler H (eds), Advances in radiation biology, New York, Academic Press, 1978, pp 211–436.
34. Hanawalt PC, Cooper PK, Ganesan AK, Smith CA: DNA repair in bacteria and mammalian cells. Ann Rev Biochem 48:783–836, 1979.
35. Laval J, Laval F: Enzymology of DNA repair. In: Montesano R, Bartsch H, Tomatis L (eds), Molecular and cellular aspects of carcinogen screening tests, Lyon, IARC Scientific Publications No 27, 1980, pp 55–73.
36. Pegg AE: Formation and metabolism of alkylated nucleosides: Possible role in carcinogenesis by nitroso compounds and alkylating agents. Adv Cancer Res 25:195–269, 1977.
37. Verly WG: Prereplicative error-free DNA repair. Biochem Pharmacol 29:977–982, 1980.
38. Grossman L: Enzymes involved in the repair of damaged DNA. Arch Biochem Biophys 211:511–522, 1981.

154

39. Lindahl T: DNA repair enzymes. Ann Rev Biochem 51:61–87, 1982.
40. Kacinski B, Rupp WD, Ludlum DB: unpublished data.
41. Erickson LC, Laurent G, Sharkey NA, Kohn KW: DNA cross-linking and monoadduct repair in nitrosourea-treated human tumour cells. Nature 288:727–729, 1980.
42. Tashima M, Sawada H, Uchino H, Nishioka H: Effect of 1,3-bis(2-chloroethyl)-1-nitrosourea on Escherichia coli DNA repair system. Gann 69:695–698, 1978.
43. Loveless A: Possible relevance of O-6 alkylation of deoxyguanosine to the mutagenicity and carcinogenicity of nitrosamines and nitrosamides . Nature 223:206–207, 1969.
44. Schendel PF, Robins PE: Repair of O^6-methylguanine in adapted Echerichia coli. Proc Natl Acad Sci USA 75:6017–6020, 1978.
45. Robins P, Cairns J: Quantitation of the adaptive response to alkylating agents. Nature 280:74–76, 1979.
46. Karran P, Lindahl T: Adaptive response to alkylating agents involves alteration *in situ* of O^6-methylguanine residues in DNA. Nature 280:76–77, 1979.
47. Pegg AE, Hui G: Formation and subsequent removal of O^6-methylguanine from DNA in rat liver and kidney after small doses of dimethylnitrosamine. Biochem J 173:739–748, 1978.
48. Olsson M, Lindahl T: Repair of alkylated DNA in Escherichia coli. Methyl group transfer from O^6-methylguanine to a protein cysteine residue. J Biol Chem 255:10569–10571, 1980.
49. Bogden JM, Eastman A, Bresnick E: A system in mouse liver for the repair of O^6-methylguanine lesions in methylated DNA. Nucleic acids Res 9:3089–3102, 1981.
50. Renard A, Verly WG, Mehta JR, Ludlum DB: Repair of O^6-ethylguanine in DNA by a chromatin factor from rat liver. Fed Proc 40:1763, 1981.
51. Mehta JR, Ludlum DB, Renard A, Verly WG: Repair of O^6-ethylguanine in DNA by a chromatin fraction from rat liver: Transfer of the ethyl group to an acceptor protein. Proc Natl Acad Sci USA 78:6766–6770, 1981.

7. Thymidylate Synthetase Inhibitors: Experimental and Clinical Aspects

ANN L. JACKMAN, TERENCE R. JONES and A. HILARY CALVERT

1. INTRODUCTION

The enzyme thymidylate synthetase (TS) which accomplishes the methylation of deoxyuridine monophosphate to thymidine monophosphate has been of interest ever since its discovery in 1957 [1]. Its crucial role in the synthesis of the only nucleotide required exclusively for DNA synthesis makes it an obvious target for antimetabolite attack. The discovery by Cohen [2] that 5-fluorodeoxyuridine monophosphate (FdUMP), a metabolite of the antipyrimidines 5-fluorouracil and 5-fluorodeoxyuridine, was a potent inhibitor of TS, coupled with the documentation of clinical antitumour activity for this drug ensured the continuing studies both of TS and antipyrimidines. The detailed and painstaking studies of the nature of the tight binding of FdUMP to TS in the presence of the cofactor $5,10\text{-}CH_2FH_4$, to produce a stable ternary complex have given us enormous insights into the mechanism of TS catalysis and have allowed the rational design of further TS-inhibitory uracil derivatives. The inhibition of TS by FdUMP was accepted for many years as the main basis for the cytotoxicity of the fluorinated pyrimidines, and only recently have the incorporations of these molecules into nucleic acids been fully considered as alternative or contributory cytotoxic events. The knowledge that FU has cytotoxic actions unrelated to TS inhibition implies that an inhibition of TS *uncomplicated by other actions* has not been evaluated as an antitumour event. Both this observation and a critical appraisal of antifolate design have led to increasing interest in TS as a locus for folate analogues. The present range of antifolate drugs are, for historical reasons, all DHFR inhibitors. Although the prototype antifolate, aminopterin, entered the clinic [3] nine years before DHFR was even discovered [4], at the time it was synthesised it was rationally designed, stemming from an application of the Fildes-Woods theory of antimetabolites [5]. Apart from their usage as drugs, aminopterin and the

F.M. Muggia (ed.), Experimental and Clinical Progress in Cancer Chemotherapy
© *1985, Martinus Nijhoff Publishers, Boston. ISBN 0-89838-679-9. Printed in the Netherlands.*

closely related methotrexate have helped in elucidating folate biochemistry. Some sixteen folate enzymes have since been discovered and their interlocking metabolic functions described [6]. This knowledge highlights TS as a locus for a new antifolate. Thus investigations of and attempts to improve upon the long established drugs FU and methotrexate started separately but in recent years have converged to bring TS firmly into focus. In this review we concentrate upon the efforts made in recent years to inhibit TS by a folate analogue, and attempt to discover whether such an analogue will indeed offer therapeutic advantages over methotrexate or FU.

ABBREVIATIONS AND CONVENTIONS

TS	Thymidylate synthetase (EC 2.1.1.45)
DHFR	Dihydrofolate reductase (EC 1.5.1.4)
FPGS	Folyl polyglutamate synthetase
FH_2	7,8-dihydrofolate
FH_4	5,6,7,8-tetrahydrofolate
$5,10\text{-}CH_2FH_4$	5,10-methylenetetrahydrofolate
dUMP	Deoxyuridylic acid
TMP	Thymidylic acid
TdR	Thymidine
FU	5-Fluorouracil
FUR	5-Fluorouridine
FUTP	5-Fluorouridinetriphosphate
FUdR	5-Fluorodeoxyuridine
FdUMP	5-Fluorodeoxyuridylic acid
FdUTP	5-Fluorodeoxyuridine triphosphate
PRPP	5-phosphoribosyl pyrophosphate
dRP	5-phosphodeoxyribosyl
Glu	L-glutamic acid
Tosyl	p-toluenesulphonyl

When refering to polyglutamates, the number given signifies the *total* number of glutamic acid residues present in the molecule.

For the convenience of keeping the number of formulae within limits, certain of the folate analogues are shown to have a 4-hydroxy group. It must be understood that such molecules normally exist as the lactam tautomer in which the oxygen is a doubly-bonded carbonyl oxygen. Other of the formulae make this clear.

2. CATALYTIC MECHANISM

2.1 *Molecular*

The elegant and painstaking studies which have led to our present understanding of the mechanism of TS catalysis have been well reviewed [7–13] and these articles should provide the reader with the historical development of this subject. The currently accepted theory of the mechanism is therefore reviewed here only in outline.

It has been established that dUMP (I) binds first to the enzyme and that a dissociated cysteine sulphydryl group of the enzyme then adds covalently to position 6 of the pyrimidine ring to produce a binary complex (II) (Scheme). This complex is an enolate anion intermediate with charge delocalised between the 4-oxo and 5-methine groups (scheme 1). The carbon atom at 5 is thus made highly nucleophilic and primed for alkylation by the electrophilic methylene group of the cosubstrate, 5,10-methylenetetrahydrofolate (III). The alkylating species is probably not the 5,10-methylene compound *per se* with its unreactive sp^3-hybridised carbon atom but a derived iminium ion at N^5 or N^{10} with a more reactive sp^2 carbon [14]. What evidence there is (15) supports the idea that protonation occurs at N^{10} with opening of the imidazolinone ring to give the 5-iminium ion (IV) and not *vice versa*. Alkylation produces the ternary complex (V) and completes the first stage of events within the active site. The second stage of catalysis is the reduction of the attached methylene group to form the thymine methyl group. In this process the hydrogen at C^5 of the pyrimidine ring is cleaved and lost (loss as tritium forms the basis of several TS radioassays) and the hydrogen at C^6 of the pteridine is transferred in its entirety [16, 17] and stereospecifically [18, 19] to give dihydrofolate (VI) and thymidylate (VII) with regeneration of the cysteine sulphydryl group. The mechanism of this reduction and concomitant fragmentation to products is unknown. Product release is ordered with FH$_2$ released before thymidylate.

As earlier alluded to, FdUMP is so close an analogue of dUMP that it can undergo the enzymic reactions leading to its incorporation into a FdUMP-5,10-CH$_2$FH$_4$-TS ternary complex analogous to (V). This complex is stable and can be considered as an analogue of the intermediate which occurs in the natural reaction. For FdUMP to progress further along the catalytic pathway would require the cleavage of the C^5-F bond, a process which does not occur, probably because the fluorine atom cannot depart carrying a positive charge in the presumed manner that the hydrogen atom departs in the natural reaction. Since FdUMP inactivates TS by taking part in the catalytic sequence it qualifies for description as a suicide or K$_{cat}$ inhibitor. FdUMP has proved a useful tool in elucidating the first stage of TS catalysis leading up to the formation of the ternary complex (V). Since the complex

158

incorporating FdUMP does not breakdown to give products little is known of the late stages of TS catalysis and this presents a major research challenge still.

2.2 *Kinetic*

In most cases the Km value for the cosubstrate $5,10\text{-}CH_2FH_4$ (III) has been determined using a mixture of diastereoisomers about the C^6 chiral centre: (d,l)- or ($\pm$)-L-$5,10\text{-}CH_2FH_4$. Such Km values fell in the range 14–45 μM (*D. pneumoniae* excepted) usually settling around 30 μM (Table 1). Only one component of this mixture is functional in the assay, this being the

Table 1. Sources and properties of bacterial, avian, viral and mammalian thymidylate synthetase ranging in purity

Source	Affinity Ligand, if so purified	Km (µM) dUMP	Km (µM) $5,10\text{-}CH_2\text{-}FH_4$ [a]	Dimer M. Wt. (Daltons)	Ref.
Calf thymus		20	38–45		83
Calf thymus		9.0	—	77,500	84
Calf thymus	N^{α}-[pteroyltetra(γ-glutamyl)]lysine–sepharose	—	—	70,000 [b]	85
Chick embryo		7.5	14	58,000	28
L. Casei resistant to dichloromethotrexate		5.2	45	67,000 [c]	21
L.Casei resistant to MTX		5.1 [d]	32	70,000 [e]	29
L. Casei resistant to MTX	5-fluoro-2'-deoxyuridine 5'-(4-aminophenylphosphate)	17 [f]	—		86 [g]
L. Casei resistant to MTX	deoxyuridylic acid	—	—	—	87 [h]
L. Casei					88 [i]
L. Casei resistant to MTX		0.7	14.0 [j]		34
L. Casei resistant to MTX	N^{α}-[pteroyltetra(γ-glutamyl)]–lysine sepharose				89
L. Casei	N^{α}-[pteroyltetra(γ-glutamyl)]lysine & N-[5,8–dideaza pteroyl)lysine				90
Ehrlich ascites		6.3	43	67,000 [b]	91
Ehrlich ascites	10-formyl-5,8-dideazafolic acid	1.3	32.2	78,500	92
Ehrlich ascites [k] resistant to FUdR	10-formyl-5,8-dideazafolic acid	1.6	39.3	68,300 [l]	93
Pig thymus form I		1.0	17 [j]		30
form II		7.4	17 [j]		
T4-phage		—	—	58,000	94
T5-phage		—	—	55,000	
T2-phage		6	20	64,400	95
D. Pneumoniae		30.8	266	36,000 [m]	73
E. Coli and Bombyx mori	tetrahydromethotrexate	—	—		96
Human Leukemic cells	methotrexate	1.8	31	76,000	35

Table 1. (Continued)

Source	Affinity Ligand, if so purified	Km (µM)		Dimer M. Wt. (Daltons)	Ref.
		dUMP	$5,10\text{--}CH_2\text{--}FH_4$ [a]		
B. Subtilis					
— Thy A gene		4			97
— Thy B gene		20			
E. Coli K12		10	14 [j]	64,000	32
E. Coli K12	10–formyl–5,8–dideazafolic acid	–	–	59,000 [n]	98
L1210 mouse leukaemia	10–formyl–5,8–dideazafolic acid			75,000	99
L1210 mouse leukaemia	10–formylfolic acid			76,000	100
L1210 mouse leukaemia	10–ethyl–5,8–dideazafolic acid	0.77	17 [o]		81
CCRF CEM human lympho-blastoid leukaemia	tetrahydromethotrexate	2.7 [p]		66,000	101
…/resistant to FUdR	methotrexate	0.90			102
HeLa cells	10–formyl–5,8–dideazafolic acid	2.0	31	73,000	103
Mouse Liver	10–methyl–5,8–didezazafolic acid				104
T4-phage	10–formyl–5,8–dideazofolic acid			64,000 [q]	105
S. Faecium resistant to MTX	N^α-[pteroyltetra(γ-glutamyl)]–lysine sepharose	8.2	30	72,000 [r]	106

[a] For($\pm$) or (d,1)–(L) $5,10\text{--}CH_2FH_4$ unless otherwise stated.
[b] Attempts to dissociate the protein into monomers failed.
[c] Later obtained crystalline (107).
[d] In the presence of Mg^{++}; 0.68 uM in its absence.
[e] Obtained crystalline. See also refs 108 and 109.
[f] Determined in phosphate buffer pH 7.2.
[g] See also ref. 110.
[h] See also ref. 111.
[i] Crystalline.
[j] (1)–(L)–$5,10\text{--}CH_2FH_4$ was used.
[k] Binds FdUMP with tenfold lower affinity.
[l] 58,300 given in paper—seemingly a printer's error.
[m] The catalytically active monomer.
[n] Obtained by genetic manipulation; the gene and its product were later sequenced (112).
[o] Obtained by halving the observed Km, found using ($\pm$)–(L)–$5,10\text{--}CH_2FH_4$.
[p] Datum from the following entry in the table.
[q] Obtained by genetic manipulation.
[r] Has RNA associated which copurifies.

natural diastereoisomer designated (1)- or (+)-L-5,10-CH$_2$FH$_4$. The unnatural diastereoisomer should *not* be assumed to be an inert ingredient. For example although not a co-substrate for *L. casei* enzyme it is an inhibitor (Ki 50 μM) binding nearly as strongly as the natural co-substrate (Km 15 μM) [20]. In a few cases the Km was determined using the pure natural diastereoisomer obtained by enzymatic reduction of dihydrofolate. The values ranged from 14 to 17 μM.

Few alternative cosubstrates are known, one being 5,11-methylenetetrahydrohomofolate (IX), the presumed reaction product of tetrahydrohomofo-

VIII   IX

late (VIII) with formaldehyde (see below). This, having an extra methylene group in the bridge, incorporates a six-membered cyclic aminal. With varying lower efficacy it serves as cosubstrate for TS from *L. Casei* [21], mouse erythrocyte [22], L1210 leukaemia cells [23], Chinese hamster ovary cells [24], and HeLa cells [24]. However, this molecule functions to inhibit TS from other sources as is noted below. Other cosubstrates for TS (*E. Coli*) are some analogues of 5,10-CH$_2$-FH$_4$ bearing amino acids other than L-glutamate. The dicarboxylic aspartate, alpha-aminoadipate and alpha-aminopimelate analogues showed activity approaching that of the natural cosubstrate [25]. So too did the lysine analogue [25] – this was as much a surprise as the later discovery [26] that tetrahydropteroyl-polylysines containing up to five residues and carrying net positive charges were also good substrates for this particular synthetase. It might here be mentioned that the separated diastereoisomers of 5,10-CH$_2$-pteroyl-D-glutamate were found inactive for *L. Casei* TS either as substrates or inhibitors [27].

The Km values for dUMP are reported to fall within the range 1–10 μM (Table 1). Thymidylate synthetase is highly specific for the pyrimidine substrate dUMP, few others are known: (1) The methylation of uridine-5'-phosphate (UMP) has been the subject of three reports. Enzyme from chick embryo accomplished this reaction though the Km was 100–1000 fold higher than that for dUMP [28]. Similar results were found with *L. Casei* enzyme [29], and with pig thymus enzyme, the latter the less efficient [30]. (2) 4-thio-dUMP weakly competed (Ki 70 μM) with dUMP (Km 5 μM) for methylation by *L. Casei* TS [31]. (3) 2'-fluoro-dUMP was methylated by the

E. Coli K12 enzyme. The Km for this analogue was 110 µM while that for dUMP was 10 µM [32].

The kinetics and mechanism of the interaction of 5FdUMP with TS has been an area of much confusion and debate. The observation that FdUMP was a weak inhibitor, competitive with dUMP, when both nucleotides were added simultaneously but a tight binding non-competitive inhibitor when FdUMP and the co-substrate were preincubated with the enzyme before the addition of dUMP is no longer a puzzle. Four papers in a short space of time were instrumental in clarifying matters. Galivan, Maley and Maley [33] used equilibrium dialysis to show that dUMP, dTMP and FdUMP competed for the same binding site and that the deoxynucleotide bound first which then allowed subsequent binding of the cosubstrate. The enzyme bound dUMP (Kd = 1.80 µM) some twentyfold more strongly than FdUMP (Kd = 37.2 µM) and these bindings were reversible in the absence of folate. Two careful kinetic studies with bacterial [34] and human enzyme [35] next showed that the mechanism was ordered sequential with dUMP binding before the cosubstrate and FH_2 being released before TMP. Danenberg and Danenberg [36] used competitive ligand binding techniques allied with classical enzyme kinetics to elucidate the order and the extent of ligand binding to bacterial TS. An important first observation was that although the TS-FdUMP-5,10-CH_2FH_4 ternary complex formed rapidly with concomitant enzyme inactivation, a slow enzyme-catalysed reversal of the complex occurred. (Denaturation of the complex removes this capability for reverse catalysis and allows the isolation of a protein with the two ligands covalently bound [37]). The first observation explained the second – that incubation of the inhibitory ternary complex with an excess of dUMP enabled recovery of the enzyme activity. However, the rate of recovery was independent of dUMP concentration, implying a first-order dissociation of FdUMP from the complex. FdUMP dissociation was suppressed by increasing concentration of the cosubstrate in a linear relationship ($t_{1/2}$ ca. 1 hr at a cosubstrate concentration of 100 µM). Conversely, the dissocation of the labelled cofactor was entirely unaffected by increased FdUMP concentrations. These data unequivocally demonstrated a sequential ordered mechanism for the formation of the TS-FdUMP-5,10-CH_2FH_4 ternary complex in which binding of the nucleotide is a prerequisite to binding of the cosubstrate (Fig. 1(a)). The use of 5-BromodUMP (a dead-end inhibitor of TS competitive with dUMP) to demonstrate substrate inhibition by the cosubstrate allowed the above conclusions to be extended to the normal enzymatic reaction in agreement with the above kinetic studies (Fig. 1(b)). A second paper from this school [38] detailed similar results for human enzyme – results which bear fundamentally upon TS inhibitor design as will be amplified later in this chapter (Section 4.4.1a).

Figure 1. Cleland diagrams.

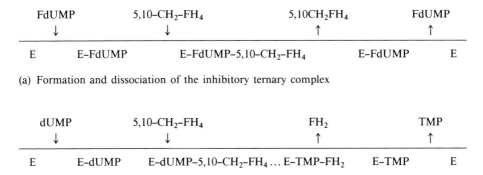

(a) Formation and dissociation of the inhibitory ternary complex

(b) The natural reaction catalysed by TS

3. INHIBITORS OF THYMIDYLATE SYNTHETASE

3.1 *Pyrimidine analogues*

TS inhibition by pyrimidine analogues of dUMP has been the subject of several recent reviews [10, 12, 39, 40]. This section, concentrating on the most recent research, will therefore be brief in preference of dealing more extensively with folate analogues in the next.

As Santi has summarised [12] a 5'-phospho-2'-deoxy-beta-D-ribosyl unit in dUMP (X, R = H) is essential if TS binding is to be preserved. In the pyrimidine unit the most potent inhibitors all have an electron-withdrawing substituent at the 5-position and this property has been recognised in a quantitative structure activity relationship (QSAR) [41]. The QSAR also showed that size was the next most important factor with smaller 5-substituents being favoured – a result which is inconsistent with the potent inhibition shown by certain 5-styryl- [42, 43] and 5-benzoquinonyl [44] derivatives of dUMP (see below). Nonetheless, a new generation of analogues (X) of 5FU has emerged with substituents such as -CHO, -CN and NO_2 in place of fluorine. Since the appearance of the reviews cited the analogue bearing the 5-ethynyl substituent ($-C \equiv CH$) has been more extensively investigated [45–47]. However, thus far these analogues have hardly progressed beyond testing as enzyme inhibitors and as inhibitors of the growth of cells in culture; none has come anywhere near a clinical trial. 5-Nitrodeoxyuridylic acid (X R = NO_2) is a potent TS inhibitor [48] but its prodrug form, 5-nitrodeoxyuridine, was ineffective against the L1210 leukaemia *in vivo*. This result was attributed to rapid catabolism of the drug by thymidine phosphorylase to the non-toxic 5-nitrouracil [49]. The interactions, some

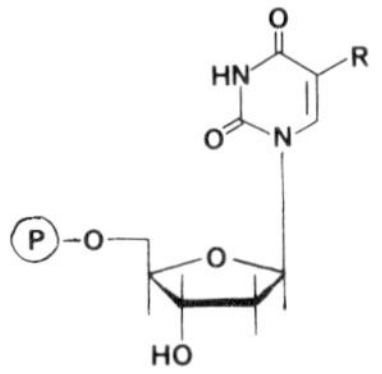

X

desirable, others not, of pyrimidine analogues with metabolising enzymes are discussed further in section 4.4.2a.

Three new and distinct substrate-based TS inhibitors have recently appeared. Kalman and Goldman have imaginatively devised a *purine* analogue which acts as a mechanism-based inhibitor. 1-(beta-D-2′-Deoxyribofuranosyl)-8-aza-purin-2-one 5′-monophosphate (XI) incorporates a triazole ring which is thought to give enhanced resonance stabilisation (structure

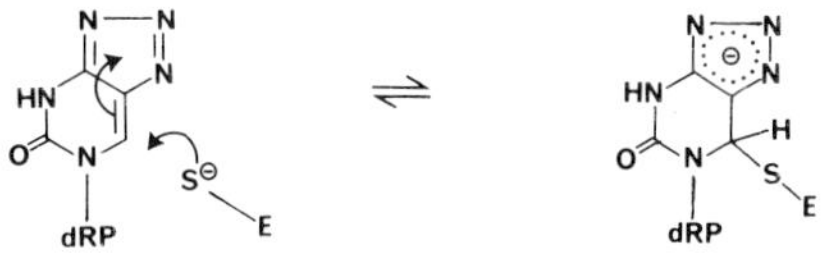

XI XII

XII) of the negative charge resulting from addition of the thiol group from the enzyme to the 6-position [50]. De Clercq and colleagues designed 5(E)-(3-azidostyryl)-2′-deoxyuridine-5′-monophosphate (XIII) as a photoactivated inhibitor of TS. According to expectation, irradiation provided the

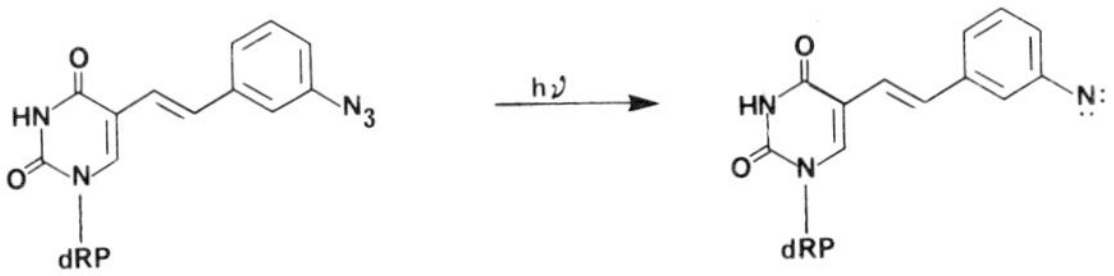

XIII XIV

nitrene (XIV) which functioned as a photoaffinity label [43]. Moreover the azide (XIII) was a light-dependent ($\lambda = 366$ nm) inhibitor of the growth of L1210, human lymphoblastoid and vaccinia cells in culture. The authors had in mind its use as an organ-specific treatment for certain dermatological disorders such as psoriasis [42]. Mertes' school has recently synthesized another new TS inhibitor, one possibly mechanism-based. 5-(p-benzoquinonyl)-2′-deoxyuridine 5′-phosphate (XV) shows time-dependent irreversible inactivation of thymidylate synthetase. The electron-withdrawing quinone substituent may promote enzymic thiol addition to the pyrimidine 6-position with the species thus resulting (XVI) then rearranging to form the more stable reduced quinone (XVII) [44].

XV   XVI   XVII

3.2 *Folate Analogues*

3.2.1 *Pteridines*

Folate molecules containing a fully aromatic, oxidised pteridine ring are weak inhibitors of thymidylate synthetase. 2-Amino-4-hydroxypteridines usually bind more strongly than their 2,4-diamino counterparts. However, in the 2,4-diamino series the corresponding 7,8-dihydro and 5,6,7,8-tetrahydro analogues and derivatives thereof inhibit more strongly. The first systematic investigations of 2,4-diaminopteridines were made by Kisliuk. With Levine [51] he showed that aminopterin (XVIIIa) weakly inhibited TS from *E. coli* ($IC_{50} = 100 \, \mu M$ in the presence of $300 \, \mu M$ ($\pm$) cosubstrate) and that dihydro- and tetrahydroaminopterin were respectively 20-fold and 10-fold better inhibitors. Referring to the last-named compound the authors pointed

XVIII   a, R=H,   Aminopterin

           b, $R=CH_3$, Methotrexate

out that insofar as the cosubstrate for the enzyme assay is formed *in situ* from FH_4 and an excess of formaldehyde – a reaction which tetrahydroaminopterin is equally capable of – it is difficult to determine whether the inhibitory species is tetrahydroaminopterin or its 5,10-methylene derivative. Horwitz and Kisliuk [52] next showed that against the same enzyme system methotrexate (XVIIIb) and its reduction products gave results in parallel to those of aminopterin. Now since methotrexate is the 10-methyl derivative of aminopterin, formation of a tricyclic 5,10-methylene derivative from tetrahydromethotrexate is not possible, suggesting that the corresponding inhibitor in the aminopterin series is not 5,10-methylenetetrahydroaminopterin. In a third paper [53] Kisliuk's school examined the interaction of formaldehyde with two ($\pm$) tetrahydropteridines in detail. The results were complicated. With tetrahydrofolate it was shown that two pairs of diastereoisomers were formed, not one pair as expected. Of these four products only one was fully enzymatically active, but it contained only 0.75 molecular equivalent of formaldehyde not 1.0. This suggested that it actually contained 5,10-methylenetetrahydrofolate complexed with half its amount of a molecule containing two tetrahydropteridines linked intermolecularly by a formaldehyde residue. Reaction of formaldehyde with tetrahydroaminopterin produced a corresponding set of four paired diastereoisomers. But none of these preformed adducts were inhibitory when added to the TS assay. Which molecular species it is that actually inhibits TS when tetrahydroaminopterin is added to the assay is still an unanswered question.

A similar story can be told for tetrahydrohomofolate (VIII). As earlier mentioned, for certain types of TS this can substitute for tetrahydrofolate in the reaction mixture which produces thymidylate from deoxyuridylate. That is a true statement, but what is only probably true is that 5,11-methylenetetrahydrohomofolate (IX) can substitute for 5,10-methylenetetrahydrofolate as cosubstrate. Considering its inhibitory action, it was originally implied that the inhibition of *E. Coli* TS was accomplished by tetrahydrohomofolate itself [54] but a subsequent paper [25] brought evidence that a reaction, presumably (VIII) to (IX), had occurred in the assay, and went on to discuss the geometry of the presumed inhibitory species (IX). A datum consistent with the 5,11-methylene compound being the inhibitor proper is that (1)-5-methyltetrahydrohomofolate (XIX) inhibits *E. coli* TS with Ki

XIX

56 µM in an assay where (1)-tetrahydrohomofolate had Ki 56 nM [24]. Here again a methyl group prohibits the formation of a tricyclic species; it could of course weaken the inhibition by some other effect so the evidence is circumstantial. In the case of tetrahydrohomofolate, as with tetrahydroaminopterin, the nature of the inhibitory species is not proven. This review will dwell no more upon the uncertainty of events within the TS assay except to caution that it contains highly reactive formaldehyde in excess and that one should keep a broad imagination when assessing the inhibition seen with any molecule loaded with amino groups. Before leaving homofolates it should be remembered that although tetrahydrohomofolate causes strong inhibition of bacterial TS with a Ki of 0.28 µM [25] this is not true for mammalian enzyme. Thus thymidylate synthetase from FR8 mouse leukaemia was inhibited by 20 to 30-fold less [55] and secondly the Ki for L1210 TS was measured as high as 42 µM [23]. Tetrahydrobishomofolate (XX) with two extra methylenes in the bridge region did not inhibit TS or serve as cosubstrate [25]. This inactivity may be attributable to the molecule (XX) *per se* since there was no spectroscopic shift observed when it was put with formaldehyde.

$CH_2-CH_2-CH_2-NH$ —⟨ ⟩— $CO-Glu$

XX

In an examination of their TS-binding properties, the tetrahydrofolic acid series and the tetrahydroaminopterin series were comprehensively explored by Slavik and Zakrzewski [56]. The best inhibitor found in the former series was C^9, N^{10}-dimethyl-FH_4 (Ki 22 μM, competitive with the cosubstrate) and in the latter series tetrahydromethotrexate (Ki 1.97 μM, noncompetitive) – neither particularly potent. Reaction of tetrahydrofolate with reagents other than formaldehyde produced tricyclic structures in which the N^5 and N^{10} atoms were linked by -CO-, -CS-, -C(=NH)- and -CH_2-CH_2- groups but all showed insignificant activity against mammalian TS [57].

In designing potential new antifolates, the medicinal chemists have turned a great deal of attention to the bridge region of the molecule (Z in XXII). DeGraw and colleagues made 10-deazaäminopterin (XXIa) which by itself was a very poor TS inhibitor but activity was improved in the dihydro and tetrahydro derivatives (IC_{50}'s 10 μM and 5.7 μM respectively) [58]. Homologues (XXIb-d) of this molecule carrying one or more 10-alkyl groups and aromatic in the pyrazine

CH_2-C —⟨ ⟩— $CO-Glu$ (with R^1, R^2)

	R^1	R^2	IC_{50} for *L. Casei* TS (μm)
XXIa	H	H	230
b	CH_3	H	280
c	C_2H_5	H	330
d	CH_3	CH_3	390

ring inhibited no better [59]. Much work has gone into the synthesis of pteridine analogues (XXII) of folic acid and aminopterin in which the bridge region is altered to contain heteroatoms other than nitrogen. Substitution by sulphur and retaining the length gave 10-thiafolic acid (XXIIa) and 10-thiaäminopterin (XXIIb) but neither was a good TS inhibitor [60]. Homologation of the bridge in (XXIIa) gave 11-thiohomofolic acid (XXIIc) which did not significantly inhibit TS; its tetrahydro analogue inhibited not at all [61]. Homologation of the bridge in (XXIIb) gave 11-thiohomoaminopterin (XXIId) which inhibited TS with IC_{50} 60 μM – roughly the same as that of methotrexate (40 μM) thus gaining but slight improvement [62]. 11-oxahomofolic acid (XXIIe) was also synthesised but neither it nor any of its

	R	Z	IC$_{50}$ for *L. Casei* TS (μM)
XXIIa	OH	CH$_2$–S	> 30
b	NH$_2$	CH$_2$–S	> 30
c	OH	CH$_2$–CH$_2$–S	*
d	NH$_2$	CH$_2$–CH$_2$–S	60
e	OH	CH$_2$–CH$_2$–O	> 40
f	NH$_2$	CH$_2$–CH$_2$–O	> 50
g	OH	CH$_2$–N(tosyl)–CH$_2$	*
h	NH$_2$	CH$_2$–N(tosyl)–CH$_2$	*
i	NH$_2$	CH$_2$	> 300

* Described in the paper as virtually inactive.

two reduction products inhibited TS at concentrations lower than 40 μM [63]. 11-Oxahomoaminopterin (XXIIf) did not significantly inhibit *L. Casei* TS at 50 μM [64]. N^{10}-tosylisohomofolic acid (XXIIg) and N^{10}-tosylisohomoaminopterin (XXIIh), radically altered in the bridge, were poor inhibitors of *L. Casei* TS [65]. Discouraged by these results with antifolates having longer chains in the bridge, Nair's group turned to produce an analogue with a shortened bridge, 10-deaza-9-noraminopterin (XXIIi), but again the TS inhibition, by the fully aromatic molecule at least, was disappointing [66].

3.2.2 *Pyridopyrimidines and Other Heterocyles*
Work in this area has been less than in the pteridine or quinazoline series. DeGraw *et al.* synthesised and tested 8-deazafolic acid (XXIII) and its reduction products against *L. Casei* TS. The IC$_{50}$ values for the parent, the

XXIII

(presumed 5,6-)dihydro- and the 5,6,7,8-tetrahydro- derivative were 14,30 and 75 μM respectively – none very potent [67]. Broom and Srinivasan, in designing bisubstrate TS inhibitors modelled upon the proposed intermediate (V) occurring during enzymic catalysis, worked in the tetrahydro-8-deazapteridine series (presumably) to avoid any problem of regioselectivity, inherent in the tetrahydrofolate series, when introducing the thyminyl residue by alkylation. The nucleoside (XXIV, R = H) was a weak inhibitor of human thymidylate synthetase, a result attributable to the fact that TS does

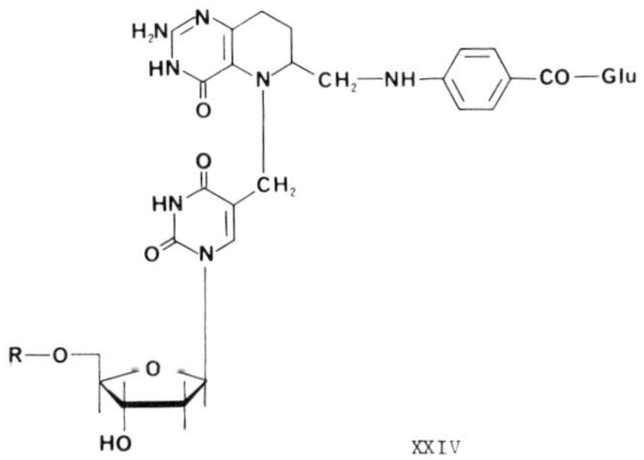

XXIV

not bind deoxyuridine. However, the nucleotide (XXIV, R = PO$_3^=$) was a potent inhibitor with Ki 70 nM [68]. This hard-won result confirms many of our ideas about TS catalysis but it is doubtful if the bisubstrate approach will give rise to a useful drug not only because of the difficult chemistry involved but also because the negatively charged phosphate group disadvantages the molecule for transport across the cell membrane. This section closes with two 7,8-dihydro-8-oxapterin analogues (XXV) shortened in the bridge. Neither inhibited · *L. Casei* · TS at concentrations up to 100 µM [69].

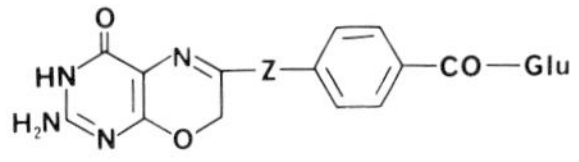

XXV, Z = nothing or CH$_2$

3.2.3 *Quinazolines*

The quinazoline nucleus has been a useful building stone in many biologically active molecules as Johne [70] has summarised. Most derivatives of this nucleus are 2,4-diaminoquinazolines synthesised by Elslager and Werbel and their colleagues at Warner-Lambert/Parke-Davis with antimalarial and antibacterial action in view and by Hynes' group in South Carolina with antitumour and antibacterial action in view. These compounds were screened enzymatically only against DHFR but not against TS and are thus excluded from this review.

TS-inhibiting quinazoline antifolates were first described by Bird, Vaitkus and Clarke in 1970 [71]. The results of these workers established that the quinazoline ring in (XXVIa) in the 2,4-diamino-10-methyl series (IC$_{50}$ for *E. Coli* TS = 2.1 µM) improved .the inhibition relative to the pteridine (XXVIb, IC$_{50}$ 70 µM) by over thirtyfold. But more important was that in the 2-amino-4-hydroxyquinazoline series (XXVII) placement of a 10-methyl substituent reduced the IC$_{50}$ from 0.75 µM (XXVIIa) to 0.098 µM (XXVIIb) – a nearly tenfold increase in inhibition. The compound (XXVIIb), also known as 10-methyl-5,8-dideazafolic acid, thus became the

	Y	R
XXVIa	CH	CH_3
b	N	CH_3
c	N	$CH_2-C\equiv CH$

R		IC_{50} for purified L 1210 TS (nM)
XXVIIa	H (AHQ)	570 [a]
b	CH_3	42 [a]
c	CH_2-CH_3	27 [a]
d	$CH_2-CH_2-CH_3$	170 [a]
e	$CH_2-CH_2-CH_2-CH_3$	3200 [a]
f	$CH_2-CH=CH_2$	69 [b]
g	$CH_2-C\equiv CH$ (CB3717)	5 [b]
h	CHO	

[a] Data from ref. 79
[b] Data from ref. 80.

most potent TS-inhibiting folate known – much more potent than tetrahydrohomofolate (VII) which had $IC_{50} = 2\ \mu M$ in a similar assay [54]. Moreover, in contrast to tetrahydrohomofolate, the inhibition by this methylated quinazoline was maintained when tested against mammalian enzyme since Carlin and coworkers [72] subsequently observed an IC_{50} of 0.14 μM for TS from mouse neuroblastoma. These authors implied that 10-methyl-5,8-dideazafolic acid (XXVIIb) was a more potent inhibitor of mammalian than of bacterial TS thinking that they had used a tenfold higher 5,10-CH_2FH_4 concentration. However, close inspection reveals that a decimal place was lost in their interpretation of Bird's data [71] and that the assay conditions were in fact virtually identical. McCuen and Sirotnak [73] examined the inhibition of TS from *Diplococcus pneumoniae* by several quinazoline analogues and confirmed that this nucleus confers good inhibitory properties.

The interesting lead of Bird and colleagues was not immediately developed by the medicinal chemists. The 10-formyl analogue (XXVIIh) seemed equipotent with (XXVIIb) but this compound was developed more as a biochemical tool [74]. The quinazoline analogues synthesised over the years in Hynes' group were eventually tested as inhibitors of bacterial (*L. Casei*) and mammalian (L1210) TS by Scanlon *et al.* [75]. Once more the general potency of this class of compound was confirmed. The finding of Bird and colleagues relating to the 10-methyl group was confirmed for the bacterial enzyme but not (in this study) for the mammalian enzyme. The introduction of a 5-methyl group in the 2-amino-4-hydroxy series (XXVIIIa → XXVIIIb) was reported to cause a slight reduction in the inhibition of the bacterial enzyme but to leave the inhibition of the mammalian enzyme unchanged. The same manoeuvre applied in the 2,4-diamino series (XXVIIIc → XXVIIId) brought about a tenfold increase in binding. The effect of inverting the bridge in 5,8-dideazafolic acid (XXVIIa or AHQ) to

	R	Y
XXVIIIa	OH	H
b	OH	CH$_3$
c	NH$_2$	H
d	NH$_2$	CH$_3$

produce the compound known as IAHQ (XXIX) was to reduce the TS inhibition by twofold for the bacterial enzyme and by fivefold for the mam-

XXIX (IAHQ)

malian enzyme. Further biological properties of IAHQ are discussed below.

Jones, meanwhile, taking note of the result of Bird and colleagues [71] and the structure of the 5,10-methylene FH$_4$ cosubstrate speculated that the methyl group might enhance the inhibition more were it located at carbon 5. The compounds (XXVIIIa) and (XXVIIIb) were made [76] and tested [77] against TS from Yoshida ascites sarcoma cells. However, the methyl group was found to reduce the inhibition by 75-fold. This result for this pair of compounds contrasted strongly with that found by Scanlon *et al.* [75] for the L1210 enzyme. Contrast was again seen with the 2,4-diamino pair (XXVIIIc) and (XXVIIId) where Scanlon and colleagues reported a tenfold improvement upon methylation [75] while Calvert and colleagues reported a 400-fold improvement [77]. Both used mammalian enzyme. Molecular models show that the 5-methyl group effectively transmits the steric bulk of the 4-substituent, be this carbonyl oxygen or amino, onto the bridge methylene group forbidding completely free rotation about the C^6-C^9 bond. This explanation may account for the different effects seen in the 2-amino-4-hydroxy series and in the 2,4-diamino series but it requires that the binding conformations differ between the series – a reasonable proposition given the recent discoveries of how methotrexate binds to DHFR.

The lead of Bird and his colleagues (compound XXVIIb) was eventually exploited by the present reviewers [78, 79]. The ethyl, propyl and butyl homologues were synthesised and tested against mammalian (L1210) and bacterial (*L. Casei*) TS. For the mammalian enzyme the IC_{50} values for the compounds XXVIIa, b, c, d and e were 570, 42, 27, 170 and 3200 nM respectively, the activity peaking with the ethyl substituent (XXVIIc). Further development illustrating the importance of the N^{10} substituent came upon introducing the unsaturated substituents allyl and propargyl into that position giving compounds (XXVIIf) and (XXVIIg) respectively [80]. The latter compound, CB3717, had an IC_{50} of 5 nM for L1210 TS and a Ki value of 4.2 nM, competitive with the cosubstrate [81]. Preliminary data from another laboratory suggest that the interaction of CB3717 with *L. Casei* TS occurs in two stages, the first of which is competitive with 5,10-CH_2FH_4. Following this initial binding, a unimolecular change takes place with a $t_{1/2}$ of about 50 min in which dUMP becomes covalently bound to the enzyme to produce a relatively stable ternary complex with $t_{1/2}$ for dissociation of about 27 hr. By contrast, the $t_{1/2}$'s for the association and the dissociation of unsubstituted compound, AHQ, are about 1 min and 25 min respectively. The $t_{1/2}$ for the dissociation of the FdUMP-5,10-CH_2FH_4-TS complex under the same conditions is about 7 hr (DV Santi, personal communication). CB3717 is the tightest binding folate inhibitor of TS yet known; its biological and clinical properties are dealt with more fully in the subsequent pages. Piper and colleagues, taking note, synthesised 10-propargylaminopterin (XXVIc) but found that although it inhibited *L. Casei* TS (IC_{50} 20 μM) better than did methotrexate (IC_50 75 μM) the enhancement was less than that observed in the 2-amino-4-hydroxyquinazoline series [82].

4. BIOCHEMICAL EFFECTS OF TS INHIBITORS

4.1 *Introduction*

We have restricted ourselves in this chapter to discussing TS inhibitors in the purest sense, that is, compounds that interact directly with the enzyme. Methotrexate is not usually included in this category since its primary site of action is on dihydrofolate reductase and it is only the consequent depletion of 5,10-methylenetetrahydrofolate (the cosubstrate for TS) which leads to a reduction in the rate of synthesis of thymidylate [176, 193]. Functionally, methotrexate is not a pure TS inhibitor since it also affects *de novo* purine synthesis and various amino acid interconversions (reviewed by 176). Nevertheless methotrexate is capable of inhibiting TS directly, albeit at high concentrations (ki ca 10^{-5} M [114]) and in some circumstances this effect may be significant. Clinically, high dose methotrexate followed by folinic acid rescue results in plasma levels theoretically high enough to cause TS inhibition [244]. Experimental evidence suggests that the effective locus of action of methotrexate may change in methotrexate-resistant cell lines with elevated DHFR levels. It is possible that in these lines the direct effect of free intracellular methotrexate on TS may become rate limiting for TMP synthesis before saturation of DHFR has occurred [115]. It is also clear that methotrexate may be converted to polyglutamate forms [116–122 and rev. by 123] which are better inhibitors of TS than is the parent compound [124–126].

Inhibition of TS whether achieved directly or indirectly has similar biochemical consequences, namely a reduction in the pool of TMP (and consequently in those of TDP and TTP) and an increase in the pool of dUMP [127–133, 153]. Direct inhibition of TS may be achieved by analogues of either the pyrimidine or the folate substrate. However, pyrimidine analogues have other biochemical effects which complicate the interpretation of results obtained in isolated cells or *in vivo* systems.

4.2 *Fluorinated Pyrimidines*

The most widely studied are the 5-fluorinated analogues of uracil and of 2'-deoxyuridine (5-fluorouracil (FU) and 5-fluorodeoxyuridine (FUdR) respectively). These compounds require metabolic activation by enzymes of normal pyrimidine metabolism in order to exert their cytotoxic effects. The pathways involved are illustrated by Fig. 2. Both compounds can be metabolised to FdUMP, a tight-binding inhibitor of TS (see section 2).

FU may also be metabolised via several other pathways, forming not only FdUMP, but other fluorinated ribo- or deoxyribonucleotides which may also interfere with cellular metabolism [reviewed by 113, 134–136]. The intrinsic differences in pyrimidine, and consequently FU metabolism, in various cell types probably account for the conflicting reports on the mode of action of FU. Incorporation of FU into RNA (via FUTP) may occur and interfere with the synthesis and function of all classes of RNA [137–141]. More recently incorporation of FU (or FUdR) into DNA has been demonstrated [142–145, 201–203]. This occurs via metabolism to FdUTP which can replace TTP as a substrate for DNA synthesis [144, 146].

These disturbances in nucleic acid metabolism may contribute to the

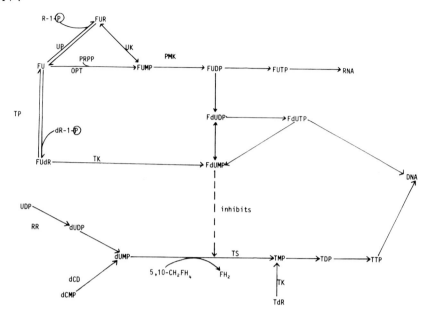

Figure 2. R-1-P Ribose-1-phosphate / dR-1-P Deoxyribose-1-phosphate / PRPP 5-Phosphoribo-syl-1-pyrophosphate / RR Ribonucleotide reductase / PMK Pyrimidine monophosphate ki-nase / UK Uridine kinase / UP Uridine phosphorylase / TK Thymidine kinase / dCD Deoxyxy-tidylate deaminase / OPT Orotate phosphoribosyl transferase / TS Thymidylate synthetase / TP Thymidine phosphorylase.

cytotoxicity of the compounds. Historically the cytotoxicity of fluorinated pyrimidines has been attributed to the inhibition of TS but a more rigorous evaluation of their loci of action has led to the realisation that different cell lines probably succumb by different mechanisms. There is now substantial evidence that FU cytotoxicity primarily or partially results from incorpora-tion into RNA in many cells/tumours [136, 147–149, 151–153 and reviewed by 134, 135, 154]. The consequences of incorporation into RNA may extend further than effects purely on RNA function since this could, in turn, lead to inhibition of DNA synthesis either by inhibition of the synthesis of key enzymes or by the production of a non-functional form of the primer RNA required for the initiation of DNA synthesis. This has been suggested by Sawyer *et al.* [136].

In vivo metabolism of FUdR to FU occurs in plasma and in the liv-er [236] and consequently the effects of this drug may be expected to be similar to those of FU. However, the extent to which FUdR owes its cyto-toxicity *in vitro* to incorporation into RNA is unclear. It is largely assumed that the one-stage activation to FdUMP by thymidine kinase generates suf-ficiently high concentrations of the TS inhibitor for this enzyme to be the cytotoxic locus.

4.3 *Folate Analogues*

Since the original 2-amino-4-hydroxy quinazoline analogue (AHQ) (Fig. XXVIIa) of folic acid was shown by Bird *et al.* [71] to inhibit TS, a large number of similar structures have been synthesised and tested. However, very few have progressed past an initial enzyme and cell culture screen. One of the most widely studied quinazoline TS inhibitors is CB3717 (Fig. XXVIIg) whose biochemical and pharmacological evaluation has led to a clinical study [127, 81, 80, 155–161, 212]. Bird's original unsubstituted quinazoline analogue of folic acid has been modified by reversing the 9–10 bridge [162, 75]. Although this analogue, IAHQ, (XXIX) seems to be a much poorer inhibitor of TS when compared with CB3717 it has some interesting properties that will be discussed in relation to its potential as an anti-tumour agent. Thus the data on three 2-amino-4-hydroxy quinazolines are available for a discussion of their biochemical properties. These are the direct quinazoline analogue of folic acid AHQ, which may be regarded as the 'parent', the corresponding compound with an iso-bridge (IAHQ) and 10-propargyl AHQ (CB3717).

4.3.1 *AHQ*

This compound is a better inhibitor of DHFR than of TS, the Ki values for the mammalian enzymes being 0.35 nM and 67 nM respectively [77], but the effective cytotoxic locus of action is nevertheless probably TS. The almost complete protection from its cytotoxicity in culture by TdR is suggestive of this, but is not conclusive [77]. Jackson *et al.* have pointed out that delayed TdR rescue is a more sensitive indicator of the cytotoxic locus than is the concurrent addition of TdR (protection) [127]. For example the cytotoxicity of methotrexate may be partially prevented by co-administration of TdR, particularly when trace amounts of reduced folates are present [127]. Delayed thymidine, however, seems not to reverse, even partially, the effects of methotrexate. These authors using a mathematical model of folate metabolism [163] also attempted to predict which enzyme became rate-limiting in the presence of antifolates that inhibited both DHFR and TS competitively. The model predicted that even if the inhibition of TS by a compound was up to 3.5 orders of magnitude weaker than its inhibition of DHFR, TS would still be rate-limiting in the dihydrofolate reduction-oxidation cycle. Although the model used enzyme levels and kinetic data from WIL2 lymphoblastoid cells there is no reason to believe that other mammalian tumour cells would differ significantly in this respect.

A mutant L1210 cell line that overproduces DHFR 160-fold (L1210/R71) and is consequently resistant to methotrexate (630-fold) is only partially cross-resistant to AHQ (75-fold) suggesting that the primary locus of this compound is not DHFR [79].

Thus it would appear that AHQ has TS as a cytotoxic locus. Bird *et al.* also tested the 10-methyl analogue of AHQ (Fig. XXVIIb) and showed that this substituent enhanced the inhibition of TS by about 10-fold [71]. These observations led to a series of TS inhibitors being synthesised and tested at The Institute of Cancer Research [79, 80], the most potent being CB3717, a compound that undoubtedly owes its anti-tumour activity to inhibition of TS and consequently is active against cells resistant to methotrexate by virtue of DHFR overproduction [80, 167].

4.3.2 *CB3717*

This compound was first described by Jones *et al.* in 1981 [80] and has since been the subject of extensive biochemical and pharmacological examination [80, 81, 127, 155–157, 161]. Its entry into phase I study in 1981 has, for the first time, allowed the clinical evaluation [158–160, 212] of an antifolate that has TS as its exclusive cytotoxic locus. No other loci are implicated in its cytotoxic action in experimental systems so that the concept of cancer cell death mediated by the induction of a thymineless state may now be tested clinically.

INHIBITION KINETICS OF CB3717 FOR TS

Initial studies of the inhibition kinetics of this compound were done using the Michaelis-Menten assumptions for the kinetic analysis. The inhibition appeared to be competitive but the data were inadequate to exclude a non-competitive element with a mixed type of inhibition. Although an increase in the Km was observed when $5,10\text{-CH}_2\text{FH}_4$ was used as the variable substrate a small decrease in the V_{max} was also apparent. However, an estimation of the Ki, assuming competitive inhibition, revealed the very low figure for this constant (~ 1 nM). It was therefore obvious that the tight-binding nature of the inhibition made this type of kinetic analysis inappropriate and possibly misleading. Zone B analysis for tight-binding inhibition was applied to CB3717 using highly purified enzyme from both L1210 cells and WIL2 human lymphoblastoid cells. CB3717 was found to be a competitive inhibitor with respect to the folate co-substrate $5,10\text{-CH}_2\text{FH}_4$, the Ki values being 4.2 nM and 4.9 nM for the two enzymes respectively [127, 81]. However, new evidence now suggests that a more stable, non-competitive complex may be formed slowly by CB3717, dUMP and TS (see section 3.2.3).

1. *Theoretical Considerations*

We have already alluded to the fact (section 4.3.1) that 2-amino-4-hydroxy quinazolines are also DHFR inhibitors but kinetic simulation using a mathematical model suggests that although TS inhibition may be very much weaker than that of DHFR (up to 3.5 orders of magnitude) the effective cytotoxic locus is still TS. Tight-binding kinetic analysis of CB3717 inhibition of DHFR reveals a relatively weak inhibition when compared with the more potent diamino compounds that inhibit this enzyme. The Ki for the L1210 enzyme was found to be 14 nM [80] while that for human enzyme was 23 nM [127]. Thus the mathematical model predicted unequivocally that the TS inhibition would be the rate-limiting event in the inhibited steady state when cells were exposed to CB3717 [127]. There is now a substantial amount of experimental data to support this prediction.

2. *Thymidine Reversal Experiments*

Thymidine alone prevented the cytotoxic effects of CB3717 against both the L1210 [80] and WIL2 [127] cells grown in culture while it only partially prevented methotrexate cytotoxicity in these cell lines [127, 164]. Even when given as a delayed rescue (8 hours) TdR reversed the effects of the drug [127]. These observations supported the hypothesis that TS was the sole locus of action. The cytotoxicity of methotrexate was not even partially reversed by delayed TdR administration as expected (see section 4.3.1).

3. *Intracellular Dihydrofolate Pools*

FH_2 did not accumulate in WIL2 lymphoblastoid cells treated with CB3717 while those treated with an equally toxic dose of methotrexate showed marked elevation (normal <0.2 µM, treated 6.8 µM) [127]. This is probably the strongest evidence to suggest that DHFR is not the cytotoxic locus of action in cells treated with CB3717.

4. *Intracellular Pyrimidine Deoxynucleotide pools*

Measurement of the pyrimidine deoxynucleotide pools has substantiated the thesis that the *de novo* synthesis of thymine nucleotides is inhibited in cells treated with CB3717. WIL2 cells exposed to an ID_{50} dose of either CB3717 or methotrexate showed a marked decrease in the mono, di and triphosphates of thymidine when compared with controls after 16 hours of treatment [127]. As predicted the level of the TS substrate, dUMP, rose dramatically, giving levels 2936% and 4455% of control for methotrexate and CB3717 respectively [127]. Elevation of the dUMP pool has been demonstrated several times previously when either methotrexate or FU (see section 4.1.1a) has been used to inhibit the *de novo* synthesis of thymidylate and does not itself establish whether the inhibition of the TS is direct or indirect.

5. *Purine Nucleotide Pools*

Measurement of the purine nucleotide pools is more informative in establishing the effective locus of CB3717. If inhibition of DHFR were rate-limiting or if CB3717 inhibited one of the two folate dependent enzymes in the *de novo* purine pathway, then a fall in the purine nucleotide pools would be expected. Jackson *et al.* compared the effects of equally toxic doses of methotrexate and CB3717 on the purine nucleotide pools in WIL2 cells grown in culture [127]. As expected, a reduction in the ATP and GTP pools was apparent following exposure to methotrexate, but this effect was not seen with CB3717. However, a decrease of the dGTP pool was observed in cells treated with either drug. This may be explained as a secondary effect of the decreased TTP pool since TTP is known to be an obligatory activator for the GDP reductase activity of ribonucleotide reductase [165, 166].

6. *Resistance Studies*

Methotrexate resistant cell lines that over produce DHFR are virtually not cross-resistant to CB3717 [80, 167], again suggesting that DHFR is not the cytotoxic locus for this compound.

A cell line with acquired resistance to CB3717 [182, 168] overproduces TS ~30 fold. This cell line is not significantly cross-resistant to methotrexate (see section 4.7).

We may conclude therefore that CB3717 has its cytotoxic effects, at least in cells grown *in vitro*, solely associated with inhibition of TS.

4.3.3 *IAHQ*

a) Kinetic

This TS inhibitor was first described by Scanlon *et al.* in 1979 [75] as an analogue of isofolic acid. The reversed configuration of the 9–10 bridge actually worsened the IC_{50} against TS when compared with its 'parent' compound (AHQ). However, recent work has established that the mode of inhibition of TS is non-competitive with respect to 5,10-CH_2FH_4 [162], unlike the other 2-amino-4-hydroxy quinazolines so far reported which are all competitive [75, 77, 81, 127]. The Ki reported was ~8 μM when 5,10-CH_2FH_4 was used as the variable substrate and 5 μM when dUMP was varied [162]. The documented uncompetitive nature of the inhibition with dUMP as the variable substrate is expected when binding of this substrate is a prerequisite for inhibitor binding and indeed the level of dUMP was suggested to be important in the promotion of such binding. The way in which the intracellular substrate levels modulate the inhibition by quinazoline antifolates is discussed in section 4.4.1. An important advance in the quinazoline antifolate field has been the synthesis of the triglutamate derivative of IAHQ. Kinetic analysis demonstrated a 10-fold improvement in the Ki when $5,10\text{-}CH_2FH_4$ was the variable substrate and a 50-fold improvement when dUMP was varied, suggesting that the ternary complex formed with the triglutamate is more stable than that found with the parent compound [162]. It would be expected (by analogy with IAHQ, methotrexate and $5,10\text{-}CH_2FH_4$) that polyglutamation of any folate-based TS inhibitor would decrease the Ki for TS. The authors point out that the cytotoxicity of IAHQ may be determined by the extent of intracellular polyglutamation.

b) Intracellular Locus
If we apply the mathematical rationale of Jackson *et al.* (see section 4.3.1) then IAHQ undoubtedly acts as a TS inhibitor (Kis for DHFR = 0.7 μM). This is supported by the fact that TdR almost completely prevented the cytotoxicity of IAHQ in HCT-8 cells [162]. In addition the reported measurements of intracellular ribonucleotide and deoxyribonucleotide pools were consistent with TS being rate-limiting for growth in L1210 cells exposed to IAHQ [162]. Studies where ^3H UdR incorporation (in drug-free medium) were used as a measure of TS activity in human colonic cells (HCT-8) after a short exposure to IAHQ suggested that the drug was in a non-effluxable form. This fact together with the knowledge that IAHQ was a substrate for folylpolyglutamate synthetase (FPGS) at μM drug concentrations was the basis for the authors' thesis that IAHQ is a 'prodrug' for the more active polyglutamated form that is the proposed active agent. It has been reported that CB3717 (personal communications, R. Moran and J. McGuire) is also a substrate for FPGS at low concentrations although substrate inhibition was noted at high concentrations. It will be interesting to establish whether this phenomenon is general for the quinazoline TS inhibitors.

4.4 *Factors Affecting TS Inhibition*
Cells lacking sensitivity to an enzyme inhibitor are frequently said to be 'resistant'. Acquired resistance is the term used to describe a reduction in the sensitivity of cell lines following prolonged exposure to the drug. Intrinsic resistance is simply a function of the normal cellular biochemistry where conditions may be unfavourable for effective inhibition. Studies of the mechanisms of intrinsic and acquired resistance of various cell lines to fluorinated pyrimidines has helped considerably in the design of folate-based inhibitors of TS. Fortuitously, some factors associated with resistance to the pyrimidine analogues may actually increase the sensitivity to the folate ana-

logues. It is now clear that the concentrations of substrates in relation to the kinetics of the reaction play an important role in determining sensitivity to TS inhibitors.

4.4.1 *Inhibition Kinetics in Relation to The Natural Substrate Concentrations*

a) dUMP Levels

Christopherson and Duggleby [170] have recently used a theoretical model to describe the protection of enzymes from tight binding inhibitors by accumulation of substrate. This capacity to generate, what they describe as 'metabolic resistance', applies to the TS reaction when inhibited by FdUMP. Until recently FdUMP was thought to bind to TS competitively in the first instance followed by an irreversible covalent binding as it becomes covalently linked to the enzyme (see section 2.4.2). However, Lockshin and Danenberg have demonstrated, using enzyme purified from CCRF-CEM human leukemic cells, that although FdUMP binds covalently this is not irreversible [38]. When the synthesis of thymidylate is inhibited, the substrate, dUMP, accumulates [130–133, 153, 171] and may effectively compete with FdUMP for enzyme binding [38, 130].

The accumulation of dUMP has been documented to occur in many cell lines and is unrelated to the mechanism by which TS is inhibited. Thus, the indirect inhibition of TS by methotrexate also results in accumulation of dUMP [127–129, 171]. The limit of this substrate build up appears to be in the mM range as levels in excess of 2 mM have been measured. Although the initial cause of the expansion of the dUMP pool is clearly an accumulation of dUMP behind the block, several secondary factors probably serve to augment this effect – including derepression of feedback inhibition of ribonucleotide reductase and derepression of deoxycytidylate deaminase activities due to a fall in the TTP level. Myers *et al.* [130] measured intracellular FdUMP levels in some tissues after FU administration to P1534 ascites tumour-bearing mice. Although TS activity was initially inhibited, recovery occurred as intracellular FdUMP levels fell and dUMP levels rose. Differential tissue recovery was related to the rate of dUMP accumulation. These authors applied a model used for the inhibition of acetylcholinesterase by di*iso*propylfluorophosphate to demonstrate that when the substrate concentration exceeded the Km the rate of inactivation of the enzyme should decrease rapidly. Their experimental data was consistent with this model. As the initial intracellular dUMP concentration and Km are more or less equivalent this effect might be expected to occur readily. In more recent work, Lockshin and Danenberg [38] have extended the theoretical modelling of TS inhibition by using data from ligand binding studies of TS isolated from CCRF-CEM human lymphoblastic leukemia cells. They demonstrated that both dUMP and inorganic phosphate (Pi) decreased the rate of association of FdUMP with TS and that the effect of dUMP and Pi together was additive. The stabilisation of FdUMP binding by $5,10\text{-}CH_2FH_4$ was also studied. At low $5,10\text{-}CH_2FH_4$ concentrations the rate of FdUMP association was slow while that of dissociation was increased. Lockshin and Danenberg were able to demonstrate that at very low $5,10\text{-}CH_2FH_4$ concentrations FdUMP dissociated more rapidly from the human than from the bacterial enzyme. The effects of increased dUMP together with low $5,10\text{-}CH_2FH_4$ on decreasing the affinity of FdUMP binding to TS was more than additive.

Accumulation of the substrate dUMP is obviously a serious problem in relation to the cytotoxicity of pyrimidine-based TS inhibitors. For this reason Moran et al. [172] have proposed that FU could be used in combination with inhibitors of ribonuceotide reductase and deoxycytidylate deaminase thereby preventing the build up of dUMP.

b) Folate Cofactor Levels

Intracellular CH_2FH_4 levels are low ($<1\,\mu M$) [173, 174] and well below the Km for this co-substrate ($\sim 17\,\mu M$) (table 1). $5,10\text{-}CH_2FH_4$ can not build up significantly in the cell as a result of the inhibition of TS since the total concentration of intracellular folates is only $\sim 3\text{–}6\,\mu M$ [174, 175] and these compounds are not synthesised de novo in mammalian systems. In addition, $5,10\text{-}CH_2FH_4$ is at a metabolic branch point and equilibration between the reduced folates would be expected. Lockshin and Danenberg [38] used the intracellular levels of dUMP, Pi and $5,10\text{-}CH_2FH_4$ present in some tissues (after TS inhibition) in their mathematical model and demonstrated that the K_D for FdUMP increased by several orders of magnitude to $> 10^{-6}$ M. This was 5 orders greater than the lowest K_D achieved when dUMP and Pi were absent and $5,10\text{-}CH_2FH_4$ was high ($75\,\mu M$). This excellent work thus described in mathematical terms how TS inhibition by FdUMP could be severely retarded by the intracellular milieu. It not only explains recovery of TS activity in the presence of free FdUMP because of the accumulation of dUMP but also supports the data of Houghton et al. [177] who correlated a lack of sufficient $5,10\text{-}CH_2FH_4$ with non-responsiveness in human colorectal adenocarcinoma xenografts. Washtein [178] however, was unable to increase the amount of ^{3}H-FdUMP binding to TS in the cell sonicates of five human G.I. gastrointestinal tumour cell lines by the addition of $5,10\text{-}CH_2FH_4$, although she did not measure the naturally occurring $5,10\text{-}CH_2FH_4$ levels.

The proportion of various polyglutamate forms of CH_2FH_4 may well be important and is not considered in the previously described mathematical model. The Km for the pentaglutamate form of this co-substrate is considerably reduced ($\sim 2\,\mu M$) [179] and the degree of polyglutamation of folates within a given cell type may help to determine sensitivity to the fluorinated pyrimidines.

c) Conclusions

We may conclude therefore from kinetic and biochemical studies that pyrimidine-based inhibitors of TS may not achieve the degree of inhibition suggested by the tight-binding nature of their active metabolite, FdUMP. The same factors may however promote more efficient inhibition by a folate-based inhibitor of TS. Elevation of the dUMP pools has been found in WIL2 human lymphoblastoid cells exposed to the TS inhibitor, CB3717 [127]. Because this antifolate interacts directly with the enzyme, and the presence of the pyrimidine substrate is a prerequisite for ternary complex formation it should follow that high dUMP levels enhance the initial binding of CB3717 to the enzyme (the kinetics of inhibitor competing with the 2nd substrate of an ordered mechanism are dealt with by Spector *et al.* [169]. A similar phenomenon has been proposed by Fernandes *et al.* in relation to the quinazoline antifolate IAHQ (see section 4.3.3). The very slow dissociation of CB3717 from the complex (see action 3.2.3) should therefore allow TS to remain inhibited for some time. If we examine the levels of the competing substrate i.e. $5,10\text{-}CH_2FH_4$ it is clear that these can never accumulate significantly. We have already established that the concentration of $5,10\text{-}CH_2FH_4$ is unlikely to exceed the Km even in a polyglutamate form.

Thus a comparison of the kinetics of the inhibition of TS by the two tight-binding inhibitors FdUMP and CB3717 shows that the concentration of CB3717 required to achieve complete TS inhibition should be lower than that of FdUMP. Inhibitor levels are the next variable to be discussed in relation to tissue sensitivity to TS inhibitors.

4.4.2 *Intracellular Inhibitor Levels*

These levels are determined by a) the pharmacodynamics and pharmacokinetics of the drug *in vivo*, b) transport into the cell, c) metabolic activation, if this is necessary, d) catabolism of either the precursor or the active species, e) efflux.

a) Fluorinated pyrimidines

As a fluorinated pyrimidine has to be administered in a nonphosphorylated form the routes for metabolic activation will therefore determine what proportion will become FdUMP. There is no evidence that the facilitated transport of these compounds is rate-limiting [113]. FU may be activated by a variety of routes, including pyrimidine phosphoribosyl transferase enzymes which form FUMP, and thymine phosphorylase which forms FUdR (see Fig. 2). The activity of the activating enzymes and levels of the various ribose, deoxyribose and phosphate donors may all determine the route by which FU is activated in a particular cell type. Although FUdR has an apparently one-step activation to FdUMP via thymidine kinase a proportion may be channelled through FU by the action of thymidine phosphorylase. In this manner FUdR may exert the additional RNA effects associated with FU. *In vivo,* as will be discussed in section 5.1. the activity of this enzyme is responsible for almost complete conversion of FUdR to FU.

Measurement of FdUMP levels in various tumours reveals wide variations and it appears that the persistence of FdUMP within the cell may be a more important determinant of sensitivity than peak levels [131, 132]. On the other hand neither may relate to response [148] as the presence of free FdUMP does not necessarily imply good ternary complex formation with TS for reasons already discussed.

FdUMP persists in some cells for longer than may be expected for a pyrimidine. As would be surmised, FdUMP is readily dephosphorylated by phosphatases and a 5′-nucleotidase. It has been shown by Ardalan [135] that the action of these enzymes on free FdUMP ultimately relieves TS of its inhibition as more and more free FdUMP dissociates from the enzyme. The low capacity of human colonic tumours to dephosphorylate FdUMP compared with that of normal intestinal mucosa has been proposed as an explanation for the efficacy of FU in some of these tumours [135]. Myers [130] proposes that the expansion of the dUMP pool as a result of TS inhibiiton may actually protect FdUMP from degradation by competing with the dephosphorylating enzymes. Myers also speculates that the incorporation of FU into RNA may form a depot form for FdUMP, allowing for prolonged TS inhibition.

b) Antifolates

Certain 2,4-diamino quinazoline analogues of folic acid (which are primarily DHFR inhibitors) appear to be transported across the cell membrane by the same system that transports methotrexate and folates, but reach higher intracellular levels than methotrexate [77]. For the 2-amino-4-hydroxy compounds no information is currently available on intracellular levels or how this correlates with sensitivity. However, certain other biochemical features of these compounds contrast sharply with those of the pyrimidine analogues and are intrinsic to their design rationale.

The lack of requirement for metabolic activation ensures that the inhibitor is not dependent on intracellular metabolism to provide the active species. This has three advantages. Firstly metabolites active at another locus are unlikely to be produced unless the inhibitory specificity of the polyglu-tamate forms (which are usually produced) differs widely from that of the parent. Secondly, tissues lacking activating enzymes will not be intrinsically resistant. The third advantage relates to the impossibility of the develop-ment of acquired resistance through deletion of activating enzymes, a known, and common cause of resistance to the fluorinated pyrimidines (sec-tion 4.7). Of course what is not built in to this arguement is the possibility of tumour selectivity based on differential activation.

Although folate-based inhibitors of TS do not require activation, the for-mation of polyglutamate forms may lead to enhanced inhibitory activity. We have already discussed how Fernandes *et al.* [162] describe the new TS inhibitor IAHQ as a prodrug that after polyglutamation (at least to the tri-glutamate) becomes an improved TS inhibitor. If polyglutamation of folate-based TS inhibitors improves their efficacy then the activity of FPGS and the proportion and inhibitory activity of each polyglutamate formed may be determinants of tissue response. As both CB3717 and IAHQ behave as TS inhibitors in culture systems we must assume that the addition of extra glutamate residues does not alter their cytotoxic locus. However, caution may be necessary when testing similar structures to ensure that the polyglu-tamated compound is not a more potent inhibitor of another folate enzyme. For example, the methotrexate pentaglutamate has a greatly increased affin-ity for MCF-7 human breast cell TS (Ki ca 2.0×10^{-8} M) when compared with methotrexate (Ki ca 1×10^{-5} M) [126] but DHFR inhibition is not apparently affected [180].

Interpretation of the effects of polyglutamation of antifolates is further complicated by the existence of polyglutamated forms of the natural folate substrates. These polyglutamated forms generally have lower Km's for the relevant enzymes [179, and reviewed by 123] and the degree of polygluta-mation may itself be affected by the presence of an antifolate [reviewed by 123].

Unlike pyrimidine inhibitors of TS, folate analogues are unlikely to be catabolised extensively. Natural folates are not synthesised *de novo* in mam-malian systems and as may be expected with a vitamin, are not easily cata-bolised. For example, *in vitro*, no catabolic products of methotrexate are described. Even *in vivo* only a small proportion of this drug is converted to metabolites. So, providing folate analogues do not have reactive substi-tuents they may be expected to be relatively stable to catabolism.

Of course lack of catabolism of free drug may result in persistence of the mono or polyglutamated forms intracellularly, the levels ultimately depend-ing on their efflux kinetics. The line dividing the advantages of drug persis-tence in the tumour cells with the disadvantages of prolonged toxicity to normal tissues may be a thin one. Extensive polyglutamation to a form unable to be effluxed may or may not be advantageous. There is conflicting evidence but generally it is accepted that the polyglutamates of methotrexate are less readily effluxed [116, and reviewed by 123].

It has been suggested in recent years that folic acid, reduced folates and methotrexate all share the same transport system [181] although the Km for folic acid is markedly higher than those for the reduced folates or methotrexate. The mechanism is active so that folates are concentrated within the cell. Thus methotrexate and other non-lipid soluble antifolates may achieve the intracellular concentrations necessary to inhibit DHFR. Very little information is currently available on the transport of the 2-amino-4-hydroxy quinazoline antifolates designed as TS inhibitors. We have recently tried to measure the transport of ^{14}C CB3717 into L1210 cells. Initial results suggested that accumulation of the drug was slow but until the higher specific activity ^{3}H label is available we are unable to examine the kinetics more thoroughly. However, the transport process appeared to be temperature dependent suggesting an active process.

Other unpublished observations suggest that in L1210 cells grown in culture, at a toxic concentration of CB3717 (50 µM), the drug may only reach 1–2 µM within 6 hours despite the fact that ^{3}H deoxyuridine incorporation is markedly reduced within 1 hour. This would suggest that the inhibition reaches a sufficiently high concentration within the cell at this time to affect TS despite the fact that equilibrium has not been reached. In this respect the apparently poor transport of the drug may be compensated for by its high affinity for TS. These results need to be substantiated but it would seem that the high dose requirement for CB3717 relates to poor transport. However, mutant cell lines which transport methotrexate poorly and consequently are resistant to this drug are not significantly cross-resistant to CB3717 [167]. This suggests that CB3717 has transport characteristics different from those of methotrexate which may bestow an advantage upon this drug.

4.4.3 *Enzyme Levels*
The level of TS in a particular tumour or normal tissue may reasonably be expected to be a determinant of the cytotoxicity of a TS inhibitor. Washtein *et al.* studied 5 gastrointestinal carcinoma lines in culture and found that those with the lower levels were more sensitive to FUdR [178]. However, *in vivo*, Houghton using colonic xenografts found that no correlation existed between sensitivity and enzyme levels, but that the factor limiting sensitivity to fluorinated pyrimidines was not enzyme levels, but rather the availability of the cosubstrate $5,10\text{-}CH_2FH_4$ [177].

4.4.4 *Discussion*
In the preceeding section we have discussed the various biochemical factors

which may modulate the inhibition of TS in tumour cells. Generally, these considerations would favour an antifolate rather than a pyrimidine analogue as a general method for inducing this inhibition. It is, however, possible that such an inhibition could be non-toxic if a sufficient source of exogenous thymidine were present to supply the substrate requirement for DNA synthesis. This possibility is the subject of the next section.

4.5 The Significance of the TdR Salvage Pathway

The presence of an active TdR salvage pathway confers upon the cell the capability to by-pass any inhibition of thymidylate synthetase. Generally cells grown in culture have virtually no TdR available to them from the medium and serum supplement. The addition of exogenous TdR to the cell suspension is therefore a valuable way to investigate the locus of action of putative TS inhibitors. TdR prevents the cytotoxicity of both CB3717 and IAHQ in culture [127, 162, 80].

It would be rather naive to consider TdR protection or reversal experiments as simply a method of by-passing the effects on TS. For example, whereas the combination of TdR and FU will indeed have this effect, thereby isolating the effects of FU on RNA metabolism, this should not be regarded as evidence that the RNA effects are or are not the cytotoxic events in cells exposed to FU alone. Indeed FU incorporation into RNA may be augmented by TdR resulting in enhanced anti-tumour activity [151].

When TdR is used to protect from FUdR toxicity in culture not only will TdR by-pass any TS inhibitor, but also it may compete with FUdR for both transport [183] and thymidine kinase [135]. The concentrations of TdR used has often exceeded that of FUdR by several orders of magnitude making the interpretation of the results inconclusive.

When reversing the effect of an antimetabolite by providing the depleted metabolite exogenously, it will clearly be necessary to provide sufficient to allow for its utilization by the cell for DNA synthesis. It can be calculated that 1 µmole of TdR is necessary to provide the thymine residues in the DNA of 10^5 murine cells. It is therefore not surprising that a high dose of thymidine is necessary for reversal of TS inhibitors in culture. As thymidine is utilised for DNA synthesis there is a progressive fall in the extracellular thymidine level [184, 185]. This, coupled with the fact that TdR is catabolised to thymine in the medium, complicates the estimation of the minimal steady state extracellular TdR concentration from which cells can salvage thymidine effectively in the presence of a block on *de novo* synthesis of thymidylate. By reducing the initial cell inoculum and monitoring the ^{14}C thymidine in the culture medium throughout the experiments Jackman *et al.* [185] have established that the critical concentration of TdR in the medium, below which L1210 cells will salvage inadequately, is approximately 0.1 μM. The implications of these results in relation to plasma TdR levels are discussed in section 5.3.

With the recent interest in human tumour cloning techniques it may be pertinent here to point out one particular problem associated with such techniques. Human tumours may be exposed to the drug under investigation in tissue culture medium containing a significant quantity of thymidine. For example CMRL 1066 has as much as $\sim 1 \times 0^{-5}$ M TdR, a quantity sufficient to protect a number of cell lines from the toxicity of TS inhibitors. Even pre-incubation in a thymidineless medium will probably not overcome this problem. For instance we know that TdR will reverse the toxicity of CB3717 to WIL2 cells in suspension culture even if it is added to the medium after many hours of exposure [127]. Unless human tumour cloning assays employ media devoid of such high quantities of salvageable precursors, it is difficult to imagine how antimetabolites such as CB3717 or IAHQ can be evaluated in these systems.

4.6 *Secondary Effects Associated With TS Inhibition*
4.6.1 *Misincorporation of Uracil into DNA*
We have already discussed how the decreased TTP pool that occurs as a result of TS inhibition may derepress feedback inhibition on other enzymes in pyrimidine metabolism (section 4.4.1a). The normal function of this regulatory role of TTP is to control its own synthesis via both *de novo* and salvage pathways. However when the *de novo* pathway is inhibited (in the absence of sufficient salvageable TdR) the effects of decreased TTP become evident. In recent years it has been proposed that the cytotoxicity of inhibitors of thymidylate synthesis may not be entirely due to a decreased TTP pool but additionally due to an increase in the dUTP:TTP ratio [186, 187, 127, 188]. Uracil is not a normal component of DNA even though dUTP may replace TTP as a substrate for DNA polymerase [189]. The reason for failure to detect uracil in DNA is twofold, first the presence of the enzyme UTPase that hydrolyses any dUTP formed back to dUMP and PPi. Second, any uracil that may be incorporated is removed by uracil – DNA glycosylase and the excision subsequently repaired by the insertion of a thymidine residue. Where TS is inhibited either directly by FUdR or CB3717 or indirectly by MTX the resultant accumulation of dUMP leads to a smaller but significant increase in dUTP levels despite the action of dUTPase [186, 190, 127]. Goulian *et al.* showed the presence of uracil in mammalian DNA after exposure to methotrexate, presumably as a consequence of a raised dUTP pool [188]. The levels of dUTP in WIL2 human lymphoblastoid cells treated with an ID_{50} dose of CB3717 or methotrexate have also been reported and were only slightly lower than the TTP levels [127]. A

similar increase in the dUTP:TTP ratio has been shown previously in methotrexate treated cells [186]. A cyclic process of futile excision and repair has been proposed to be a possible mechanism by which such drugs exert their cytotoxic effects [186]. However, Jackson *et al.* failed to demonstrate potentiation of CB3717 by the addition of deoxyuridine. Further, the inhibition of dUMP accumulation by pyrazofurin or PALA did not antagonise the cytotoxicity of CB3717 [127]. These results do not therefore support the hypothesis that uracil misincorporation into DNA contributes to the cytotoxicity of TS inhibitors. However, this subject is still under intensive investigation and recently dUDP-GLc-NAc has been identified in human lymphoid cells treated with methotrexate [191]. It is assumed that this is formed from dUTP and offers an alternative pathway for limiting the accumulation of dUTP (the other being dUTPase). Whether cells deficient in one or both of these enzymes may more readily succumb to the proposed cytotoxic effects of misincorporation of uracil into DNA is as yet unknown.

4.6.2 *Modulation of The TdR Salvage Pathway*
It has been suggested that the high levels of dUMP found in cells where TS is inhibited may compete with thymidylate for thymidylate kinase [186]. Similarly the documented increase in intracellular levels of the corresponding nucleoside, deoxyuridine, after methotrexate or FUdR treatment [171] may compete with TdR for thymidine kinase. The net effect of these two changes could be inhibit TdR salvage although preliminary evidence suggests that the addition of a high concentration (100 µM) of extracellular deoxyuridine does not interfere with the salvage of 1 µM thymidine in the presence of a cytotoxic dose of CB3717 (unpublished observation, A.L. Jackman and G.A. Taylor).

In conclusion, inhibition of TS results not only in a fall in the TTP pool, but a general disturbance in deoxypyrimidine metabolism. Whether these disturbances participate in the efficacy of the TS inhibitors *in vitro* or *in vivo* is not clear.

4.7 *Resistance*
The development of resistance to antimetabolites is a common problem in patients receiving treatment. Although the causes of acquired resistance to agents such as methotrexate or FU are well defined experimentally, they are not so well studied in man. Perhaps the most intensively investigated mechanism of resistance is the overproduction of DHFR in cells exposed to methotrexate [reviewed by 192, 193]. This has been shown to be associated with amplification of the DHFR gene in cells grown *in vitro* [reviewed by 193]. An increase in DHFR has been measured in the cells of patients

receiving methotrexate and recently amplification of the DHFR gene has been documented in one patient who exhibited this type of resistance [194].

Resistance to methotrexate in experimental tumours may also be the result of reduced membrane transport, or the production of an altered enzyme with a decreased affinity for methotrexate [reviewed by 192].

Experimental resistance to FU has been associated with the deletion of the activating enzymes uridine kinase [195], nucleoside phosphorylase [196], uracil phosphoribosyl transferase [197] and pyrimidine monophosphate kinase [135]. An altered TS enzyme with lower affinity for FdUMP has also been reported [231].

Resistance to FUdR is normally associated with deletion of thymidine kinase [198] so that the active metabolite FdUMP is not formed. A small overproduction of TS by a cultured hepatoma cell line has been reported by Priest et al. [199]. Overproduction of TS has also been documented by Baskin et al. [200] although the authors point out that the relatively small increase in enzyme (8-fold) does not correlate with the very high degree of resistance observed suggesting that another unidentified mechanism is also present. As FUdR administered in vivo is converted to FU by the action of thymidine phosphorylase, acquired clinical resistance to the fluorinated pyrimidines is likely to occur by the same mechanisms as those described for FU resistance in experimental systems. Thus there are a number of diverse mechanisms by which cells may develop resistance to the fluorinated pyrimidines.

Most antifolates are active inhibitors in the absence of metabolic activation, although increased inhibitory activity may be expected as the result of the formation of polyglutamates. Deletion of FPGS has not been documented as a cause of resistance (indeed it seems to be a lethal lesion to the cell) [reviewed by 123] therefore we may expect resistance to folate-based TS inhibitors to be mediated either by a defect in cell membrane transport or by a change in the quantity or kinetics of the target enzyme, TS. Several L1210 monoclonal sub-lines with acquired resistance to CB3717 have been developed [168]. These lines overproduce TS by about 30-fold and purification and kinetic analysis of the enzyme indicated that the form of the enzyme was identical to that of the parent line [168, 182]. The cells maintain their resistant properties in the absence of CB3717 (> 300 cell doublings).

We therefore have examples of several types of acquired resistance to antimetabolites that have their cytotoxic loci associated completely or in part to inhibition of the de novo synthesis of thymidylate. The study of the mechanisms of resistance and studies of cross-resistance with other drugs have been useful in elucidating the loci of action of compounds designed as

TS inhibitors. A number of cell lines with acquired resistance to methotrexate, by virtue of overproduction of DHFR demonstrated practically no cross-resistance to CB3717 although they did to other DHFR inhibitors [167, 80]. These observations are consistent with the concept that DHFR is not the locus for CB3717. Further, two cell lines resistant to methotrexate by virtue of a transport defect have been reported not to be significantly cross-resistant with CB3717 [167], suggesting that it may be transported by a different route from methotrexate.

The L1210 cell lines with acquired resistance to CB3717 due to a 30fold overproduction of TS are not significantly cross-resistant to methotrexate. The small overproduction of DHFR (~5fold) probably accounts for the minimal amount of cross-resistance observed (Table 2). These cell lines were also not cross-resistant to either FU or FUdR suggesting that TS was not a locus of action of either of these latter compounds in these cells. This observation is particularly hard to reconcile with the literature on FUdR cytotoxicity to other cell lines. The authors are currently examining various biochemical parameters in these cells in order to establish the mechanism by which the fluorinated pyrimidines act in both the parent and resistant L1210 cell lines.

5.   IN VIVO STUDIES OF THYMIDYLATE SYNTHETASE INHIBITORS

5.1 *Pharmacokinetics and Metabolism of 5-Flourouracil and 5-Fluorodeoxyuridine*
5.5.1 *5-Fluorouracil*
Following an intravenous bolus some clinical studies have demonstrated a monophasic decay of the plasma levels with a half life of 10–20 min [204–

Table 2. Cross-resistance studies with an L1210 cell line with acquired resistance to CB3717

Compound	ID_{50} in culture (at 48 hrs) (μM)		L1210 R/L1210 S
	L1210 (S)	L1210 (R) [1]	
CB3717	5	> 1000	> 200
AHQ	5	500	100
Methotrexate	0.011	0.070	6.4
FU	0.84	1.3	1.5
FUdR	0.0026	0.0025	1.0

[1] L1210 (R) – overproduces TS ~ 30 fold and DFHR ~ 5 fold. Thymidine kinase activity is unchanged.
Data of D.L. Alison and A.L. Jackman

206] while in others it was biphasic with half lives of approximately 8 and 40 minutes [207, 208]. It is possible that the plasma half life may be prolonged slightly at the end of a 5-day course. It is notable that little variation between patients [204–206] was apparent, and that evidence that retention was associated with toxicity was scant. It appears that the pharmacokinetics of FU are dose dependent [207–209] due to saturation of the enzyme dihydrouracil dehydrogenase which is responsible for the initial degradation of FU to 5,6-dihydro-5-fluorouracil [210]. This catabolism is the major route of elimination of FU and largely takes place in the liver. Plasma levels of FU have been reported to be raised in patients with hepatic metastases [204]. Clearly the important determinant of FU toxicity and therapeutic effect will relate to the levels of phosphorylated species retained within the cell. Evidence exists to suggest that these may form a depot, from which FU may be slowly released causing a third plasma half life [211].

5.1.2 5-Fluorodeoxyuridine
The pharmacokinetics of this compound are less studied than those of FU. There is no doubt that FUdR is converted rapidly to FU in cancer patients, primarily by hepatic metabolism although thymidine phosphorylase activity has also been detected in human plasma [236].

5.2 Pharmacokinetics and Metabolism of CB3717
The clinical and experimental pharmacology of the quinazoline CB3717 have been reported in abstract form. Following a one hour intravenous infusion in man, plasma decay was biphasic with mean half lives of 70 min and 9 hours. Metabolites were not detected in urine or plasma, but the desglutamyl derivative was found in faeces [212]. A similar pattern was seen in rats. In this species it was possible to demonstrate that the desglutamyl metabolite was not formed in the faeces of rats following gut sterilisation with neomycin, suggesting that this metabolite is formed by bacteria [161]. In many ways the reported pharmacokinetics and metabolism of CB3717 are similar to those of methotrexate [154] with the chief differences being: (1) the beta half life of CB3717 is somewhat longer, (2) CB3717 is cleared less in the urine (ca 25%) and more in the bile (ca 75%) [212] and (3) the protein binding of CB3717 is higher than that of methotrexate. It may be speculated that a drug with a relatively long persistence in the plasma is more likely to be distributed to poorly vascularised areas than is one which is rapidly degraded.

5.3 Plasma Nucleosides
The plasma levels of thymidine have been reported to fall in patients following the administration of methotrexate [213]. It is clearly important to document the changes in plasma nucleoside levels following the administra-

tion of antimetabolites since they affect the availability of 'salvage' precursors. Jackman and Taylor measured the levels of thymidine and deoxyuridine in mice treated with CB3717. Following a single dose of CB3717 plasma deoxyuridine levels rose ca. 6-fold peaking after 4 hours, but declined to normal within 24 hours [155, 156]. This is most probably the result of an increase in intracellular dUMP such as is observed following TS inhibition *in vitro* [127]. Plasma thymidine levels also rose slightly initially but rapidly returned to normal. When CB3717 was administered for 5 consecutive days the plasma thymidine level measured 24 hours after each dose fell progressively and reached a nadir 24 hours after the final injection recovering by three days thereafter. The level at the nadir was dose dependent and at the highest dose used (200 mg/kg) was approximately one third of the pre-treatment level [185]. Even at the nadir, the plasma thymidine level (~ 0.47 µM) in mice still exceeded the normal levels reported for man (~ 0.1 µM).

In view of the large differences observed in normal plasma TdR levels between mice (> 1 µM) [156, 239, 185] and man (0.1 µM) [156, 240–242] it seems that the results of experimentation on rodents should be extrapolated to man only with great caution. If the experiments concern fluorinated pyrimidines the possible interactions of plasma nucleosides with FU and its metabolites are many and vary in different test systems (see 6.1). In the case of folate-based TS inhibitors man may be intrinsically more sensitive, particularly if TdR levels fall during treatment. This is concluded from *in vitro* TdR salvage experiments briefly described in section 4.5. These experiments also predicted that TS inhibitors should be inactive in mice because of the high TdR levels circulating in these animals. CB3717 is not toxic to the normal proliferating tissues of mice (gut and bone marrow) when given at maximally tolerated doses. In general, the antitumour effect of this compound against murine tumours is modest or absent (see section 5.4). The one exception is the L1210 tumour used at the Institute of Cancer Research. This tumour is exceptionally responsive to CB3717 but the antitumour activity of the drug can be completely prevented by co-administration of TdR, an observation consistent with the locus of action of the drug. The antitumour activity of TS inhibitors is the subject of the next section.

5.4 *Antitumour Studies*
5.4.1 *CB3717*
CB3717 (~ 100 mg/kg) was used in a daily $\times 5$ schedule (starting three days after i.p. tumour innoculation) and was curative to the L1210 tumour carried at the Institute of Cancer Research [80]. These results were subsequently confirmed [185, and unpublished communications]. The 80–100% cure rate obtained was significantly better than the 0–20% rate obtained when methotrexate was administered at the optimal dose (4 mg/kg daily $\times 5$).

Even when the tumour was innoculated i.v. and CB3717 injected i.p. a very substantial antitumour response was obtained at 240 mg/kg (~40% cures) [155]. Other tumours reported were either partially responsive (eg PC6 plasmacytoma [155], or the L1210 tumour carried at the NCI) or non-responsive (eg TLX/5 lymphoma) [155]. The antitumour results are summarised in Table 3. All *in vitro* tumours (animal and human) so far tested have been similarly sensitive to CB3717, the ID_{50} values ranging between 1 and 5 μM [80, 127, 167, 243].

We have already suggested in the previous section that caution must be used in interpreting data obtained in rodents. Not only may the activity against tumours (rodent or human xenografts) be prevented by circulating TdR, but also the toxicity to normal tissues.

5.4.2 IAHQ

This compound is reported to be active against the colon tumour 38. At 85 mg/kg injected on days 2 and 10 after subcutaneous tumour innoculation 6 out of 10 mice were tumour free at day 90.

Table 3. Antitumour activity of CB3717 in murine systems

Tumour	Tumour innocula-tion	Drug route	Drug schedule	Result (at optimal dose)	Ref.	Activity relative to methotrexate (at optimal dose)
L1210–ICR subline	IP	IP	daily × 5	80–90% cures	80,185	better
L1210–ICR subline	IV	IP	daily × 5	40% cures	155	better
L1210–NCI subline	IP	IP	daily × 5	<10% ILS	1*	—
L1210–NCI subline	IP	IP	daily × 9	~40% ILS	2*,3*	worse
TLX–5 lymphoma	SC	IP	daily × 5	<22% ILS	155	worse
TLX–5 lymphoma	IP	IP	daily × 5	<25% ILS	1*	worse
ADJ/PC6 plasmacytoma	SC	IP	daily × 5	80% inhibit. of tumour growth	155	better
P388	IP	IP	daily × 5	minimal ILS	3*	worse
Colon 38	SC	IP	days 1,9	40% inhibit.	3*	—

* Refs.: 1 Unpublished observation AL Jackman
    2 Personal communication M. Wolpert, NCI
    3 Personal communication Dr. Atassi, Inst. Jules Bordet, Brussels

The ID_{50} concentration of IAHQ against several cell lines grown in culture was similar to that of CB3717 or AHQ i.e. $\sim 5\,\mu M$ [162]. However IAHQ was more toxic to HCT-8 cells (a human colon adenocarcinoma cell line), the ID_{50} being $0.5\,\mu M$.

6. CLINICAL PROPERTIES OF TS INHIBITORS

6.1 *Pyrimidine Analogues*
6.1.1 *5-Flurouracil*
5-Fluorouracil (FU) was introduced into clinical practice shortly after its discovery by Heidelberger and his co-workers in 1957 and has remained a widely used drug since that time. It is now extensively used as a single agent for the palliative treatment of metastatic gastro-intestinal tumours, particularly those of the colon and rectum. It is also used in combination therapy for the treatment of carcinoma of the breast, pancreas and head and neck. It is perhaps surprising that FU, unlike other antimetabolites, has never found a place in the treatment of leukaemias or in any other 'curative' schedule. However, the clinical role of FU, whether alone or in combination, may not have been fully evaluated. For example, recent reports [214] show that a 50% complete response rate may be achieved in head and neck tumours by the combination of fluorouracil and cisplatinum. If these results are reproducible they may well represent a significant advance not only in the treatment of head and neck tumours, but also in our utilisation of FU in combination therapy in general.

FU was designed, in part, to interfere with the methylation of the uracil moiety to form the thymine moiety (later defined as the reaction catabolised by TS) and until recently was indeed thought to act as such. Newer experimental evidence (see section 4.2) suggests that its cytotoxicity is frequently not due to TS inhibition, but rather due to its incorporation into nucleic acids. Clinically, studies of the co-administration of thymidine have demonstrated that the maximal tolerated dose of FU is decreased rather than increased by thymidine, again arguing against TS being the only locus responsible for producing the cytotoxic effects of the drug in man [215–217]. For these reasons, only the clinical applications of FU in which an attempt has been made to exploit the interaction of the drug with TS will be considered in more detail. The sequenced combination of methotrexate and FU and the use of FU in combination with folinic acid are examples of such applications.

a) Methotrexate – 5-Fluorouracil Combinations
A number of pieces of evidence exist to suggest that if methotrexate and FU

are used in combination, synergistic cytotoxicity may be achieved if exposure to methotrexate preceeds that to FU. Tattersall *et al.* argued that prior exposure to FU would prevent the depletion of tetrahydrofolate pools (meditated by TS catalysis) by the subsequent administration of methotrexate and that consequently the combination would be antagonistic [128]. They therefore advocated the reverse sequence and also showed an enhanced antitumour effect for the simultaneous combination against the L1210 tumour *in vivo*. More recently the concept has been explored in some detail by the group at Yale University. They were able to show that the methotrexate, particularly in its polyglutamate forms, was able to enhance the binding of FU to TS in the same manner as the normal cofactor 5,10-CH_2FH_4 [218]. Further, methotrexate treatment, due to its inhibition of *de novo* purine synthesis, led to an increase in the intracellular phosphoribosylpyrophosphate pool and consequently an increase in the activation of FU to the nucleotide form [219]. Increased levels of FUTP and dUMP were noted. Incorporation of FU into RNA was also increased. It was suggested that synergistic toxicity to the bone marrow would not occur owing to the reliance of this tissue on salvage pathways for purine synthesis [220].

The clinical efficacy of sequential methotrexate and FU has been evaluated in a number of studies of breast cancer, head and neck cancer and gastrointestinal cancer [221–227]. A wide range of methotrexate doses (40–1500 mg/m^2) FU doses (300–1500 mg/m^2) and time intervals (1–24 hours) have been employed. The reported response rates are 14–53% (breast cancer), 64 and 71% (head and neck cancer) and 0–80% (gastrointestinal cancer). The results of the two head and neck studies were particularly promising because a large number of complete responses (54% and 31%) were reported. Unfortunately these latter results have not been confirmed by two prospective randomised studies. Browman *et al.* randomised 79 patients to receive sequential or simultaneous treatment and documented a higher response rate in the simultaneous group, although this difference was not significant [228]. Coates *et al.* made a three way comparison of methotrexate – FU simultaneously or in either sequence and were unable to show any advantage for sequential therapy [229]. A number of explanations are available to explain this failure. Certain of the metabolic disturbances induced by methotrexate, notably the increase in the dUMP pool and the decrease of the tetrahydrofolate pools are inimical to the binding of 5-fluorouracil. One could also argue that an exposure to methotrexate sufficient to lead to the formation of amounts of methotrexate polyglutamates large enough to substitute for the 5,10-CH_2FH_4 would already have led to a virtual cessation of TS catalysis due to cofactor depletion, so that the subsequent binding of FdUMP had no additional function. The clinical protocols used in the sequential combinations have all employed folinic acid rescue, albeit given some hours after the FU. However, the possibility that the high response rates observed were not due to the proposed synergistic interaction of FU with folinic acid and (see below) cannot be completely excluded. Finally Tattersall has suggested that plasma purine levels in the region of the tumour may be higher than was thought and that the preservation of *de novo* purine synthesis via the salvage pathways prevents the depletion of PRPP [230]. The difficulty in making accurate ad hoc prediction of synergy or antagonism for drug combinations even in an area where an enormous amount of background knowledge is available, emphasizes the need for the further development of mathematical models.

b) 5-Fluorouracil – Folinic Acid Combinations

Ample biochemical evidence exists to suggest that the binding of FdUMP, the metabolite of FU, to TS may frequently be inadequate to achieve a rate-limiting inhibition of this step. One of the factors prejudicing the binding *in vivo* may be the low levels of the cofactor $5,10\text{-}CH_2FH_4$ necessary for binding (see 4.4.1). This suggests that the increase of folate cofactors may enhance the binding of FdUMP to such an extent that TS becomes the primary locus. A number of clinical studies have attempted to exploit this phenomenon by administering folinic acid concurrently with FU. Machover *et al.* [232] studied thirty patients with advanced colorectal and gastric tumours. FU was given at a dose of $400 \text{ mg/m}^2/\text{day}$ for 5 days and folinic acid at $200 \text{ mg/m}^2/\text{day}$. Nine of 16 patients who had received no previous chemotherapy responded to treatment, and, remarkably 3/14 patients who were resistant to FU given as a single agent responded. Toxicity was primarily haemotological and mucosal.

6.1.2 *5-Fluorodeoxyuridine (FUdR)*

This drug, the deoxynucleoside of 5-fluorouracil, has received less clinical attention, probably because its rapid conversion to FU in plasma [236] has meant that its clinical effects are similar to those of FU [233], even though its cytotoxicity *in vitro* is considerably greater than that of FU (see table 2). A number of groups have used FUdR by intrahepatic arterial perfusion in an attempt to subject hepatic metastases to its toxic effects directly [234–237]. Consistently high response rates ($> 50\%$) for metastases from gastrointestinal tumours have been noted following either FU or FUdR administration. It is of interest to note that the degree of toxicity to the normal hepatic tissue as evidenced by a rise in the peripheral aspartate aminotransferase activities is greater following FUdR administration than following FU (52% and 10% of patients respectively). The chief side effect seen clinically with a folate TS inhibitor has been elevated transaminase levels.

6.2 *Folate Analogue – CB3717*

Only one folate analogue designed as an inhibitor of thymidylate synthetase has, to the knowledge of the authors, been evaluated clinically. This is the N^{10}-propargyl-5,8-dideaza analogue of folic acid, CB3717. Clinical results to date are reported only in preliminary abstract form [238]. A phase I clinical trial was commenced in September 1981 and 88 patients received 225 treatments. Doses were dissolved in 250 ml of 0.15 M $NaHCO_3$ (pH 9.0) and infused over 1 hour every 3 weeks. The starting dose of 140 mg/m^2 was escalated to 550 mg/m^2. Reversible hepatic toxicity associated with malaise occurred in 66/80 assessable patients of whom 29 had normal liver function tests prior to treatment. Thirty eight experienced rises in alanine transaminase levels to >2 times the normal laboratory range and 15 had elevations to 1–2 times normal values. Rises in alkaline phosphatase levels also occurred. A self-limiting rash appeared in 10 patients and radiation recall was seen in 2. Leukopaenia developed in 11 patients (WBC $<3 \times 10^9/L$). The nadir was 9–12 days followed by recovery at 14–16 days. Neither the incidence nor the severity of any of these toxicities was dose-related. Renal toxicity, detected by a fall in ^{51}Cr EDTA clearance values was observed in 3 patients at doses ≥ 400 mg/m^2. It was anticipated that the maximum tolerated dose would be in the region of 600 mg/m^2 with renal toxicity being dose-limiting. Responses to treatment occurred at doses ≥ 200 mg/m^2 in 55 evaluable patients and were: ovary 1 CR, 1 PR, 3 MR/12; breast 2 PR, 1 MR/8; adenocarcinoma lung 1 PR, 4 MR/7; mesothelioma 1 PR/5; bowel 2 MR/4 (CR = complete response, PR = partial response, MR = minor response). A dose of 400 mg/m^2 caused only mild toxicity and it was anticipated that the recommended phase II dose using that particular schedule of administration would be in this range.

In this clinical study definite signs of antitumour activity have been seen in patients resistant to methotrexate and 5-fluorouracil in the doses used in the 'CMF' protocol thus demonstrating that the approach of designing a folate inhibitor aimed at a different locus can, by whatever mechanism, overcome clinical resistance. The presence of dose-limiting nephrotoxicity, probably related to the deposition of the drug in the tubules demonstrates the need for more potent analogues with a lower dose requirement.

7. FINAL COMMENTS

The idea of utilising TS as a cytotoxic locus was conceived many years ago. However, this enzyme has proved more difficult both to study and to inhibit than DHFR. The technology necessary to purify and study homogenous human TS has only been developed during the past few years. During the same space of time specific inhibitors of the enzyme have been character-

198

ised. The compounds developed appear to have different toxicities and anti-tumour effects compared to either methotrexate or FU. In particular it is notable that mucosal toxicity has not been reported for the 2-amino-4-hydroxyquinazolines. The experimental antitumour spectrum of these qui-nazolines at first sight appears to be more limited, although different, from that of methotrexate. However, recent advances in our understanding of the interaction of the inhibitors and the intracellular and extracellular pools of nucleotides and nucleosides suggest that placing too much reliance upon murine screens may be unwise.

Clinically, the one compound evaluated which may reasonably be ex-pected to act as a pure TS inhibitor *in vivo* does indeed seem to be showing antitumour activity. This activity has been seen both in patients whose tumours had previously been resistant to methotrexate or FU and in patients with tumours not normally sensitive to either of these drugs. Only time and further effort will tell whether compounds of this class form a useful addition to the pharmacopoeia.

REFERENCES

1. Friedkin M, Kornberg A: The enzymatic conversion of deoxyuridylic acid to thymidylic acid and the participation of tetrahydrofolic acid. In: The chemical basis of heredity, McElroy WD, Glass B (eds). Baltimore: The John Hopkins Press, pp 609–614, 1957.
2. Cohen SS, Flaks JG, Barner HD, Loeb MR, Lichtenstein J: The mode of action of 5-fluorouracil and its derivatives. Proc Natl Acad Sci USA 44:1004–1012, 1958.
3. Farber S, Diamond LK, Mercer RD, Sylvester RF, Wolff JA: Temporary remissions in acute leukaemia in children produced by folic acid antagonist, 4-aminopteroyl-glutamic acid (aminopterin). New Eng J Med 238:787–793, 1948.
4. Futterman S: Enzymatic reduction of folic acid and dihydrofolic acid to tetrahydrofolic acid: J Biol Chem 288:1031–1038, 1957.
5. Woods DD: The relation of p-aminobenzoic acid to the mechanism of the action of sul-phanilamide. Brit J Exptl Pathol 21:74–90, 1940.
6. Blakley RL: The biochemistry of folic acid and related pteridines. Amsterdam: North Holland publishing Company, 1969.
7. Friedkin M: Thymidylate synthetase, Adv Enzymol 38:235–292, 1973.
8. Danenberg PV: Thymidylate synthetase – a target enzyme in cancer chemotherapy. Biochim Biophys Acta 473:73–92, 1977.
9. Danenberg PV, Lockshin A: Fluorinated pyrimidines as tight-binding inhibitors of thymi-dylate synthetase. Pharmac Ther 13:69–90, 1981.
10. Lewis JR CA, Dunlap RB: Thymidylate synthetase and its interaction with 5-fluoro-2'-deoxyuridylate. In: Topics in molecular pharmacology, Burgen ASV, Roberts GCK (eds). Amsterdam: Elsevier/North Holland Biomedical Press, 1981, pp 169–219.
11. Maley F, Maley GF: Studies on identifying the locus of action of fluorouracil. In: Mole-cular actions and targets for cancer chemotherapeutic agents, Sartorelli AC, Lazo JS, Ber-tino JR (eds). New York: Academic Press, pp 265–283, 1981.
12. Santi DV: Inhibition of thymidylate synthetase: Mechanism, methods and metabolic con-

sequences. In: Molecular actions and targets for cancer chemotherapeutic agents, Sartorelli AC, Lazo JS, Bertino JR (eds). New York: Academic Press, pp 285–300, 1981.

13. Danenberg PV, Lockshin A: Thymidylate synthetase – substrate complex formation. Mol Cellul Biochem 43:49–57, 1982.

14. Jencks WP: Mechanism and catalysis of simple carbonyl group reactions. Prog Phys Org Chem 2:63–128, 1964.

15. Pogolotti Jr AL, Ivanetich KM, Sommer H, Santi DV: Thymidylate synthetase: Studies on the peptide containing covalently bound 5-fluoro-2′-deoxyuridylate and 5,10-methylenetetrahydrofolate. Biochem Biophys Res Comm 70:972–978, 1976.

16. Pastore EJ, Friedkin M: The enzymatic synthesis of thymidylate. J Biol Chem 237:3802–3810, 1962.

17. Blakley RL, Ramasastri BV, McDougall BM: The biosynthesis of thymidylic acid. J Biol Chem 238:3075–3097, 1963.

18. Tatum C, Vederas J, Schleicher E, Benkovic SJ, Floss H: Stereospecifity of thymidylate synthetase. J Chem Soc Chem Comm:218–220, 1977.

19. Slieker LJ, Benkovic SJ: Synthesis of (6R,11S)- and (6R,11R)-5,10-methylene[11-^{1}H,^{2}H]tetrahydrofolate. Stereochemical paths of serine hydroxymethyltransferase, 5,10-methylenetetrahydrofolate dehydrogenase, and thymidylate synthetase catalysis. J Am Chem Soc 106:1833–1838, 1984.

20. Leary RP, Gaumont Y, Kisliuk RL: Effects of the diastereoisomers of methylenetrahydrofolate on the reaction catalysed by thymidylate synthetase. Biochem Biophys Res Comm 56:484–488, 1974.

21. Crusberg TC, Leary R, Kisliuk RL: Properties of thymidylate synthetase from dichloromethotrexate-resistant *Lactobacillus casei*. J Biol Chem 245:5292–5296, 1970.

22. Reid VE, Friedkin M: Thymidylate synthetase in mouse erythrocytes infected with *Plasmodium berghei*. Mol Pharmacol 9:74–80, 1973.

23. Scanlon KJ, Cashmore AR, Moroson BA, Dreyer RN, Bertino JR: Inhibition of serine metabolism by tetrahydrohomofolate in L1210 mouse leukemia cells. Mol Pharmacol 19:481–490, 1981.

24. Taylor RT, Hanna ML: 5-Methyltetrahydrohomofolate: A substrate for cobalamin methyltransferases and an inhibitor of cell growth. Arch Biochem Biophys 163:122–132, 1974.

25. Plante LT, Crawford EJ, Friedkin M: Enzyme studies with new analogues of folic acid and homofolic acid. J Biol Chem 242:1466–1475, 1967.

26. Plante LT, Crawford EJ, Friedkin M: Polyglutamyl and polylysyl derivatives of the lysine analogues of folic acid and homofolic acid. J Med Chem 19:1295–1299, 1976.

27. Kisliuk RL, Strumpf D, Gaumont Y, Leary RP, Plante L: Diastereoisomers of 5,10-methylene-5,6,7,8-tetrahydropteroyl-D-glutamic acid. J Med Chem 20:1531–1533, 1977.

28. Lorenson MY, Maley GF, Maley F: The purification and properties of thymidylate synthetase from chick embryo extracts. J Biol Chem 242:3332–3344, 1967.

29. Dunlap RB, Harding NGL, Huennekens FM: Thymidylate synthetase from amethopterin-resistant *Lactobacillus casei*. Biochemistry 10:88–97, 1971.

30. Gupta VS, Meldrum JB: Purification and properties of thymidylate synthetase from pig thymus. Can J Biochem 50:352–362, 1972.

31. Kalman TI, Bloch A, Szekeres GL, Bardos TJ: Methylation of 4-thio-2′-deoxyuridylate by thymidylate synthetase. Biochem Biophys Res Comm 55:210–217, 1973.

32. Haertlé T, Wohlrab F, Guschlbauer W: Thymidylate synthetase from *Escherichia coli* K12. Eur J Biochem 102:223–230, 1979.

33. Galivan JH, Maley GF, Maley F: Factors affecting substrate binding in *Lactobacillus casei* thymidylate synthetase as studied by equilibrium dialysis. Biochemistry 15:356–362, 1976.

34. Daron HH, Aull JL: A kinetic study of thymidylate synthetase from *Lactobacillus casei*. J Biol Chem 253:940–945, 1978.
35. Dolnick BJ, Cheng YC: Human thymidylate synthetase derived from blast cells of patients with acute myelocytic leukemia. J Biol Chem 252:7697–7703, 1977.
36. Danenberg PV, Danenberg KD: Effect of 5,10-methylenetetrahydrofolate on the dissociation of 5-fluoro-2'-deoxyuridylate from thymidylate synthetase: evidence for an ordered mechanism. Biochemistry 17:4018–4024, 1978.
37. Langenbach RJ, Danenberg PV, Heidelberger C: Thymidylate synthetase: mechanism of inhibition by 5-fluoro-2'-deoxyuridylate. Biochem Biophys Res Comm 48:1565–1571, 1972.
38. Lockshin A, Danenberg PV: Biochemical factors affecting the tightness of 5-fluorodeoxyuridylate binding to human thymidylate synthetase. Biochem Pharmacol 30:247–257, 1981.
39. Santi DV: Perspectives on the design and biochemical pharmacology of inhibitors of thymidylate synthetase. J Med Chem 23:103–111, 1980.
40. De Clercq E, Balzarini J, Torrence PF, Mertes MP, Schmidt CL, Shugar D, Barr PJ, Jones AS, Verhelst G, Walker RT: Thymidylate synthetase as target enzyme for the inhibitory activity of 5-substituted 2'-deoxyuridines on mouse leukaemia L1210 cell growth. Mol Pharmacol 19:321–330, 1981.
41. Wataya Y, Santi DV, Hansch C: Inhibition of *Lactobacillus casei* thymidylate synthetase by 5-substituted 2'-deoxyuridylates. Preliminary structure-activity relationship. J Med Chem 20:1469–1473, 1977.
42. De Clercq E, Balzarini J, Chang CT-C, Bigge CF, Kalaritis P, Mertes MP: 5(e)-(3-Azidostyryl)-2'-deoxyuridine 5'-phosphate is a photo-activated inhibitor of thymidylate synthetase. Biochem Biophys Res Comm 97:1068–1075, 1980.
43. De Clercq E, Balzarini J, Descamps J, Bigge CF, Chang CT-C, Kalaritis P, Mertes MP: Antiviral, antitumour and thymidylate synthetase inhibition studies of 5-substituted styryl derivatives of 2'-deoxyuridine and their 5'-phosphates. Biochem Pharmacol 30:495–502, 1981.
44. Maggiora L, Chan CT-C, Hasson ME, Bigge CF, Mertes MP: 5-p-Benzoquinonyl-2'-deoxyuridine 5'-phosphate: A possible mechanism-based inhibitor of thymidylate synthetase. J Med Chem 26:1028–1036, 1983.
45. Barr PJ, Nolan PA, Santi DV, Robins MJ: Inhibition of thymidylate synthetase by 5-alkynyl-2'-deoxyuridylates. J Med Chem 24:1385–1388, 1981.
46. Danenberg PV, Bhatt RS, Kundu NG, Danenberg KD, Heidelberger C: Interaction of 5-ethynyl-2'-deoxyuridylate with thymidylate synthetase. J Med Chem 24:1537–1540, 1981.
47. Barr PJ, Robins MJ, Santi DV: Reaction of 5-ethynyl-2'-deoxyuridylate with thiols and thymidylate synthetase. Biochemistry 22:1696–1703, 1983.
48. Maggiora L, Chang CT-C, Torrence PF, Mertes MP: 5-Nitro-2'-deoxyuridine 5'-phosphate: A mechanism-based inhibitor of thymidylate synthetase. J Am Chem Soc 103:3192–3198, 1981.
49. Washtien WL, Santi DV: Mechanism of action of 5-Nitro-2'-deoxyuridine. J Med Chem 25:1252–1255, 1982.
50. Kalman TI, Goldman D: Inactivation of thymidylate synthetase by a novel mechanism-based enzyme inhibitor: 1-(beta-D-2'-Deoxyribofuranosyl)8-azapurin-2-one 5'-monophosphate. Biochem Biophys Res Comm 102:682–689, 1981.
51. Kisliuk RL, Levine MD: Properties of reduced derivatives of aminopterin. J biol Chem 239:1900–1904, 1964.
52. Horwitz SB, Kisliuk RL: Reduced derivatives of methotrexate. J Med Chem 11:907–908, 1968.

53. Horwitz SB, Kwok G, Wilson L, Kisliuk RL: Diastereoisomers of formaldehyde derivatives of tetrahydrofolic acid and tetrahydroaminpterin. J Med Chem 12:49–51, 1969.

54. Goodman L, DeGraw J, Kisliuk RL, Friedkin M, Pastore EJ, Crawford EJ, Plante LT, Al-Hahas A, Morningstar Jr JF, Kwok G, Wilson L, Donovan EF, Ratzan J: Tetrahydrohomofolate, a specific inhibitor of thymidylate synthetase. J Am Chem Soc 86:308–309, 1964.

55. Livingston D, Crawford EJ, Friedkin M: Studies with tetrahydrohomofolate and thymidylate synthetase from amethopterin-resistant mouse leukemia cells. Biochemistry 7:2814–2818, 1968.

56. Slavik K, Zakrzewski SF: Inhibition of thymidylate synthetase by some analogs of tetrahydrofolic acid. Mol Pharmacol 3:370–377, 1967.

57. Temple JrC, Bennett Jr LL, Rose JD, Elliott RD, Montgomery JA, Mangum JH: Synthesis of pseudo cofactor analogues as potential inhibitors of the folate enzymes. J Med Chem 25:161–166, 1982.

58. DeGraw JI, Kisliuk RL, Gaumont Y, Baugh CM, Nair MG: Synthesis and antifolate activity of 10-deazaminopterin. J Med Chem 17:552–553, 1974.

59. DeGraw JI, Brown VH, Tagawa H, Kisliuk RL, Gaumont Y, Sirotnak FM: Synthesis and antitumour activity of 10-alkyl-10-deazaminopterins. A convenient synthesis of 10-deazaminopterin. J Med Chem 25:1227–1230, 1982.

60. Kim YH, Gaumont Y, Kisliuk RL, Mautner HG: Synthesis and biological activity of 10-thia-10-deaza analogs of folic acid, pteroic acid and related compounds. J Med Chem 18:776–780, 1975.

61. Nair MG, Chen SY, Kisliuk RL, Gaumont Y, Strumpf D: Folate analogues altered in the C^9-N^{10} bridge region: 11-thiohomofolic acid. J Med Chem 22:850–855, 1979.

62. Nair MG, Chen SY, Kisliuk RL, Gaumont Y, Strumpf D: Folate analogues altered in the C^9-N^{10} bridge region. synthesis and antifolate activity of 11-thiohomoaminopterin. J Med Chem 23:899–903, 1980.

63. Nair MG, Saunders C, Chen SY, Kisliuk RL, Gaumont Y: Folate analogues altered in the C^9-N^{10} bridge region. 11-Oxahomofolic acid, a potential antitumour agent. J Med Chem 23:59–65, 1980.

64. Nair MG, Bridges TW, Henkel TJ, Kisliuk RL, Gaumont Y, Sirotnak FM: Folate analogues altered in the C^9-N^{10} bridge region. Synthesis and antitumour evaluation of 11-oxahomoaminopterin and related compounds. J Med Chem 24:1068–1073, 1981.

65. Nair MG, O'Neal PC, Baugh CM, Kisliuk RL, Gaumont Y, Rodman M: Folate analogues altered in the C^9-N^{10} bridge region: N^{10}-tosylisohomofolic acid and N^{10}-tosylisohomoaminopterin. J Med Chem 21:673–677, 1978.

66. Nair MG, Rozmyslovicz MK, Kisliuk RL, Gaumont Y, Sirotnak FM: The nor-analogues of folic acid. In: Chemistry and Biology of Pteridines, Blair JA (ed). Berlin: de Gruyter 1983, pp 121–126.

67. DeGraw JI, Kisliuk RL, Gaumont Y, Baugh CM: Antimicrobial activity of 8-deazafolic acid. J Med Chem 17:470–471, 1974.

68. Broom AD, Srinivasan A: Synthesis of an 8-deaza analog of the intermediate in the thymidylate synthetase reaction. In: Chemistry and Biology of Pteridines, Blair JA (ed). Berlin: de Gruyter, 1983, pp 445–449.

69. Nair MG, Salter OC, Kisliuk RL, Gaumont Y, North G: Folate analogues. Synthesis and biological evaluation of two analogues of dihydrofolic acid possessing a 7,8-dihydro-8-oxapterin ring system. J Med Chem 26:1164–1168, 1983.

70. Johne S: Search for pharmaceutically interesting quinazoline derivatives: Efforts and results (1969–1980). Prog Drug Res 26:259–341, 1982.

71. Bird OD, Vaitkus JW, Clarke J: 2-Amino-4-hydroxyquinazolines as inhibitors of thymidylate synthetase. Mol Pharmacol 6:573–575, 1970.

202

72. Carlin SC, Rosenberg RN, VandeVenter L, Friedkin M: Quinazoline antifolates as inhibitors of growth, dihydrofolate reductase and thymidylate synthetase of mouse neuroblastoma cells in culture. Mol Pharmacol 10:194–203, 1974.
73. McCuen RW, Sirotnak FM: Thymidylate synthetase from *Diplococcus pneumoniae*. Properties and inhibition by folate analogues. Biochim Biophys Acta 384:369–380, 1975.
74. Scanlon KJ, Rode W, Hynes JB: Use of a new biospecific absorbent for affinity chromatography to purify thymidylate synthetase from mouse leukemia cells, L1210. Proc Am Assoc Cancer Res 19:136, 1978.
75. Scanlon KJ, Moroson BA, Bertino JR, Hynes JB: Quinazoline analogues of folic acid as inhibitors of thymidylate synthetase from bacterial and mammalian sources. Mol Pharmacol 16:261–269, 1979.
76. Jones TR: 5-Substituted quinazoline antifolates. Eur J Cancer 16:707–711, 1980.
77. Calvert AH, Jones TR, Dady PJ, Grzelakowska-Sztabert B, Paine RM, Taylor GA, Harrap KR: Quinazoline antifolates with dual biochemical loci of action. Biochemical and biological studies directed towards overcoming methotrexate resistance. Eur J Cancer 16:713–722, 1980.
78. Jones TR, Calvert AH, Jackman AL, Brown SJ, Harrap KR: 2-Amino-4-hydroxy quinazoline analogues of folic acid as thymidylate synthetase inhibitors. Brit J Cancer 40:318–319, 1979.
79. Calvert AH, Jones TR, Jackman AL, Brown SJ, Harrap KR: An approach to the design of antimetabolites active against cells resistant to conventional agents illustrated by quinazoline antifolates with N^{10}-substitutions. In: Human Cancer, Its Characterization and Treatment, Davis W, Harrap KR, Stathopoulos G (eds). Amsterdam: Excerpta Medica, 1980, pp 272–283.
80. Jones TR, Calvert AH, Jackman AL, Brown SJ, Jones M, Harrap KR: A potent antitumour quinazoline inhibitor of thymidylate synthetase: Synthesis, biological properties and therapeutic results in mice. Eur J Cancer 17:11–19, 1981.
81. Jackman AL, Calvert AH, Hart LI, Harrap KR: Inhibition of thymidylate synthetase by the new quinazoline antifolate CB3717; Enzyme purification and kinetics. In: Adv Exptl Med Biol 165B. De Bruyn CHMM, Simmonds HA, Müller MM (Eds): Plenum, pp 375–378, 1984.
82. Piper JR, McCaleb GS, Montgomery JA, Kisliuk RL, Gaumont Y, Sirotnak FM: 10-Propargylaminopterin and alkyl homologues of methotrexate as inhibitors of folate metabolism. J Med Chem 25:877–880, 1982.
83. Jenny E, Greenberg DM: Further studies on thymidylate synthetase from calf thymus. J Biol Chem 238:3378–3382, 1963.
84. Horinishi H, Greenberg DM: Purification and properties of thymidylate synthetase from calf thymus. Biochim Biophys Acta 258:741–752, 1972.
85. Dwivedi CM, Kisliuk RL, Maley GF: Structural studies of calf thymus thymidylate synthetase. In: Chemistry and Biology of Pteridines, Blair JA (ed). Berlin: de Gruyter, 1983, pp 639–644.
86. Whiteley JM, Jerkunica I, Deits T: Thymidylate synthetase from amethopterin-resistant *Lactobacillus casei*. Purification by affinity chromatography. Biochemistry 13:2044–2050, 1974.
87. Dananberg PV, Langenbach RJ, Heidelberger C: Purification of thymidylate synthetase from *L. casei* by affinity chromatography. Biochem Biophys Res Comm 49:1029–1033, 1972.
88. Galivan JH, Maley GF, Maley F: The effect of substrate analogs on the circular dichroic spectra of thymidylate synthetase from *Lactobacillus casei*. Biochemistry 14:3338–3344, 1975.

89. Plante LT, Gaumont Y, Kisliuk RL: N^{α}-[Pteroyltetra(γ-glutamyl)]-lysine as a ligand for the purification of thymidylate synthetase by affinity chromatography. Prep Biochem 8:91–98, 1978.

90. Plante LT: Antifolate inhibitors of thymidylate synthetase as ligands for affinity chromatography. In: Chemistry and Biology of Pteridines, Kisliuk RL, Brown GM (eds). New York: Elsevier/North Holland, 1979, pp 267–271.

91. Fridland A, Langenbach RJ, Heidelberger C: Purification of thymidylate synthetase from Ehrlich ascites carcinoma cells. J Biol Chem 246:7110–7114, 1971.

92. Jastreboff M, Kedzierska B, Rode W: Properties of thymidylate synthetase from Ehrlich ascites carcinoma cells. Biochem Pharmacol 31:217–223, 1982.

93. Jastreboff MM, Kedzierska B, Rode W: Altered thymidylate synthetase in 5-fluorodeoxyuridine-resistant Ehrlich ascites carcinoma cells. Biochem Pharmacol 32:2259–2267, 1983.

94. Capco GR, Krupp JR, Mathews CK: Bacteriophage-coded thymidylate synthetase: Characteristics of the T4 and T5 enzymes. Arch Biochem Biophys 158:726–735, 1973.

95. Galivan J, Maley GF, Maley F: Purification and properties of T2 bacteriophage-induced thymidylate synthetase. Biochemistry 13:2282–2289, 1974.

96. Rode W, Zielińska ZM, Slavik K, Slavíková V: Purification of thymidylate synthetase by means of affinity chromatography on tetrahydroamethopterin-aminoethyl-sepharose. Biochem Soc Trans 4:925–927, 1976.

97. Neuhard J, Price AR, Schack L, Thomassen E: Two thymidylate synthetases in *Bacillus subtilis*. Proc Natl Acad Sci USA 15:1194–1198, 1978.

98. Belfort M, Maley GF, Maley F: Characterization of the *Escherichia coli* thyA gene and its amplified thymidylate synthetase product. Proc Natl Acad Sci USA 80:1858–1861, 1983.

99. Rode W, Scanlon KJ, Hynes J, Bertino JR: Purification of mammalian tumour (L1210) thymidylate synthetase by affinity chromatography on stable biospecific absorbent. J Biol Chem 254:11538–11543, 1979.

100. Banerjee CK, Bennett Jr L, Brockman RW, Sani BP, Temple Jr C: A convenient procedure for purification of thymidylate synthetase from L1210 cells. Anal Biochem 121:275–280, 1982.

101. Lockshin A, Moran RG, Danenberg PV: Thymidylate synthetase purified to homogeneity from human leukemic cells. Proc Natl Acad Sci USA 76:750–754, 1979.

102. Bapat AR, Zarow C, Danenberg PV: Human leukemic cells resistant to 5-fluoro-2'-deoxyuridine contain a thymidylate synthetase with lower affinity for nucleotides. J Bio Chem 258:4130–4136, 1983.

103. Rode W, Dolnick BJ, Bertino JR: Isolation of a homogeneous preparation of human thymidylate synthetase from HeLa cells. Biochem Pharmacol 29:723–726, 1980.

104. Priest DG, Doig MT, Hynes JB: Purification of mouse liver thymidylate synthetase by affinity chromatography using 10-methyl-5,8-dideazafolate as the affinant. Experientia 37:119–120, 1981.

105. Belfort M, Moelleken A, Maley GF, Maley F: Purification and properties of T4 phage thymidylate synthetase produced by the cloned gene in an amplification vector. J Biol Chem 258:2045–2051, 1983.

106. Rao KN, Kisliuk RL: Association of RNA with thymidylate synthetase from methotrexate-resistant *streptococcus faecium*. Proc Natl Acad Sci USA 80:916–920, 1983.

107. Leary RP, Kisliuk RL: Crystalline thymidylate synthetase from dichloromethotrexate-resistant *Lactobacillus casei*. Prep Biochem 1:47–54, 1971.

108. Lyon JA, Pollard AL, Loeble RB, Dunlap RB: Thymidylate synthetase: An improved purification procedure and description of some spectral properties. Cancer Biochem Biophys 1:121–128, 1975.

204

109. Dunlap RB: TMP synthetase from *Lactobacillus casei*. Meth Enzymol 51:90–97, 1978.
110. Whiteley JM: 5-Fluoro-2'-deoxyuridylate-agarose in the affinity-chromatographic purification of thymidylate synthetase. Meth Enzymol 51:98–104, 1978.
111. Danenberg PV, Langenbach RJ, Heidelberger C: Structures of reversible and irreversible complexes of thymidylate synthetase and fluorinated pyrimidine nucleotides. Biochemistry 13:926–933, 1974.
112. Belfort M, Maley G, Pedersen-Lane J, Maley F: Primary structure of the *Escherichia coli* thyA gene and its thymidylate synthetase product. Proc Natl Acad Sci USA 80:4914–4918, 1983.
113. Chabner BA: Pyrimidine antagonists. In: Pharmacologic Principles of Cancer Treatment. Chabner BA (ed) WB Saunders Co, 1982.
114. Harrap KR, Hill BT, Furness ME, Hart LI: Sites of action of amethopterin: Intrinsic and acquired resistance. Ann NY Acad Sci 186:312–324, 1971.
115. Jackson RC, Niethammer D: Acquired methotrexate resistance in lymphoblasts resulting from altered kinetic properties of dihydrofolate reductase. Eur J Cancer 13:567–575, 1977.
116. Rosenblatt, Whitehead VM, Vera N, Pottier A, Dupont M, Vuchich MJ: Prolonged inhibition of DNA synthesis associated with the accummulation of methotrexate polyglutamates by cultured tumour cells. Mol Pharmacol 14:1143–1147, 1978.
117. Whitehead VM: Synthesis of methotrexate polyglutamates in L1210 murine leukemia cells. Cancer Res 37:408–412, 1977.
118. Schilsky RL, Baily BD, Chabner BA: Methotrexate polyglutamate synthesis by cultured human breast cancer cells. Proc Natl Acad Sci USA 77:2919–2922, 1980.
119. Galivan J: Transport and metabolism of methotrexate in normal and resistant cultured rat hepatoma cells. Cancer Res 39:735–743, 1979.
120. Poser RG, Sirotnak FM, Chello PL: Differential synthesis of methotrexate polyglutamate in normal proliferative and neoplastic mouse tissues *in vivo*. Cancer Res 41:4441–4446, 1981.
121. Fry DW, Yalowich JC, Goldman ID: Rapid formation of polygamma-glutamyl derivatives of methotrexate and their association with dihydrofolate reductase as assessed by HPLC in the Ehrlich ascites tumour cell *in vitro*. J Biol Chem 257:1890–1896, 1982.
122. Baugh CM, Krumdieck C, Nair MG: Polygammaglutamyl metabolites of methotrexate. Biochem Biophys Res Comm 52:24–27, 1973.
123. Covey JM: Polyglutamate derivatives of folic acid coenzymes and methotrexate. Life Sciences 26:665–678, 1980.
124. Szeto DW, Cheng Y-C, Rosowsky A, Yu C-S, Modest EJ, Piper JR, Temple JrC, Elliott RD, Rose JD, Montgomery JA: Human thymidylate synthetase-III effects of methotrexate and folate analogues. Biochem Pharmacol 28:2633–2637, 1979.
125. Bertino JR, McGuire JJ: Folates and cancer chemotherapy. In: Chemistry and Biology of Pteridines. Berlin: de Gruyter, pp 263–274, 1983.
126. Jolivet J, Drake JC, Chabner BA: Inhibition of human thymidylate synthetase (TS) by methotrexate polyglutamates (MTXPGs). Proc AACR 24:276, 1983.
127. Jackson RC,Jackman AL, Calvert AH: Biochemical effects of a quinazoline inhibitor of thymidylate synthetase, CB3717, on human lymphoblastoid cells. Biochem Pharmacol 32:3783–3790, 1983.
128. Tattersall MHN, Jackson RC, Connors TA, Harrap KR: Combination chemotherapy: The interaction of methotrexate and 5-fluorouracil. Europ J Cancer 9:733–739, 1973.
129. Jackson RC: Modulation of methotrexate toxicity by thymidine: sequence dependent biochemical effects. Mol Pharmacol 18:281–286, 1980.
130. Myers CE, Young RC, Chabner BA: Biochemical determinants of 5-fluorouracil response *in vivo*. The role of deoxyuridylate pool expansion. J Clin Invest 56:1231–1238, 1975.

131. Klubes P, Connelly K, Cerna I, Mandel HG: Effects of 5-fluorouracil on 5-fluorodeoxyuridine 5'-monophosphate and 2-deoxyuridine 5'-monophosphate pools, and DNA synthesis in solid mouse L1210 and rat Walker 256 tumours. Cancer Res 38:2325–2331, 1978.
132. Ardalan B, Buscaglia MD, Schein PS: Tumour 5-fluorodeoxyuridylate concentration as a determinant of 5-fluorouracil response. Biochem Pharmacol 27:2009–2013, 1978.
133. Maybaum J, Cohen MB, Sadee W: *In vivo* rates of pyrimidine nucleotide metabolism in intact mouse T-lymphoma (S-49) cells treated with 5-fluorouracil. J Biol Chem 256:2126–2130, 1981.
134. Myers CE: The pharmacology of the fluoropyrimidines. Pharm Revs 33·1–15, 1981.
135. Ardalan B, Cooney D, Macdonald JS: Physiological and pharmacological determinants of sensitivity and resistance to 5-fluorouracil in lower animals and man. Adv in Pharmacol and Chem 17:289–321, 1980.
136. Sawyer RC, Stolfi RL, Nayak R, Martin DS: Mechanism of cytotoxicity of 5-fluorouracil chemotherapy of two murine solid tumours. In: Nucleosides and Cancer Treatment. Australia: Academic Press, pp 309–337, 1981.
137. Kufe DW, Major PP: 5-fluorouracil incorporation into human breast carcinoma RNA correlates with cytotoxicity. J Biol Chem 256:9802–9805, 1981.
138. Hadjiolova KV, Naydenova ZG, Hadjiolov AA: Inhibition of ribosomal RNA maturation in Friend erythroleukemia cells by 5-fluorouridine and toyocamycin. Biochem Pharmacol 30:1861–1863, 1981.
139. Wilkinson DS, Cihak A, Pitot HC: Inhibition of ribosomal ribonucleic acid maturation in rat liver by 5-fluoroorotic acid resulting in the selective labelling of cytoplasmic messenger ribonucleic acid. J Biol Chem 246:6418–6427, 1971.
140. Wilkinson DS, Pitot HC: Inhibition of ribosomal ribonucleic acid maturation in Novikoff hepatoma cells by 5-fluorouracil and 5-fluorouridine. J Biol Chem 248:63–68, 1973.
141. Carrico CK, Glazer RI: Effects of 5-fluorouracil on the synthesis and translation of polyadenylic acid-containint RNA from regenerating rat liver. Cancer Res 39:3694–3701, 1979.
142. Danenberg PV, Heidelberger C, Mulkins MA, Peterson AR: The incorporation of 5-fluoro-2'-deoxyuridine into DNA of mammalian tumour cells. Biochem Biophys Res Comm 102:654–658, 1981.
143. Kufe DW, Major PP, Egan EM, Loh E: 5-Fluoro-2'-deoxyuridine incorporation in L1210 DNA.J Biol Chem 256:8885–8888, 1981.
144. Caradonna SJ, Cheng Y-c: The role of deoxyuridine triphosphate nucleotidohydrolase, uracil-DNA glycosylase, and DNA polymerase alpha in the metabolism of FUdR in human tumour cells. Mol Pharmacol 18:513–520, 1980.
145. Major PP, Egan E, Herrick D, Kufe DW: 5-fluorouracil incorporation in DNA of human breast carcinoma cells. Cancer Res 42:3005–3009, 1982.
146. Tanaka M, Yoshida S, Saneyoshi M, Yamaguchi T: Utilization of 5-fluoro-2'-deoxyuridine triphosphate and 5-fluoro-2'-deoxycytidine triphosphate in DNA synthesis by DNA polymerases alpha and beta from calf thymus. Cancer Res 41:4132–4135, 1981.
147. Laskin JD, Evans RM, Slocum HK, Burke D, Hakala MT: Basis for natural variation in sensitivity to 5-fluorouracil in mouse and human cells in culture. Cancer Res 39:383–390, 1979.
148. Houghton JA, Houghton PJ, Wooten RS: Mechanism of induction of gastrointestinal toxicity in the mouse by 5-fluorouracil, 5-fluorouridine and 5-fluoro-2'-deoxyuridine. Cancer Res 39:2406–1423, 1979.
149. Piper AA, Fox RM: Differential metabolism of fluorouracil (FU) in cultured human T and B lymphocyte cell lines: modulation of sensitivity by purine nucleosides and bases. In: Nucleosides and Cancer Treatment. Australia: Academic Press, 1981, pp 251–265.
150. Houghton JA, Houghton PJ: Elucidation of pathways of 5-fluorouracil metabolism in xenografts of human colorectal adenocarcinoma. Eur J Cancer 19:807–815, 1983.

151. Spiegelman S, Nayak R, Sawyer R, Stolfi R, Martin D: Potentiation of the antitumour activity of 5-FU by thymidine and its correlation with the formation of (5FU) RNA. Cancer 45:1129–1134, 1980.

152. Evans RM, Laskin JD, Hakala MT: Assessment of growth-limiting events caused by 5-fluorouracil in mouse cells and human cells. Cancer Res 40:4113–4122, 1980.

153. Maybaum J, Ullman B, Mandel HG, Day JL, Sadee W: Regulation of RNA- and DNA-directed actions of 5-fluoropyrimidines in mouse T-lymphoma (S-49) cells. Cancer Res 40:4209–4215, 1980.

154. Chabner BA: Antimetabolites. In: Cancer Chemotherapy: The EORTC Cancer Chemotherapy Annual 2. Pinedo HM (ed) Excerpta Medica, 1980, pp 1–26.

155. Jackman AL, Calvert AH, Taylor GA, Harrap KR: Biological properties of the new quinazoline inhibitor of thymidylate synthetase, CB3717. In: The Control of Tumour Growth and its Biological Bases. Davis W, Maltoni C, Tanneberger St (eds). Berlin: Akademie-Verlag, 1983, pp 404–410.

156. Taylor GA, Jackman AL, Calvert AH, Harrap KR: Plasma nucleoside and base levels following treatment with the new thymidylate synthetase inhibitor, CB3717. In: Adv Exptl Med Biol 165B. De Bruyn CHMM, Simmonds HA, Müller MM (Eds): Plenum, pp 379–382, 1984.

157. Jackman AL, Taylor GA, Calvert AH, Newell DR, Harrap KR: Biochemical disturbances observed *in vitro* and *in vivo* following inhibition of thymidylate synthetase by CB3717. Brit J Cancer 46:505–506, 1982.

158. Calvert AH, Jackman AL, Alison DL, Siddik ZH, Newell DR, Newlands ES, Taylor GA, Harrap KR: Clinical and experimental studies with a folate based inhibitor of thymidylate synthetase. Proc 13th Int Cancer Congress, Seattle (1983) in press.

159. Calvert AH, Alison DL, Harland SJ, Jackman AL, Mooney CJ, Smith IE, Harrap KR: Phase I studies with CB3717. Brit J cancer 48:116–117, 1983.

160. Alison DL, Calvert AH: Early clinical studies with CB3717 at the Royal Marsden Hospital. In: Cancer Chemotherapy and Selective Drug Development. Harrap KR, Davis W, Calvert AH (Eds): Martinus Nijhoff, p 535, 1984.

161. Newell DR, Siddik ZH, Calvert AH, Jackman AL, Alison DL, McGhee KG, Harrap KR: Pharmacokinetic and toxicity studies with CB3717. Proc Am Assoc Cancer Res 23:181, 1982.

162. Fernandes DJ, Bertino JR, Hynes JB: Biochemical and antitumour effects of 5,8-dideazaisopteroylglutamate, a unique quinazoline inhibitor of thymidylate synthetase. Cancer Res 43:1117–1123, 1983.

163. Jackson RC: Int J Bio-Med Comput 11:197, 1980.

164. Tattersall MHN, Jackson RC, Jackson STM, Harrap KR: Factors determining cell sensitivity to methotrexate: studies of folate and deoxyribonucleoside triphosphate pools in five mammalian cell lines. Europ J Cancer 10:819–826, 1974.

165. Chang C-H, Cheng Y-C: Effects of nucleoside triphosphates on human ribonucleoside reductase from Molt-4F cells. Cancer Res 39:5087–5092, 1979.

166. Moore EC, Hulbert RB: J Biol Chem 24:4802, 1966.

167. Diddens K, Niethammer D, Jackson RC: Human cells resistant to methotrexate: cross resistance and collateral sensitivity to the non-classical antifolates trimetrexate, metoprine, homofolic acid and CB3717. In: Chemistry and Biology of Pteridines, Blair JA (ed). Berlin/New York: deGruyter, 1983, pp 953–957.

168. Jackman AL, Alison DL, Calvert AH, Harrap KR: Increased thymidylate synthetase activity in L1210 cells resistant to CB3717. Brit J Cancer 48:133–134, 1983.

169. Spector T, Cleland WW: Meanings of Ki for conventional and alternate-substrate inhibitors. Biochem Pharmacol 30:1–7, 1981.

170. Christopherson RI, Dugglegy RG: Metabolic resistance: the protection of enzymes against

drugs which are tight-binding inhibitors by the accumulation of substrate. Europ J Biochem 134:331–335, 1983.

171. Jackson RC: The regulation of thymidylate biosynthesis in Novikoff hepatoma cells and the effects of amethopterin, 5-fluorodeoxyuridine, and 3-deazauridine. J Biol Chem 253:7440–7446, 1978.
172. Moran RG, Danenberg PV, Heidelberger C: Therapeutic response of leukemic mice treated with fluorinated pyrimidines and inhibitors of deoxyuridylate synthesis. Biochem Pharmacol 31:2929–2935, 1982.
173. Houghton JA, Schmidt C, Houghton PJ: The effect of derivatives of folic acid on the fluorodeoxyuridylate thymidylate synthetase covalent complex in human colon xenografts. Europ J Cancer Clin Oncol 18:347–354, 1982.
174. Moran RG, Werkheiser WC, Zakrzewski SF: Folate metabolism in mammalian cells in culture. J Biol Chem 251:3569–3575, 1976.
175. Jackson RC, Harrap KR: Studies with a mathematical model of folate metabolism. Arch Biochem Biophys 158:827–841, 1973.
176. Chabner BA: Methotrexate. In: Pharmacologic Principles in Cancer Treatment. Chabner BA (ed). USA: WB Saunders CO, 1982, pp 229–255.
177. Houghton JA, Maroda SJ, Phillips JO, Houghton PJ: Biochemical determinants of responsiveness to 5-fluorouracil and its derivatives in xenografts of human colorectal adenocarcinomas in mice. Cancer Res 41:144–149, 1981.
178. Washtien WL: Thymidylate synthetase levels as a factor in 5-fluorodeoxyuridine and methotrexate cytotoxicity in gastrointestinal tumour cells. Mol Pharmacol 21:723–728, 1982.
179. Dolnick BJ, Cheng Y: Human Thymidylate synthetase II. derivatives of pteroylmono- and-polyglutamates as substrates and inhibitors. J Biol Chem 253:3563–3567, 1978.
180. Clendeninn NJ, Cowan KH, Kaufman BT, Nadkarni MV, Chabner BA: Dihydrofolate reductase (DHFR) from a methotrexate resistant human breast cancer cell line: purification, properties and binding of methotrexte (MTX) and polyglutamates. Proc Am Assoc Cancer Res 24:276, 1983.
181. Huennekens FM, Suresh MR, Grimshaw CE, Jacobsen DW, Quadros Et, Vitols KS, Henderson GB: Transport of folate and pterin compounds. In: Chemistry and Biology of Pteridines Blaie JA (ed). Berlin/New York: deGruyter, 1983, pp 1–22.
182. Jackman AL, Alison DL, Calvert AH, Barrie SE, Harrap KR: Studies with mutant L1210 cell lines that have acquired resistance to CB3717. In: Cancer Chemotherapy and Selective Drug Development. Harrap KR, Davis W, Calvert AH (Eds): Martinus Nijhoff, p 527, 1984.
183. Plagemann PGW, Erbe J: The deoxyribonucleoside transport systems of cultured Novikiff rat hepatoma cells. J Cell Physiol 83:337–344, 1974.
184. Leyva A, Nederbragt H, Lankelma J, Pinedo HM: Methotrexate cytotoxicity: Studies on its reversal by folates and nucleosides. Cancer Treat Rep 65:45–54, 1981.
185. Jackman AL, Taylor GA, Calvert AH, Harrap KR: Modulation of Anti-Metabolite effects. Biochem Pharmacot 33:3269–3275, 1984.
186. Goulian M, Bleile B, Tseng BY: The effect of methotrexate on levels of dUTP in animal cells. J Biol Chem 255:10630–10637, 1980.
187. Sedwick WD, Kutler M, Brown OE: Antifolate-induced misincorporation of deoxyuridine monophosphate into DNA: Inhibition of high molecular weight DNA synthesis in human lymphoblastoid cells. Proc Natl Acad Sci USA 78:917–921, 1981.
188. Goulian M, Bleile B, Tseng BY: Methotrexate-induced incorporation of uracil into DNA. Proc Natl Acad Sci USA 77:1956–1960, 1980.
189. Dube DK, Kunkel TA, Seal G, Loeb LA: Distinctive properties of mammalian DNA polymerases. Biochim Biophys Acta 561:369–382, 1979.

208

190. Bestwick RK, Moffet DGL, Sipiro C, Mathews CK: Differential effects of methotrexate or fluorodeoxyuridine upon mitochondrial and cellular nucleotide pools. In: Chemistry and Biology of Pteridines, Blair JA (ed). Berlin/New York: deGruyter, 1983, pp 311–315.

191. Peterson MS, Ingraham HA, Goulian M: 2'-deoxyribosyl analogues of UDP-n-acetylglucosamine in cells treated with methotrexate or 5-fluorodeoxyuridine. J Biol Chem 258:10831–10834, 1983.

192. Bertino JR: Towards improved selectivity in cancer chemotherapy: The Richard and Hilda Rosenthal Foundation Award Lecture. Cancer Res 39:293–304, 1979.

193. Jolivet J, Curt GA, Clendeninn NS, Chabner BA: Antimetabolites. In: Cancer Chemotherapy: The EORTC Cancer Chemotherapy Annual 4, Pinedo HM (ed), 1982, pp 1–28.

194. Dower WJ, Schimke RT: Human dihydrofolate reductase (DHFR) gene amplification after (MTX) treatment. Proc Am Ass Cancer Res 24:280, 1983.

195. Reichard P, Skold O, Klein G, Revesz I, Magnussom P-H: Studies on resistance against 5-fluorouracil. Cancer Res 22:235–243, 1962.

196. Kasbekar DK, Greenberg DM: Studies on tumour resistance to 5-fluorouracil. Cancer Res 23:818–824, 1963.

197. Reyes P, Hall TC: Synthesis of 5-fluorouridine 5'-phosphate by a pyrimidine phosphoribosyltransferase of mammalian origin-II. Correlation between the tumour levels of the enzyme and the 5-fluorouracil-promoted increase in survival of tumour-bearing mice. Biochem Pharmacol 18:2587–2590, 1969.

198. Umeda M, Heidelberger C: Comparative studies of fluorinated pyrimidines with various cell lines. Cancer Res 28:2529–2538, 1968.

199. Priest DG, Ledford BE: Increased TS in 5-fluorodeoxyuridine resistant cultured hepatoma cells. Biochem Pharmacol 29:1549–1553, 1980.

200. Baskin F, Carlin SC, Kraus P, Friedkin M, Rosenberg RN: Experimental chemotherapy of mouse neuroblastoma. Mol Pharmacol 11:105–117, 1975.

201. Kufe DW, Scott P, Fram R, Major P: Biologic effects of 5-fluoro-2'-deoxyuridine incorporation in L1210 deoxyribonucleic acid. Biochem Pharmacol 32:1337–1340, 1983.

202. Cheng YC, Nakayama K: Effects of 5-fluoro-2'-deoxyuridine on DNA metabolism in HeLa cells. Mol Pharmacol 23:171–174, 1983.

203. Ingraham HA, Tseng BY, Goulian M: Nucleotide levels and incorporation of 5-fluourouracil and uracil into DNA of cells treated with 5-fluorodeoxyuridine. Mol Pharmacol 21:211–216, 1982.

204. Cohen JL, Irwin LE, Marchal GJ, Darvey H, Bateman JR: Clinical pharmacology of oral and intravenous 5-fluorouracil. Cancer Chemother Rep part 1 58:723–731, 1974.

205. Sitar DS, Shaw DH, Thirlwell MP, Ruedy JR: Disposition of 5-fluorouracil after intravenous bolus doses of a commercial formulation. Cancer Res 37:3981–3984, 1977.

206. McMillan WE, Wolberg WH, Welling PG: Pharmacokinetics of fluorouracil in humans. Cancer Res 38:3479–3482, 1978.

207. Kirkwood JM, Ensminger W, Rosowsky a, Papthanasopoulos n, Frei E III: Comparison of pharmacokinetics of 5-fluorouracil with concurrent thymidine infusion in a phase I trial. Cancer Res 40:107–113, 1980.

208. Garrett ER, Hurst GH, Green RJ: Kinetics and mechanisms of drug action on microorganisms XXIII. Microbial kinetic assay for fluorouracil in biological fluids and its application to human pharmacokinetics. J Pharm Sci 66:1422–1429, 1977.

209. Finch RE, Bending MR, Lant AF: Plasma levels of 5-fluorouracil after oral and intravenous administration in cancer patients. Brit J Clin Pharmacol 7:613–614, 1979.

210. McDermott BJ, Van den Berg HW, Murphey RF: Nonlinear pharmacokinetics for the elimination of 5-fluorouracil after intravenous administration in cancer patients. Cancer Chemother Pharmacol 9:173–178, 1982.

211. Finn C, Sadee W: Determination of 5-fluorouracil (NSC 19893) plasma levels in rats and

man by isotope dilution-mass fragmentography. Cancer Chemother Rep 59:279–286, 1975.

212. Alison DL, Newell DR, Calvert AH: Pharmacokinetic studies in humans with CB3717 (N-(4-(2-amino-4-hydroxy-6-quinazolinyl)methyl)prop-2-ynylamino)benzoyl)-L-glutamic acid. Brit J Cancer 48:126, 1983.

213. Howell SB, Mansfield SJ, Taetle R: Significance of variation in serum concentration for the marrow toxicity of MTX. Cancer Chemother Pharmacol 5:221–226, 1981.

214. Kish J, Drelichman A, Jacobs J, Hoschner J, Kinzie J, Loh J, Weaver A, Al Sarraf M: Clinical trial of cisplatin and 5-FU as initial treatment for advanced squamous carcinoma of the head and neck. Cancer Treat Rep 66:471–474, 1982.

215. Ohnuma T, Roboz J, Waxman S, Mandel E, Martin DS, Holland JF: Clinical pharmacologic effects of thymidine and 5-FU. Cancer Treat Rep 64:1169–1177, 1980.

216. Woodcock TM, Martin DS, Damin LAM, Kerneny NE, Young CW: Combination clinical trials with thymidine and fluorouracil: A phase I and clinical pharmacologic examination. Cancer 45:1135–1143, 1980.

217. Au JLS, Rustum YM, Ledesma EJ, Mittleman A, Creaven PJ: Clinical pharmacological studies of concurrent infusion of 5-fluorouracil and thymidine in the treatment of colorectal carcinomas. Cancer Res 42:2930–2937, 1982.

218. Fernandes DJ, Bertino JR: 5-Fluorouracil-methotrexate synergy: enhancement of 5-fluorodeoxyuridylate binding to thymidylate synthetase by dihydropteroylpolyglutamates. Proc Natl Acad Sci USA 77:5563–5667, 1980.

219. Cadman EC, Heimer R, Davis L: Enhanced 5-fluorouracil formation after methotrexate administration: explanation for drug synergism. Science 250:1135–1137, 1979.

220. Lajthe LG, Vane JR: Dependence of bone marrow cells on the liver for purine supply. Nature 182:191–192, 1958.

221. Tisman G, WU SJG: Effectiveness of intermediate-dose methotrexate and high dose 5-fluorouracil as sequential combination chemotherapy in refractory breast cancer and as primary therapy in metastatic adenocarcinoma of the colon. Cancer Treat Rep 64:829–835, 1980.

222. Gerwitz AM, Cadman E: Preliminary report on the efficacy of sequential methotrexate and 5-fluorouracil in advanced breast cancer. Cancer 47:2552–2555, 1981.

223. Ringborg U, Evert G, Kinnman J, Landquist PG, Strander H: Sequential methotrexate-5-fluorouracil treatment of squamous cell carcinoma of the head and neck. Cancer 1983, (in press).

224. Pitman SW, Kowal DC, Papac RJ, Bertino JR: Sequential methotrexate-5-fluorouracil. A highly active drug combination in advanced squamous cell carcinoma of the head and neck. Proc Am Assoc Cancer Res 21:607, 1980.

225. Wienerman B, Schacter B, Schipper H, Bowman D, Levitt M: Sequential methotrexate and 5FU in the treatment of colorectal cancer. Cancer Treat Rep 66:1553–1555, 1982.

226. Cantrell JE, Brunet R, Lagarde C, Schein PS, Smith FP: Phase II study of sequential methotrexate-5FU therapy in advanced measurable colorectal cancer. Cancer Treat Rep 66:1563–1565, 1982.

227. Bertino JR: Clinical application of the scheduled combination of methotrexate and 5-fluorouracil. In: The Chemotherapy of Breast, Gastrointestinal and Head and Neck Cancer. Current Status and Potential Role of Methotrexate and 5-Fluorouracil. Bertino JR (ed), USA: Pharma Libri, 1983.

228. Browman GP, Archibald SD, Young JEM, Hryniuk WM, Russell R, Kiehl K, Levine MN: Prospective randomised trial I hour sequential versus simultaneous methotrexate plus 5-fluorouracil in advanced and recurrent squamous cell head and neck cancer. J Clin Oncol 1983, in press.

229. Coates et al.: J Clin Oncol, 1983, in press.

230. Tattersall MHN: Antimetabolite combinations possessing enhanced efficacy. In: Cancer Chemotherapy and Selective Drug Development. Harrap KR, Davis W, Calvert AH (Eds): Martinus Nijhoff, p 19–32, 1984.
231. Heidelberger C, Kalder G, Mukherjee KI: Studies on fluorinated pyrimidines XI. *In vitro* studies on tumour resistance. Cancer Res 202:903–909, 1960.
232. Machover D, Schwarzenberg L, Goldschmidt E, Tourani JM, Michalski B, Hayat M, Dorval T, Misset JL, Jasmin C, Maral R, Mathe G: Treatment of advanced colorectal and gastric adenocarcinoma with 5-FU combined with high does folinic acid: a pilot study. Cancer Treat Rep 66:1803–1807, 1982.
233. Gilman AG, Goodman LS, Gilman A. (eds): The Pharmacologic Basis of Therapeutics. New York: Macmillan Publishing Co. Inc., 1980, pp 1278–1280.
234. Patt YZ, Chuang VP, Wallace S, Benjamin RS, Fuqua R, Mauligit GM: Hepatic arterial chemotherapy and occlusion for palliation of primary hepatocellular and unknown neoplasm in the liver. Cancer 51:1359–1363, 1983.
235. Oberfield RA, McCaffrey JA, Polio J, Clouse ME, Hamilton TH: Prolonged and continuous percutaneous intra-arterial hepatic infusion chemotherapy in advanced metastatic liver adenocarconoma for colorectal primary. Cancer 44:414–423, 1979.
236. Ensminger WD, Rosowsky A, Raso V, Levin DC, Glode M, Come S, Steele G, Frei E III: A clinical pharmacological evaluation of hepatic arterial indusions of 5-fluoro-2'-deoxyruridine and 5-fluorouracil. Cancer Res 38:3784–3792, 1979.
237. Reed ML, Vaitkevicius VK, Al-Sarraf M, Vaughan CB, Singhakowinta A, Sexon-Parte M, Izbicki R, Baker L, Stratsma GW: The practicality of chronic hepatic artery infusion therapy of primary and metastatic hepatic malignancies. Cancer 47:402–409, 1981.
238. Alison DL, Mooney CJ, Robinson B, Smith IE, Wiltshaw E, McElwain TJ, Calvert AH: Phase I clinical trial of CB3717 ((N-(4-(N-((2-amino-4-hydroxy-6-quinazolinyl)methyl)prop-2-ynylamino)benzoyl)-L-glutamic acid). Proc 4th NCI-EORTC Symp on New Drugs in cancer Therapy 1983, in press.
239. Straw JA, Talbot DC, Taylor GA, Harrap KR: Some observations on the reversibility of methotrexate toxicity in normal proliferating tissues. J Natl Cancer Inst 58:91–97, 1977.
240. Ensminger WD, Frei E III: The prevention of methotrexate toxicity by thymidine infusions in humans. Cancer Res 37:1857–1863, 1977.
241. Dady PJ, Taylor GA, Muindi JFR, Calvert AH, Smith IE, Smyth JF, Harrap KR: Methotrexate with thymidine, inosine and allopurinol rescue: A phase I clinical study. Cancer Treat Rep 65:37–43, 1981.
242. Pinedo HM, Zaharko DS, Bull JM, Chabner BA: The reversal of methotrexate cytotoxicity to mouse bone marrow cells by leucovorin and nucleosides. Cancer Res 36:4418–4478, 1976.
243. Nair MG, Salter DC, Kisliuk RL, Gaumont Y, North G, Sirotnak FM: Folate analogues. 21. Synthesis and antifolate and antitumour activities of N^{10}-(cyanomethyl)-5,8-dideazafolic acid. J Med Chem 26:605–607, 1983.
244. Goldie JH, Price LA, Harrap KR: Methotrexate toxicity: Correlation with duration of administration, plasma levels, dose and excretion pattern. Europ J Cancer 8:409–414, 1972.

8. Autologous Bone Marrow Transplantation (ABMT) and High-Dose Chemotherapy in Small Cell Lung Cancer

J. GORDON McVIE

INTRODUCTION

Chemotherapy is accepted as the logical therapy for small cell lung cancer. The heterogeneity of this tumor combined with a fast doubling time and propensity to early metastatic spread make it a formidable opponent. Whereas combinations of cytostatic drugs have achieved impressive response rates in the last 10 years, when these response rates are dissected down into complete and less than complete only the former have been shown to benefit the patient [1]. Results have been reported in an incorrect and confusing manner in the majority of trials leading to overoptimism based on an overall response and 'median survival' times. As is too often the case with early reporting of results, the final results reveal the stark reality of long term survival statistics. Only a small number of patients treated with combination chemotherapy plus or minus local radiotherapy will achieve meaningful long term survival which may or may not be termed as cure. Those patients almost always have limited disease (that is limited to the thorax) and achieve complete remission rather quickly after chemotherapy. The converse is true that few patients with extensive disease have rarely achieved long term survival and no patient who only achieved partial remission survived 5 years. It seems an appropriate aim therefore to improve the complete remission rate and thereby long term survival; the usual mechanism has been to increase the dose or dose rate of chemotherapeutic agents or else give them with another modality viz radiotherapy.

The dose limiting toxicity of many cytotoxic drugs is myelosuppression. Early attempts to increase the dose of drugs used in an induction scheme for small cell lung cancer resulted in an increased early mortality due to sepsis and intercurrent bleeding. The long term results of this aggressive therapy have been encouraging [2]. The best long term results to date were achieved in a study reported by Johnson who employed radiotherapy combined with

F.M. Muggia (ed.), Experimental and Clinical Progress in Cancer Chemotherapy
© *1985, Martinus Nijhoff Publishers, Boston. ISBN 0-89838-679-9. Printed in the Netherlands.*

the first course of chemotherapy [3]. Again the price paid for long term survival was heavy early mortality. It must be said of the last study however, that the cause of death is not clearly documented and therefore it cannot be said that myelosuppression was the only element involved.

The ability to aspirate large volumes of bone marrow from patients, to suitably prepare it and freeze it in liquid nitrogen so that on thawing it remains viable and indeed can repopulate an aplastic bone marrow has been learned by the experiments of allogeneic bone marrow transplantation in acute leukemia [4]. The application of this technology to rescue a patient from high doses of myelosuppressive therapy by reinfusing his own stored bone marrow was initially greeted with a wave of enthusiasm. This overoptimism has given way to a more moderate realism as is typical of the evolution of a new methodology in clinical practice.

The first experience showed that a limited number of drugs are appropriate for the technique, that a limited number of patients are fit for high-dose therapy and even given the best possible conditions that the procedure is not without risk. Its worth can only be evaluated with the emergence of comparative clinical trials.

Problems related to the choice of drugs were the emergence of organ toxicity other than bone marrow at high dose. The problems related to patient selection were that they were treated frequently at the end of the therapeutic line, in other words in poor general condition with previous exposure to multiple forms of therapy and on the whole drug-resistant disease. There does seem to be an argument for further evaluation of carefully selected high dose chemotherapy in equally well selected subgroups of patients with small cell lung cancer. The current methodology (summarized in table 1) and the preliminary results will be sketched in this article.

SCHEDULING OF THERAPY

There have been two ways of regarding the optimal timing of high dose therapy. The first school claims that the best chance of success is to present

Table 1. Procedures

1. Patient selection
2. Marrow aspiration
3. Marrow storage ± clean-up
4. Treatment
5. Reinfusion
6. Supportive care

the highest possible dose of chemotherapy in first line in order to prevent the emergence of resistant clones, by exposure to sub optimal drug doses. The argument against this technique is that this involves aspiration of bone marrow from untreated patients in whom the likelihood despite vigorous staging and current immunohistological advances may very well have cancer cells in the bone marrow, which then survive freezing and thawing and then will replicate on reinfusion. Improvements in the evolution of specific monoclonal antibodies which may attack single cells in a bone marrow aspirate may further narrow selection of patients for such a technique. These antibodies may also be used as described later to 'clean up' the bone marrow after aspiration before reinfusion. Souhami and his colleagues treated a number of patients with high dose cyclophosphamide supported by ABMT in newly presenting limited disease patients [5]. Although they noted a satisfactory number of complete and partial responses indicating that even with one drug given in an appropriate dosage a predictable cell kill would result, the eventual relapse pattern was not affected by this therapeutic modality and the long term results are disappointing. However, the importance of this study was the demonstration of feasibility of the technique and the group have now gone on to underline this by repeating the technique twice several weeks apart in an attempt to reproduce the same cell kill twice in succession and thereby perhaps cure some patients. The results of the second study are not yet mature.

The more conventional application of ABMT and high dose chemotherapy has been as a so called 'late intensification' manœuvre. Norton and Simon proposed a mathematical model based on failure of current conventional chemotherapy to achieve elimination of minimal residual disease [6]. Their supposition was that minimal residual disease, contrary to the dogma of the cell kineticist was more resistant to chemotherapy than large volume disease. They argued therefore that minimal residual disease when achieved by conventional means should be treated by megadose chemotherapy. They pointed out that in reality this was frequently not possible because of the gradual deterioration in bone marrow reserve leading to ever decreasing doses of drugs. A variety of groups have therefore chosen patients with small cell lung cancer who have achieved either complete remissions with conventional chemotherapy or else partial responses of around 90 % tumor shrinkage. The lessons of the first years of ABMT have been learned by most investigators and further patient selection is based on performance status and vitality and reserve of organs at risk (e.g. liver and lung). It was to be expected that bone marrow aspirated after 3 or 4 courses of chemotherapy would contain less granulocyte and erythrocyte precursor cells than prior to this therapy and that has proved to be the case. This however has not been a limitation on the ability of bone marrow to repopulate at this late stage in treatment. There remains also the risk of residual bone marrow metastatic cells and it is to be hoped that monoclonals may be of benefit in this situation.

METHODOLOGY OF ABMT

Marrow is usually aspirated under general anaesthetic due to the time required to receive around a liter of bone marrow. The precise volume required needs to be controlled during the operation by concomitant cell counts. Most centers aim to aspirate around 2×10^8 nucleated cells/kg body weight. Lately this has been achieved under local anaesthetic, accompanied by heavy sedation; the mean duration of the procedure described is one hour and 40 minutes; the mean number of bone marrow punctures was 50, facilitated by the use of a newly developed pistol (Carmitto) which gave considerably more efficient bone marrow suction and avoided operator fatigue [7]. The patient usually requires in addition blood transfusion, although some groups process the bone marrow through a continuous flow centrifuge and reinfuse the harvested red cells within a couple of hours of bone marrow aspiration. The aspirated marrow can then be cryopreserved or if it is to be used within two or three days it can be stored at 4 °C. Although there is some dispute over the length of time that marrow can be maintained at this temperature – claims for percentage viability of progenitor cells range from 40 % after 24 hours [8] to 97 % after 4 days [9] the clinical evidence supports the feasibility of the technique after 72 hours [10]. This means in practice that drug clearance should have been effected within 72 hours to avoid late cytotoxic damage to the reinfused bone marrow. Whereas cryopreservation techniques allow marrow to be stored for a year or more the technique is not devoid of problems. Care has to be taken to eliminate granulocytes which otherwise on thawing will clump or form DNA gels. Further it is necessary to use a protective agent such as dimethyl sulphoxide prior to freezing and this substance has then to be administered to the patient. Side effects have been reported from this compound although on the whole it has been surprising well tolerated.

Mention was made above of the possibility of detecting small numbers of tumor cells in bone marrow aspirates. Preliminary communications have emerged relating to the detection of small numbers of positively staining cells in 'early' breast cancer patients using monoclonal antibodies derived against milk fat globule [11]. Although a variety of groups claim to have produced monoclonal antibodies for small cell lung cancer these claims remain to be tested and therefore their application remains at the present time hypothetical. Using the model developed in studies of leukaemia it seems more than probable that a tumor specific antibody could be used not only to detect metastatic cells but also if appropriately armed to kill cells *in vitro*. Many of the derived antibodies are not cytotoxic per sé however, and therefore require to be linked to toxins such as ricin or abrin or else to a cytotoxic drug. It is highly likely, in order to expect an efficient marrow 'clean-up' in a small cell lung specimen that again, akin to the acute leukaemia situation, a cocktail of monoclonal antibodies will be required tailor made to the variety of heterogeneous clones typical of these diseases.

A novel method of presenting a mixture of antibodies to cells *in vitrovitro* might be the use of carriers such as microspheres.

Kemshead at al have described interesting microspheres which contain magnetite and are coated with goat anti-mouse immunoglobulin [12]. These complexes are mixed with bone marrow which has been incubated with a panel of monoclonal antibodies (mouse antihuman). Tumor cells which have interacted with one of the monoclonal antibodies will then be attached to the microsphere via the goat anti-mouse immunoglobulin. The mixture of bone marrow, antibodies and microspheres is then passed through a magnetic field which separates out the microspheres due to the core of magnetite, allowing purified bone marrow to pass unhindered. There are now several instances of applications of this technique in patients, and reconstitution of bone marrow has been achieved in neuroblastoma patients, indicating survival of sufficient marrow stem cells.

In the absence of specific monoclonal antibodies against small cell lung cancer it is possible to apply cytostatic drugs *in vitro* in order to achieve pure bone marrow (see Table 2). Most experience to date has been achieved with active metabolites of cyclophoshamide such has 4-hydroxycyclophosphamide and 4-hydroxyperoxycyclophosphamide [13]. There is as yet no data on the application of these two drugs *in vitro* to small cell lung cancer bone marrow but the experience gained from leukemia (both animal models and clinical practice) is that the technique is feasible and that short incubation with these drugs *in vitro* leads to depletion of tumor cells and relative preservation of normal myeloid and erythroid precursors.

Table 2. Marrow clean-up

1. Physical-elutriation
2. Cytotoxic antibodies – single or cocktails
3. Antibody – toxin complexes
4. Antibody – microsphere – metal complexes
5. Cytotoxic drugs

CLINICAL RESULTS

The drugs which have received most attention are cyclophosphamide and etoposide (VP16–213). The ideal drug should show a steep dose response curve in small cell lung cancer. The dominant toxicity of the drug should of course be bone marrow. Problems with cyclophosphamide have included cardiotoxicity, probably minimized by dividing the dose of the drug over a 24-hour period, and urotoxicity which can be prevented successfully now by the co-administration of 2-mercaptoethane sulphonate [14]. Etoposide has been associated with stomatitis and gastrointestinal toxicity, occasional hypotension, fever, neuropathy and skin rashes. The other drugs used are BCNU (carmustine) noted above to produce both lung and hepatotoxicity in high dose and melphalan extensively used following the pilot studies by McElwain [15]. The principal toxicity of high dose melphalan is to the gastrointestinal and mucous membranes. Whereas all of these drugs are quickly cleared or metabolized from plasma it is possible that significant levels of active drug or metabolite remain in target organs explaining the later appearance of non-myeloid toxicity. Melphalan for instance has been shown in dog studies to remain circulating in the enterohepatic circulation several days after clearance from plasma. Whereas this is irrelevant from the point of view of causing further toxicity to reinfused bone marrow, it may well be the explanation for the marked dose limiting gastrointestinal toxicity associated with high doses of this drug.

Each of these drugs as a single agent may be effective without resort to bone marrow transplantation. Phase I studies of etoposide have reached a dose of higher than 2 grams/m^2 and anti-tumor activity has been seen in patients resistant to conventional doses [16]. Of particular interest is the report from Postmus et al. (personal communication) of two partial responses in brain metastases from primary small cell lung cancer appearing in previously radiated brain tissue. High dose cyclophosphamide has also been given without autologous bone marrow by Smith who demonstrated almost identical recovery kinetics of white cells and platelets after a dose of 7 g/m^2 administered over 12 hours; it was accompanied by 2-mercaptoethane sulphonate in a group of small cell lung patients not rescued with bone marrow as a group of controls when bone marrow was given back at day 3 [17]. Combination chemotherapy using conventional doses is also not ameliorated by the use of autologous bone marrow transplantation. Glode, et al. studied 10 patients with small cell lung cancer treated with 3 courses of cyclophosphamide, vincristine, doxorubicin and BCNU [18]. The toxicity measured after the first two courses of chemotherapy was compared with that following on the third course chemotherapy when the same doses of drugs were given but followed by autologous bone marrow infusion 40 hours after drug delivery. This group could detect no difference between the degree of myelosuppression or the time to blood count nadirs or the time to recovery. They warned that serial examination of bone marrow indicated gradual decline in granulocyte-macrophage precursors and that this would limit the use of the technique later than 3 or so courses of therapy. Conventional doses of chemotherapy were used and it is not surprising that conventional anti-tumor effect was noted.

Combination high-dose chemotherapy leads to marked toxicity and delayed recovery of bone marrow in the absence of bone marrow support [19]. Full supportive care is required including attention to nutritional intake, blood product requirements and bacterial profiles to assist appropriate antibiotic choice when necessary. Prophylaxis against infection ranges from simple hygiene applied to patients nursed in an open ward to the other extreme of reversed barrier nursing, sterile food and total gut sterilization. There is an expert group who have in the past advocated selective gut contamination with non-absorbable antibiotics but recently failure of this technique (51% infections) in patients undergoing autologous bone marrow transplantation for small cell lung cancer has been reported [20]. There is also evidence which suggests that cotrimoxazole alone or with non-absorbable antibiotics may be the optimal prophylaxis in this group of immuno- and myelosuppressed patients.

The anti-tumor results achieved by the few pilot studies reported to date are summarized in Table 3. The study referred to above in which cyclophos-

Table 3. Preliminary results of ABMT in small cell lung cancer

Ref.	Number of patients	Regime	Timing	Marrow storage	Median survival (wks)	% Longterm survival	Treated related deaths
5	25	C,R.T.	Ind	cryo	69	TE	1
18	10	BCDV	Con	cryo −10°C	48	0	2
21	23	C	Con	4°C	44	0	1
	22	CE	Con	4°C	48	TE	0
22	8	CE,R.T.	Con	cryo	—	0	2
23	5	BMP	Rel	cryo	—	0	1
24	13	BCE	Con	cryo	TE	TE	0
25	5	E	Con	cryo	—	0	0
	3	CE	Con	cryo	—	0	0
26	14	CDEV, R.T.	Ind	cryo	47	0	0

B = BCNU; C = Cyclophosphamide; D = Doxorubicin; E = Etoposide; M = melphalan; P = Procarbazine; V = Vincristine; R.T. = Radiotherapy; cryo = cryopreserved; TE = too early.
Ind = induction; Con = consolidation; Rel = relapse.

phamide was used as initial treatment achieved 12 complete remissions in 21 patients (18 limited disease, and 3 extensive). The median duration of response was 39 weeks despite routine radiotherapy to the primary tumor after assessment of response to the single agent therapy. Few groups have achieved conversion of patients in partial remission after conventional chemotherapy into complete remission. This may of course reflect the aggressiveness of the induction therapy. Soukop et al. used a non-aggressive induction regimen and in 23 patients treated with high-dose cyclophosphamide and autologous bone marrow rescue achieved a median survival of 2.3 months at a cost of 3 drug related deaths [21]. Then they treated 23 patients with high-dose cyclophosphamide and etoposide and radiotherapy following a more aggressive drug induction regimen, but despite this a high relapse rate was once again seen. Only two patients were disease-free 12 months after the manoeuvre. The group in the NCI combined high-dose cyclophosphamide with 2000 rads in 5 fractions over 5 days to the primary tumor and cranial radiation. 8 Patients were treated all of whom had extensive disease and none survived longer than 15 months [22]. This was a bad prognosis group including 5 partial remissions, one of whom went into complete remission with high-dose therapy but this lasted only 3 months. Three patients achieved complete remission but relapsed 8-15 months later. A French study was reported earlier in which the high-dose chemotherapy used was BCNU, procarbazine and melphalan, followed on day 6 with autologous bone marrow. Haematological recovery was acceptable in all patients and 3 partial remissions and 2 complete remissions were noted in 10 patients. There was one toxic death due to cardiorespiratory failure 15 days following high-dose chemotherapy. One of the few interesting trials which is testing the value of high-dose chemotherapy and ABMT as consolidation therapy is being conducted in the Ludwig Institute in Brussels. This group randomizes patients who have achieved complete or partial response after 3 courses of vincristine, cyclophosphamide, doxorubicin and methotrexate and 2 courses of cisplatin-etoposide to receive high-dose cyclophosphamide, etoposide and BCNU or conventional maintenance chemotherapy. In an interim report they showed that the technique was feasible, that a large number of patients would be required to evaluate the contribution of high-dose chemotherapy and ABMT and that the results in treating extensive disease patients were sombre.

Toxicity consisted mainly of gastritis and colitis associated with myelosuppression and they confirmed that bone marrow repopulation was possible despite a 50% drop in hemopoietic cells/ml of bone marrow aspirate due to the induction therapy. This group have reported conversion of several partial remissions in patients (all limited disease) into complete remission by this technique and have already reported a few relapses in the limited group and very many in the extensive disease group. It is to be hoped that at least one other similar study will be carried out in order to fully assess the cost benefit of this experimental technique. Mention has been made above of the cost to the patient in toxicity, but what has not been alluded to is the financial cost of high-doses of expensive chemotherapeutic agents, general anaesthetic for bone marrow aspiration, preservation and the cost of supportive care hospitalisation due to bone marrow aplasia. If promising results are achieved with trials such as described above then there remain a backlog of questions relevant to refinement of the technique. These relate to optimalisation of the drug dosage and delivery system, improvement of bone marrow clean-up, and evolution of more effective pharmacological rescue techniques to ensure inactivation of residual cytostatic drug. Examples of the last might be extra-corporeal circulation, administration of sulf-hydryl groups or enzymes such as carboxypeptidase which quickly and efficiently emasculate methotrexate. All such refinements require to be tested eventually in randomized trials and it cannot be too frequently stressed that reporting of such trials should focus on the assessment of long term survival rather than response rate and median survivals.

CONCLUSION

The application of ABMT as a salvage system after megadose chemotherapy has proved feasible in small cell lung cancer. No long term patient benefit has yet been demonstrated in any of the preliminary studies reported uptill now. Toxicity in organs other than bone marrow proves the limiting factor in escalation of drug doses. The best short term results (temporary remissions with minimal toxicity) have been seen in patients treated for limited disease (or already in complete remission) who have a good performance status. Many ways of improving effectiveness of the technique and lowering the morbidity exist at least in theory, and therefore the final assessment of its relevance to lung cancer must be postponed.

REFERENCES

1. Comis RL: Small cell carcinoma of the lung. Cancer Treat Rev 9:237–258, 1982.
2. Cohen MH, Creaven PI, Fossieck JR, Broder LE, Selawry OS, Johnston AV, Williams CL, Minna JD: Intensive chemotherapy of small cell bronchogenic carcinoma. Cancer Treat Rep 61:349–354, 1977.
3. Johnston RE, Brereton HD, Kent CH: Total therapy for small cell carcinoma of the lung. Ann Thorac Surg 25:510–515, 1978.
4. Thomas ED, Buckner CD, Clift RA, Fefer A, Johnson FL, Neiman PE, Sale GE, Sanders JE,

Singer JW, Shulman H, Storb R, Weiden PL: Marrow transplantation for acute non-lymphoblastic leukaemia in first remission N Eng J Med 301:597–599, 1979.

5. Souhami RL, Harper PG, Linch D, Trask C, Goldstone AH, Tobias AH, Spiro SG, Geddes DM, Richards JD: High-dose cyclophosphamide with autologous marrow transplantation as initial treatment of small cell carcinoma of the bronchus. Cancer Chemother Pharmacol 8:31–34, 1982.

6. Norton L, Simon R: Tumour size sensitivity to therapy and design of treatment schedules. Cancer Treat Rep 61:1307–1317, 1977.

7. de Vries EGE, Meinesz AF, Daenen S, Mulder NH, Postmus PE, Sleijfer DTh, Vriesendorp R: Bone marrow harvest without general anesthesia for autologous bone marrow transplantation. In: Autologous Bone Marrow Transplantation and Solid Tumours. McVie JG, Dalesio O, Smith IE (eds). New York, Raven Press, 1984.

8. McElwain TT, Hedley DW, Burton G, Clink HM, Gordon MY, Jarman M, Juttner CA, Millar JL, Milsted RAV, Prentice G, Smith IE, Spence D, Woods M: Marrow autotransplantation accelerates haematological recovery in patients with malignant melanoma treated with high-dose melphalan. Br J Cancer 40:72–80, 1979.

9. Delforge A, Range-Collard E, Stryckmans P, Spiro T, Malarme MA: Granulocyte-macrophage progenitor cell preservation at 4°C. Br J Haemat 53:49–54, 1983.

10. Tansey P, Burnett AK, Hill C, Alcorn MJ, Singer CRJ: Haematological reconstitution following supralethal chemoradiotherapy using autologous bone marrow stored at 4°C. Exp Haemat 11 (suppl. 13):173, 1983.

11. Redding WH, Coombes RC, Neville AM, Ormerod M, Powles TJ, Ford HT, Gazet JC: Detection of marrow micrometastasesin primary breast cancer. Proc of 3rd EORTC Breast Cancer Working Conference, 111:10, 1983.

12. Kemshead JT, Gibson FJ, Ugelstad J, Rembaum A: A flow system for the *in vitro* separation of tumour cells from bone marrow using monoclonal antibodies and magnetic microspheres. Proc Am Assoc Cancer Res 24:217, 1983.

13. Korbling M, Fliedner TM, Uckun F, Hunstein W: Elimination of residual tumor cells from the autologous stem cell graft by chemoseparation. In: Autologous Bone Marrow Transplantation and Solid Tumors. McVie JG, Dalesio O, Smith IE (eds). New York, Raven Press, 1984.

14. Scheaf W, Oklein H, Brock N: Controlled studies with an antidote against the urotoxicity of oxazophorines. Cancer Treat Rep 63:501–505, 1979.

15. McElwain TJ, Hedley DW, Gordon MY, Jarman M, Millar J, Pritchard J: Hich-dose melphalan and non-cryopreserved autologous bone marrow treatment of malignant melanoma and neuroblastoma. Exp Hemat 7:360–371, 1979.

16. Wolff SN, Fer MF, McKay C, Hainsworth J, Hawde KR, Greco FA: High-dose VP16 and autologous bone marrow transplantation for advanced malignancies – a phase I study. Proc Am Assoc Cancer Res 23:134, 1982.

17. Smith IE, Evans BD, Harland SJ, Millar JL: Autologous bone marrow rescue is unnecessary after very high dose cyclophosphamide. Lancet 1:8, 1983.

18. Glode LM, Robinson WA, Hartmann DW, Klein JJ, Thomas MR, Morton N: Autologous bone marrow transplantation in the therapy of small cell carcinoma of the lung. Cancer Res 43:4270–4275, 1982.

19. Gale RP, Graze PR, Wells J, Ho W, Cline MJ: Autologous bone marrow transplantation in patients with cancer. Exp Haematol (suppl. 5), 7:35–39, 1979.

20. Postmus PE, de Vries-Hospers HG, Sleijfer DTh, van Imhoff GW, Meinesz AF, Vriesendorp R, Mulder NH, de Vries EGE: Failure of selective gut decontamination with non-absorbable antibiotics in preventing infections in patients treated with high-dose chemotherapy and autologous bone marrow transplantation. In: Autologous bone Marrow Transplantation and Solid Tumors. McVie JG, Dalesio O, Smith IE (eds), New York, Raven Press, 1984.

21. Soukop M, Ahmedza S, Banham S, Burnett A, Cunningham D, Dorward A, Hutcheon A, Lucie N, Kaye S, Stevenson R, Tansey T: Late Intensification chemotherapy in small cell lung cancer. In: Autologous Bone Marrow Transplantation and Solid Tumors. McVie JG, Dalesie O, Smith IE (eds), New York, Raven Press, 1984.
22. Ihde DC, Lichter AS, Deisseroth AB, Bunn P, Carney DN, Cohen MH, Makuch RW, Johnston-Early A, Minna JD: Late intensive combined modality therapy with autolous bone marrow infusion in extensive stage small cell lung cancer. Proc Am Assoc Clin Oncol 2:198, 1983.
23. Pico JL, Beaujean F, Debré M, Carde P, LLE Chevalier T, Hayat M: High-dose chemotherapy with autologous bone marrow transplantation in small cell lung carcinoma in relapse. Proc Am Soc Clin Oncol 2:206, 1983.
24. Syman M, Bosly A, Humblet Y, Delaunois L, Steyaert J, Francis C, Machiels J, Prignot J: Late intensification the apy and autologous bone marrow transplantation in small cell lung cancer. Proc 13th Internat Congress Chemother 232:20-24, 1983.
25. Mulder NH, Meinesz AF, Sleijfer DTh, Postmus PE, de Vries EGE, Smit Sibinga CTH, Vriesendorp R: High-dose etoposide with or without cyclophosphamide and autologous bone marrow transplantation in solid tumours. In: Autologous Bone Marrow Transplantation and solid tumors. McVie JG, Dalesio O, Smith IE (eds), New York, Raven press, 1984.
26. Farha P, Spitzer G, Valdivieso M, Zander A, Verma D, Minnhaar G, Vellekoop L, Dicke K, Bodey G: Treatment of small cell bronchogenic carcinoma with high-dose chemotherapy and autologous bone marrow transplantation. Proc AACR and ASCO 22:496, 1981.

9. Chemotherapy in Osteosarcoma: Advances and Controversies

NORMAN JAFFE

During the past decade, major advances have been reported in the treatment of osteosarcoma [1–9]. These derive principally from the application of chemotherapy in the management of the primary tumor, as an adjuvant to prevent pulmonary metastases, and in multidisciplinary strategies to eradicate established disease. These developments, however, have not been without controversy [10–13]. The latter emerged principally from a comparison of the results of the new investigations with historical controls. This communication will outline the impact of chemotherapy in osteosarcoma and examine the controversial issues.

Until the beginning of the past decade, osteosarcoma was considered a chemo-resistant tumor [14]. The primary tumor was generally treated by amputation and the cure rate rarely exceeded 20% [15]. The mortality was due to pulmonary metastases. These were not demonstrable on conventional radiographs at diagnosis but usually appeared 6 to 9 months after surgery. This suggested that pulmonary micrometastases were present in at least 80% of such patients. The consistency of this experience prompted the use of these reports as historical controls as a basis of comparison with new therapies. The historical control series included a report from the Mayo Clinic in which diagnosis and treatment were accomplished with frozen section biopsy, ablative surgery and a two tourniquet technique [16].

In the 1970s, three major chemotherapeutic agents were shown to be effective in metastatic osteosarcoma. These comprised high dose methotrexate with citrovorum factor 'rescue' [1], Adriamycin [6], and Cisdiamminedichloroplatinum II [7]. This provided the impetus to administer chemotherapy as adjuvant treatment after surgical ablation of the primary tumor. The intent was to destroy the pulmonary micrometastases. This strategy produced a 3-year disease-free survival of 50–80% [1–9] (Figure 1). This appears statistically significant when compared to historical controls. Only a small number of investigators suggested that adjuvant chemotherapy had not produced any major impact [10–13].

F.M. Muggia (ed.), Experimental and Clinical Progress in Cancer Chemotherapy
© *1985, Martinus Nijhoff Publishers, Boston. ISBN 0-89838-679-9. Printed in the Netherlands.*

224

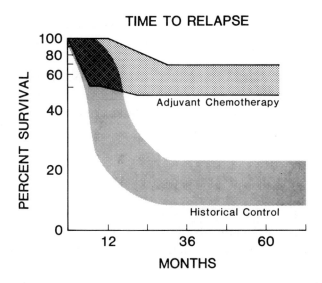

Figure 1. Disease free survival in patients treated with adjuvant chemotherapy. Life table analysis abstracted and constructed from references 1–9 and 18.

The historical control series is abstracted and constructed from references 15, 16, and 26–28.

The improvement in survival with adjuvant chemotherapy was instrumental in devising new approaches to the treatment of the primary tumor. Principally these comprised transmedullary amputation, limb salvage, (surgical resection and endoprosthetic replacement) and rotationplasty [17–19]. Concurrently, new investigative approaches were adopted: thus, in contrast to historical controls, the absence of pulmonary metastases was now confirmed by pulmonary tomography and occasionally computerized axial tomography. In some centers more intensive investigations, comprising radionuclide bone scanning and computerized axial tomography of the primary lesion were also employed.

Limb salvage was considered to be a seminal advance. To enhance the safety of the surgical procedure Rosen advocated the use of preoperative chemotherapy [18]. Subsequently, it was administered preoperatively to all patients. The intent was to identify a potentially effective postoperative chemotherapeutic agent for adjuvant treatment. Thus, the agent found to be effective preoperatively was retained postoperatively as adjuvant treatment and bolstered with additional agents. Alternatively, if ineffective, it was discarded and replaced by other therapy. Utilizing this approach, the improved survival initially reported with chemotherapy was augmented and sustained [3, 18].

However, the contention that improved survival could be attributed to chemotherapy, did not go unchallenged. A randomized study by the Mayo

Clinic revealed a disease-free survival of approximately 40% in patients treated by amputation and prophylactic whole lung radiotherapy [21]. This report was later supported by claims of a 'natural' improvement in survival over the ensuing five years and that it was not necessary to assume that chemotherapy was responsible for this improvement [22]. These authors reported that prior to 1969, survival had remained constant, around 20% (cf historical controls); however, between 1969 and 1972, a trend toward improved survival occurred, and between 1972 and 1974, survival with amputation only was 50%.

A number of factors were considered to have contributed to the foregoing result although none, either singularly or in concert, could account for the dramatic change. These impressions eventually prompted the Mayo Clinic to launch a randomized study to confirm the published efficacy of high dose methotrexate. This study failed to demonstrate an advantage with methotrexate and a 'no treatment' control arm. Survival in each was approximately 50% [11].

The study by the Mayo Clinic prompted additional attempts to refute the advances achieved with chemotherapy and invalidate the use of historical controls. Thus, it was claimed that pulmonary tomography could identify (and exclude) more patients with metastases at diagnosis. This could unintentionally bias the selection of patients treated with adjuvant chemotherapy. Further it was considered that osteosarcoma was now possibly being diagnosed earlier in its course as opposed to the several previous decades. This was based on the supposition to that medical attendants in the 1930s–1950s, were reluctant to refer patients to major medical centers for immediate treatment once osteosarcoma had been diagnosed or suspected. This implied an earlier referral pattern, and treatment of less advanced disease. In this context, earlier diagnosis and treatment are usually associated with a more favorable outcome and could thus account for the altered survival reported by the Mayo Clinic. Finally, it was stated that improvements in surgical technique could possibly also be invoked in attaining more favorable results [12].

The foregoing dispute lead to the contention that clinical trials with concurrent controls would probably be necessary to demonstrate the stated efficacy of adjuvant chemotherapy. In the absence of such trials, many patients could be subjected to unnecessary, costly and often dangerous treatment. These concepts culminated in a publication 'Is It Ethical Not to Conduct a Prospectively Controlled Randomized Trial in Osteosarcoma?' in which a randomized controlled (surgery only) clinical trial was proposed [12].

In contrast to the above, it was maintained that historical controls should still receive appropriate recognition [23, 24]. This was based upon the fact that the outcome for patients with osteosarcoma treated with amputation

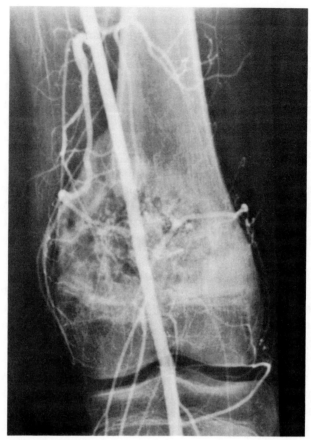

Figure 2. Left femural anteriogram in a patient with osteosarcoma of the left distal femur. There is a large hypervascular lytic area with early venous shunting.

alone prior to the 1970s, had been constant: survival, derived from published reports exceeding a patient population of over 1000, was approximately 20%. Further, statistical computations were available to compensate and adjust for differences when comparing historical control patients with current studies [23]. Thus, while it was possible that histology, tumor size, location, age, and other factors could influence the outcome of individual patients with osteosarcoma [25], such biological variables assumed less significance when similar or identical results in large numbers were reported by investigators throughout the world.

The possibility of a 'spontaneous' change in the disease free survival as reported by the Mayo Clinic was also challenged. Thus, disease free survival over several consecutive years was evaluated by the M.D. Anderson Hospital and Tumor Institute, Sidney Farber Cancer Institute, Memorial Sloan-

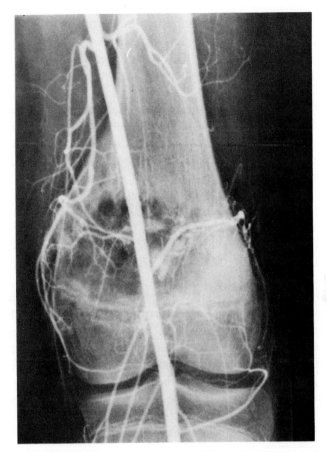

Figure 3. Following four courses of intra-arterial Cis-diamminedichloroplatinum II, the left femural arteriogram reveals decreased tumor neovascularity and almost a complete absence of tumor stain.

Kettering Cancer Center and the Instituto Orthopedico Rizzoli in Bologna. These 'changes' could not be substantiated [9, 26–28]. Further, examination of the 'improved survival' reported by the Mayo Clinic reveals that several groups of patients received a variety of adjuvant regimens in addition to surgery [22].

The contention that full lung tomography could invalidate historical controls can also be refuted. The detection of metastases at diagnosis by this means has varied from 1.9 to 9.3% [28–30]. One series reported that the incidence of unsuspected metastases on conventional radiographs was only escalated by 2.4% with pulmonary tomography [31]. Viewed from a different perspective only 2.7% of tomographic studies were helpful in identifying additional pulmonary metastases in childhood cancer [32]. Similar low diagnostic yields were reported in other malignancies [32, 33]. Thus, an unintentional case selection bias because of the absence of lung tomography in historical controls appears unlikely. These remarks also pertain to the detection of metastases by bone scanning: the incidence at presentation has varied from 1.8 to 7.7% [34–37].

There is, unfortunately, little information relating the use of computerized axial tomography in osteosarcoma. It is possible that it may improve the identification of pulmonary metastases in patients considered to be free of disease by conventional radiographs or pulmonary tomography. However, it remains to be reported that this instrument will indeed change the staging categories of patients, and to what degree if any, it will render the use of historical controls invalid. Preliminary data do not support this contention in osteosarcoma or Wilms' tumor [29, 38]. Computerized axial tomography was apparently not adopted as a standard investigative procedure in the improved survival reported by the Mayo Clinic over the past decade [22].

There is also no evidence that surgical treatment of the primary tumor has been responsible for the altered survival. On the contrary, chemotherapy has had a major impact in modifying surgical techniques. Thus, there has been an accelerating tendency to employ less radical ablative procedures. These comprise transmedullary amputation, rotationplasty and resection for limb salvage [17–19]. Pre-operative chemotherapy, by inducing tumor destruction, enhances the safety of these surgical procedures and reduces the incidence of local recurrence. The latter is also reduced by the continued application of postoperative treatment. The utility of pre-operative chemotherapy in preparation for rotationplasty for an osteosarcoma of the distal femur is illustrated in Figures 2 and 3 and the post-operative result in Figures 4 and 5.

Improvements in survival due to chemotherapy have also been observed in patients with metastatic disease. Thus, most patients who relapse while receiving adjuvant chemotherapy have a reduced number of pulmonary metastases and/or a delay in their appearance [9, 39–43]. This has been a major element in facilitating retrieval of the relapsed patient by thoracotomy and other measures. This is clearly illustrated in Table 1 generated from the M.D. Anderson Hospital and Tumor Institute [41]. During this period, the medical attendants responsible for the treatment of osteosarcoma were relatively stable and the conceptual development and enthusiasm for treatment of patients only accelerated after the 1970s when the new pattern of pulmonary metastases induced by chemotherapy emerged.

There is additional evidence to indicate changes in the natural history of osteosarcoma induced by chemotherapy. An increasing number of patients on adjuvant chemotherapy have developed extra pulmonary metastases to

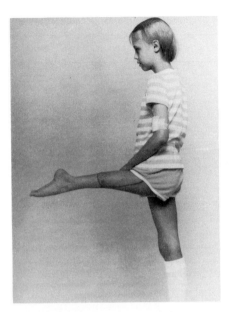

Figure 4. Post operative appearance of the patient following a successful rotationplasty. The operation involved amputation of the femur several centimeters above the known upper extent of tumor. The tibia was then excised distal to the proximal physis. The intervening skin and soft tissue were also excised and the tibia rotated through 180° prior to fixation to the proximal femoral stump. Pathological examination of the resected specimen revealed over 90% tumor destruction.

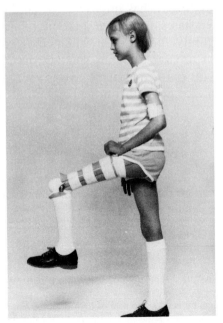

Figure 5. Prosthesis applied to rotationplasty. A functional new 'knee' has been created.

Table 1. Impact of year of diagnosis and time to metastases in post metastatic survival

Year of diagnosis	Patients	Survival
A. 1970 or earlier	62	4
B. 1971 or later	44	27
p = 0.002 (A vs. B)		

Time of metastases	Patients	Survival
A. 0	19	1
B. 1–12 mos.	73	13
C. 13+mos.	14	7
p = 0.002 (A vs. C)		
p = 0.005 (B vs C)		
p = 0.45 (A vs B)		

Modified from Sutow, W.W., Herson, J. and Perez, C., Ref. 41.

bone, spine, brain, heart and other unusual sites [44–48]. Unfortunately, at times this has not been entirely in the patients' best interests. This phenomenon can be attributed to the heterogenous nature of the tumor, partially effective chemotherapy, and prolongation of survival.

The foregoing clearly indicates that chemotherapy has had a major impact in osteosarcoma. In essence, it has improved the cure rate, altered the pattern of pulmonary metastases, facilitated multidisciplinary intervention, and enhanced the opportunity for local resection and functional restoration. There does not appear to have been any spontaneous change in the natural history of the disease (as claimed by the Mayo Clinic). Any improvement in survival must therefore be attributed principally to the use of effective chemotherapy.

ACKNOWLEDGMENTS

This study is supported in part by Grant # CA-03713 and CA-09070 from the National Institutes of Health.

REFERENCES

1. Jaffe N: Recent advances in the chemotherapy of metastatic osteogenic sarcoma. Cancer 30:1627–1631, 1972.
2. Jaffe N, Link M, Traggis D, *et al.*: The role of high dose methotrexate in osteogenic sarcoma. Sarcomas of soft tissue and bone in childhood. Natl Cancer Inst Monogr 56:201–206, 1981.

3. Rosen G, Caparros B, Huvos AG, et al.: Preoperative chemotherapy for osteogenic sarcoma: Selection of postoperative adjuvant chemotherapy based on the response of the primary tumor to preoperative chemotherapy. Cancer 49:1221–1230, 1982.
4. Sutow WW, Gehan EA, Vietti TJ, et al.: Multidrug chemotherapy in primary treatment of osteosarcoma. J Bone Jt Surg 58-A:629–633, 1976.
5. Pratt C, Shanks E, Hust O, et al.: Adjuvant multiple drug chemotherapy for osteosarcoma of the extremity. Cancer 39:51–57, 1979.
6. Cortes EP, Holland JF, Wang JJ, et al.: Amputation and adriamycin in primary osteosarcoma. N Engl J Med 291:998, 1974.
7. Ochs JJ, Freeman AI, Douglass HO, Jr, et al.: Cis-dichloro-diammine platinum (II) in advanced osteogenic sarcoma. Cancer Treat Rep 62:239–245, 1978.
8. Ettinger IJ, Douglass HO, Jr, Higby DG, et al.: Adjuvant Adriamycin and Cis-diammine-dichloroplatinum (Cis-platinum) in primary osteosarcoma. Cancer 47:248–254, 1981.
9. Campanacci M, Bacci G, Bertori F, et al.: The treatment of osteosarcoma of the extremities: Twenty years experience at the Institute Ortopedico Rizzoli. Cancer 48:1569–1581, 1982.
10. Carter SK: The dilemma of adjuvant chemotherapy for osteogenic sarcoma. Cancer Clin Trials 3:29–36, 1980.
11. Edmonson JH, Green SJ, Ivins JC, et al.: Methotrexate as adjuvant treatment for primary osteosarcoma. N Engl J Med 303:642–645, 1980.
12. Lange B, Levine AS: Is it ethical not to conduct a prospectively controlled trial of adjuvant chemotherapy in osteosarcoma? Cancer Treat Rep 66:1699–1704, 1982.
13. Brostrom LA, Apairsi T, Ingimarsson SN, et al.: Can historical controls be used in current clinical trials in osteosarcoma? Metastasis and survival in a historical and concurrent group. Int J Radiat Oncol Biol Phys 6:1717–1721, 1980.
14. Jaffe N: Osteogenic sarcoma: State of the art with high-dose methotrexate treatment. Clin Orthop 120:95–102, 1976.
15. Friedman MA, Carter SK: The therapy of osteogenic sarcoma: current status and thoughts for the future. J Surg Oncol 4 5/6):482, 1972.
16. Dahlin DC, Coventry MB: Osteogenic sarcoma: A study of 600 cases. J Bone Joint Surg 49-A:101–110, 1967.
17. Jaffe N, Traggis DG, Cohen D, et al.: The impact of high dose methotrexate on the management of osteogenic sarcoma. Vol. 10. XII International Cancer Congress. Pergamon Press Oxford, pp 175–179, 1979.
18. Rosen G, Marcove RC, Caparros B, et al.: Primary osteogenic sarcoma. The rationale for preoperative chemotherapy and delayed surgery. Cancer 43:2163–2177, 1979.
19. Jaffe N, Knapp J, Chuang VP, et al.: Osteosarcoma: Intra-arterial treatment of the primary tumor with Cis-diammine-dichloroplatinum II (CDP). Angiographic, pathologic and pharmacologic studies. Cancer 51:402–407, 1983.
20. Eilber FR, Morton DL, Grant TT: En bloc resection and allograft replacement for osteosarcoma of the extremity. In: Bone tumors in children. Jaffe N (ed). PSG Publishing Co., Inc., Littleton, Mass., 1979, pp 159–167.
21. Rab CT, Ivins JC, Childs RE, et al.: Elective whole lung irradiation in the treatment of osteogenic sarcoma. Cancer 38:939–942, 1976.
22. Taylor WF, Ivins JG, Dahlin D, et al.: Osteogenic sarcoma experience at the Mayo Clinic 1963–1974 in immunotherapy of cancer. In: Terry, Windhorst, immunotherapy of cancer. Present status of trials in man. pp 257–269, Raven Press, New York, 1978.
23. Gehan EA, Sutow WW, Uribe-Botero T, et al.: Osteosarcoma. The M. D. Anderson experience 1950–1974. In: Terry, Windhorst, immunotherapy of cancer. Present status of trials in man, pp 271–282, Raven Press, New York, 1978.
24. Jaffe N, van Eys J, Gehan EA: Response to 'Is it ethical not to conduct a prospectively controlled trial of adjuvant chemotherapy in osteosarcoma?' Cancer Treat Rep 67:743–744,

1982.

25. Dahlin DC: Osteosarcoma of bone and a consideration of prognostic variables. Cancer Treat Rep 62:193–197, 1978.

26. Mike V, Marcove RC: Osteogenic sarcoma under the age of 21. Experiences at Memorial Sloan-Kettering Cancer Center. In: Terry, Windhorst, Immunotherapy of cancer. Present status of trials in man, pp 283–292, Raven Press, New York, 1978.

27. Gehan EA, Sutow WW, Uribe-Botero T, et al.: Osteosarcoma. The M. D. Anderson experiencel 1950–1974. In: Terry, Windhorst, Immunotherapy of cancer. Present status of trials in man, Raven Press, New York, pp 271–282, 1978.

28. Frei E, III, Blum R, Jaffe N: Sarcoma: Natural history and treatment. In: Immunotherapy of cancer. Present status of trials in man. Terry WD, Windhorst D (eds). Raven Press, New York, 1978, pp 245–255.

29. Muhm JR, Pritchard DJ: Computer tomography for the detection of pulmonary metastases in patients with osteogenic sarcoma. Proc Am Assoc Cancer Res 593, 1980.

30. Rosenberg SA, Chabner BA, and Young RC: Treatment of osteogenic sarcoma. Effect of adjuvant high dose methotrexate after amputation. Cancer Treat Rep 63:739–751, 1979.

31. Bacci G, Picci P, Galderoni P, et al.: Full-lung tomograms and bone scanning in the initial work-up of patients with osteogenic sarcoma. A review of 126 cases. Eur J Cancer Clin Oncol 18:967–971, 1982.

32. Cohen M, Provisor A, Smith WL, et al.: Efficacy of whole lung tomography on diagnosing metastases from solid tumors in children. Radiology 141:375–378, 1981.

33. Gordon RE, Mettler FA, Jr, Wicks J, et al.: Chest x-rays and full lung tomograms in gynecologic malignancy. Cancer 52:559–562, 1983.

34. Goldman AB, Becker MH, Braunstein P, et al.: Bone scanning osteogenic sarcoma. Correlation with surgical pathology. Radiology 142:83–90, 1975.

35. Goldstein H, McNeil BJ, Zufall E, et al.: Changing indications for bone scintigraphy in patients with osteosarcoma. Radiology 135:177–180, 1980.

36. McKillop JH, Etcubanas E, Goris ML: The indications for and limitations of bone scintigraphy in osteogenic sarcoma: a review of 55 patients. Cancer 48:1133–1138, 1981.

37. McNeil BJ, Cassady JR, Geiser CF, et al.: Fluorine-18 bone scintigraphy in children osteosarcoma or Ewing's sarcoma. Radiology 109:627–631, 1973.

38. Wilimas J, Hammon E, Champion J, et al.: The value of computerized tomography (CT) as a routine follow-up procedure for patients with Wilms' tumor. Am Soc Clin Oncol 2:80, 1983 (Abstr 34).

39. Pratt C, Shanks E, Hustu O, et al.: Adjuvant multiple drug chemotherapy for osteosarcoma of the extremity. Cancer 39:51–57, 1979.

40. Eilber FR, Grant T, Morton DL: Adjuvant therapy for osteosarcoma: Preoperative and postoperative treatment. Cancer Treat Rep 62:213–216, 1978.

41. Sutow WW, Herson J, Perez C: Survival after metastases in osteosarcoma. Sarcomas of soft tissue and bone in childhood. NCI Monograph 56:227–231, 1981.

42. Jaffe N, Smith E, Abelson HT, et al.: Osteogenic sarcoma: alterations in the pattern of pulmonary metastases with adjuvant chemotherapy. J Clin Oncol 1(4):251–254, 1983.

43. Picci P, Calderoni P, Cagnano R, et al.: The hypothetical change in the natural history of osteosarcoma. Chemioterapia (The Journal of the Mediterranean Society of Oncology). In press.

44. Jaffe N: Current concepts in the management of disseminated malignant bone disease in children. Can J Surg 20:537–539, 1977.

45. McCarten KM, Jaffe N, Kirkpatrick JA: The changing radiographic appearance of osteogenic sarcoma. Ann Radiol 23:203–220, 1980.

46. Danziger J, Wallace S, Hardel S, et al.: Metastatic osteogenic sarcomas to the brain. Cancer 43:707–710, 1979.

47. Giuliano AE,Eilber FR: Changing patterns of metastases of osteosarcoma. Am Soc Clin Oncol 2:229, 1983 (Abstr. 894).
48. Das L, Farooki ZO, Hakami MN, *et al.*: Asymptomatic intracardiac metastases from osteosarcoma: A case report with literature review. Med Pediatr Oncol 11(3):164–166, 1983.

10. Current Issues in the Evaluation and Treatment of Epithelial Carcinoma of the Ovary

UZIEL BELLER and JAMES SPEYER

1. INTRODUCTION

Epithelial ovarian carcinoma is one of the most lethal malignancies of the female genital organs. Significant advances in our understanding of the natural history of this disease, careful initial staging and aggressive surgical and chemotherapeutic management, have improved the short term course for many of these patients. However, a number of major questions remain for the medical team involved in the management of these patients (gynecologic, medical and radiation oncologists), in order to improve the overall cure rate.

This chapter will attempt to address some of these issues and questions encountered in the evaluation and treatment of the patient with advanced epithelial ovarian carcinoma.

2. ARE CURRENT STAGING METHODS OPTIMAL?

Staging of ovarian carcinoma is conventionally done surgically and determined by thorough evaluation of intraabdominal organs followed by pathologic and cytologic study of removed tissues and fluids. The FIGO staging system, revised in 1979 [1] (Table 1), is now the accepted system for defining the stage of disease.

Non-invasive pre-operative staging has now been evaluated in several clinical studies. The use of Radiography, Ultrasonography, Lymphangiography and CAT scanning has been reviewed [1–6]. Whereas bone and liver-spleen scans were shown to make little contribution to preoperative evaluation of the extent of involvement, CAT scanning and lymphangiography can reveal important selective information regarding the presence of subclinical metastatic disease [7–9]. Clearly, a grossly positive scan or evidence of

F.M. Muggia (ed.), Experimental and Clinical Progress in Cancer Chemotherapy
© *1985, Martinus Nijhoff Publishers, Boston. ISBN 0-89838-679-9. Printed in the Netherlands.*

Table 1. FIGO (International Federation Gynecology and Obstetrics staging classification of ovarian cancer of epithelial type)

Stage	Definition
I.	Growth limited to ovaries
a.	Growth limited to one ovary; no ascites. (i) No tumor on external surface; capsule intact. (ii) Tumor on external surface or capsule ruptured or both.
b.	Growth limited to both ovaries; no ascites. (i) No tumor on external surface; capsule intact. (ii) Tumor on external surface or capsule(s) ruptured or both.
c.	Tumor stage is IA or IB, plus ascites* or malignant cells in peritoneal washings.
II.	Growth involving one or both ovaries, with pelvic extension.
a.	Extension or metastases or both to uterus or tubes or both.
b.	Extension to other pelvic tissues.
c.	Tumor stage IIA or IIB, plus ascites* or malignant cells in peritoneal washings.
III.	Growth involving one or both ovaries, with intraperitoneal metastases outside the pelvis or positive retroperitoneal nodes or both. Tumor limited to true pelvis, with histologically proven malignant extension to small bowel or omentum.
IV.	Growth involving one or both ovaries, with distant metastases. Pleural effusion must contain malignant cells to indicate stage IV disease. Parenchymal liver metastases indicate stage IV disease.
Special category	Unexplored cases thought to be of ovarian carcinoma.

* Peritoneal effusion that, in the opinion of the surgeon, is pathologic or clearly exceeds normal amounts or both.

extraabdominal disease, indicate stage III or IV disease. Our own experience with restaging patients shows that an abdominal pelvic CAT scan can reveal significant information as to the status of the liver surface and parenchyma, ascites, the retroperitoneal lymphatics, metastatic peritoneal nodules and the character of a pelvic mass. In addition, the use of contrast material enables one to obtain a visualization of kidneys and ureters, an important consideration for the surgeon. Thus, if CAT scan of the abdomen and pelvis is done, little additional information will be gained by the often routine preoperative IVP and Barium Enema. In fact the use of air insuflation of the rectogismoid during CAT scanning further renders Barium Enema unnecessary. On the other hand a negative CAT scan does not exclude even extensive intraperitoneal dissemination. Recently a series by Brenner *et al.* [10] was reported in which 49 patients underwent computerized tomography prior to second look surgery. Twenty four of 39 patients (61%) reported to have normal CAT scan, were found to have residual tumor at laparotomy.

There were no false positive examinations. Of the 24 patients, microscopic (positive washings or random biopsy), minimal (<2 cm) or gross (>2 cm) disease was found in 8, 7, and 9 patients respectively. The role of non invasive staging is certainly increased in the setting of restaging and follow up during the course of treatment. It will be addressed later in this chapter.

Therefore, non-invasive evaluation should not replace initial exploration for the purpose of accurate staging and surgical treatment. Only a surgical exploration can obtain the necessary information for staging. Since initiation of therapy is based on findings at surgery, and therapy preferably begun as soon as possible [11, 12], preoperative work up should not delay exploration for too long.

Though the current FIGO staging system correlates well with prognosis, there are problems with its use. The first is understaging in early disease. In Stages I, II the disease is limited to the ovaries or pelvic organs respectively, without extrapelvic involvement. However, several clinical studies have shown that in approximately 25% of the cases the disease may be up staged to III or IV. Studies by Fuks [13], Piver [14], Rubin [15], Day [16] and others [17-19] have all stressed and confirmed the existing problem of understaging. This is probably the main cause for the observed 60% five years survival in Stage I disease. This also accounts for the recurrence outside the pelvic port when these patients are treated with pelvic irradiation.

In order to decrease the rate of understaging, one must meticulously follow the recommended steps for surgical exploration as suggested by Wharton and Herson [20] and others [16, 18, 21-23]. Using clinical and surgical judgement the entire potential area of spread of ovarian carcinoma should be explored. This includes, in addition to hysterectomy and bilateral oophorectomy, a partial omentectomy, biopsies of peritoneal surfaces (suspicious & normal), paraortic lymph node biopsies and washings of the quadrants of the posterior parietal peritoneum. These procedures make laparoscopy (peritoneoscopy) an insufficient tool for staging purposes. However, for restaging following chemotherapy the procedure can be helpful as we shall discuss further.

It should be noted that more accurate staging should improve the statistical estimate of prognosis of all groups. Stage I and II prognosis will improve because the previously missed cases with disease outside the pelvis will be excluded. In addition, upstaging of patients with small occult extrapelvic disease, with a generally favorable prognosis, should improve the overall outcome of the Stage III and IV patients. These changes in stage distribution should be considered when evaluating the results of more recent non-randomized therapeutic trials with modestly improved survival.

It is expected that in the near future our evaluation modalities will include tumor specific antibodies based on differentiation antigens and produced by monoclonal cell lines. Identification of tumor markers with this technique will enable us to better detect the presence of tumor before or after surgery and thus improve our staging accuracy [24–26, 108].

A second area of concern is Stage III patients. The anatomic and prognostic rationale on which the staging system is designed leaves us with a rather large category. While Stages I and II are subdivided into eight groups but comprise a quarter of the patient population, Stage III is not divided but includes close to two thirds of the patients with varying amounts of tumor burden, subtypes and degree of differentiation [27]. Should these prognostic factors be added to the staging system?

One includes in Stage III both a patient with tumor limited to one ovary and microscopic metastasis to the omentum, and a patient suffering from diffuse peritoneal involvement, including large tumor masses and ascites. These two patients may well have a different prognosis, prior to and after surgery.

The relationship between tumor mass and prognosis is well known [11] and will be dealt with also in the following sections. Some clinical investigators have suggested that the adverse effect of tumor mass on the prognosis should be expressed in the staging system. Dembo and Bush [28] have recently published a multivariant analysis of 430 patients by prognostic categories including stage, age, tumor type, tumor grade and residual tumor after surgery. Factors that have been evaluated by others [27, 29–33]. In general, they have suggested two main groups, Good Prognosis and Poor Prognosis, as shown in Table 2.

Group B comprises patients in Stage IV and those in Stage II, III with large residual tumor masses, and therefore bearing Poor Prognosis. The low risk in Group A includes Stages Ia, and Ib disease with well differentiated tumors. Stages Ic, II, III are located into Group A, Intermediate or High risk, based on integration of factors such as extent of surgical debulking,

Table 2. Classification by prognostic category

	FIGO stage	Percent of total	Percent 5 year survival rate
A. Good prognosis	I & II, III Debulked	55	61
a. Low-risk		6	96
b. Intermediate		37	67
c. High risk		12	25
B. Poor prognosis	IV & II, III Bulky	45	8

(After Dembo and Bush [28]).

tumor type, cell differentiation and age. Such analysis would indicate that more accurate prognostication and decision making concerning treatment can be achieved than by using only FIGO stage. Investigators have separated Stage III patients by residual tumor after surgery as in the trial by Fuks, in which cases are separated to IIIA and IIIB [34]. For these reasons Homsley [35] suggested a substaging of Stage III patients according to tumor mass, grade and ascites.

Though in most trials patients are stratified by tumor burden after initial surgery it might be informative to document tumor volume prior to cytoreductive surgery as well. We believe that better prognostication of the ovarian cancer patient should include substaging of Stage III by the volume and spread of tumor at the time of initial exploration as well as after debulking surgery. Even though this is not part of the FIGO system, the data should presently be collected and evaluated in order to properly determine its efficacy as a predictor of response to chemotherapy and survival, as done by Dembo and Bush.

The role of tumor differentiation as expressed by tumor grade was evaluated in the past especially at the Mayo Clinic and the NCI. Malkasian *et al.* [36], Smith *et al.* [27], both showed that there is a correlation between tumor grade and prognosis. Recently Ozols *et al.* [30, 31] evaluated the importance of tumor differentiation in advanced ovarian cancer treated with Hexa-CAF or L-PAM. Using the modified Broder's criteria it was revealed that Grades 2 and 3 tumors respond and survive longer than Grade 4. It is their conclusion that tumor grade should be evaluated in further studies as a separate prognostic stratification. Hernandez *et al.* [37] from the Johns Hopkins Hospital evaluated tumor cell heterogeneity in ovarian cancer following multiagent chemotherapy. Biopsies of 34 patients were reviewed by light microscopy after treatment. Progression of grade was seen in four cases and a change in composition developed in five instances. Since these changes occurred during treatment and no patient had improvement of histology, it appears that this is further evidence for the role of tumor grade in predicting response to chemotherapy.

A different view was presented lately by Cohen *et al.* and Bruckner *et al.* [38, 39] from Mt. Sinai Hospital in New York. When cis-Platinum containing regimens were studied, the rate of negative second look operation was not dependent upon the cell characteristics. Poorly differentiated tumor had 42% negative second look, moderately differentiated 35% and well differentiated 46%. The durability of these regressions however are not assessed by these data.

With regard to tumor type, within each stage, the histologic type (serous, mucinous, endometrioid or clear cell) may also play a role in response to therapy and prognosis. Dembo *et al.* [28] showed that well differentiated serous tumors, mucinous, endometroid and clear cell tumors should be separated from undifferentiated serous tumors. Goldhirsch *et al.* [40] recently evaluated Stage III, IV patients treated by cis-Platinum, Melphalan (I.V.) and Hexamethylmelamine. They observed reduced response to chemotherapy in the clear-cell histological type compared to the other types, and concluded that stage for stage histology should be considered a prognostic factor.

Bulk disease, cell type and grade are all important factors in defining the prognosis of this patient population. Most current data do not yet support the notion that advances in chemotherapy have rendered these factors negligible. Consideration should therefore begin to address the incorporation of residual bulk and tumor grade into the FIGO system. At a minimum, clinical trials should be stratified for these factors, and a breakdown by categories should be included in the reporting of data. Finally, analysis of the data as performed by Dembo and Bush should be repeated and rendered possible.

3. HOW SIGNIFICANT IS INITIAL 'DEBULKING'?

In recent publications doubts have been raised concerning the importance of this now established procedure. The cytoreductive operation, aimed at decreasing tumor burden prior to initiation of chemotherapy has been studied for many years apparently confirming the original studies of Griffiths *et al.* [32, 41, 42]. In a recent review of the literature Young *et al.* [43], have demonstrated, by combining five clinical trials (233 patients) in which pathologic response was reported, that residual disease after initial laparotomy had a significant influence on response to combination chemotherapy. When residual disease measured <3 cm, pathologic complete response rate was 69% (range 30–100%) compared to 11% (4–16%) when the residual was >3 cm. On the other hand Cohen *et al.* [38] reported on the findings at 'second look' in 73 patients treated with 6 different protocols. When analyzed in relation to residual tumor at initial surgery, the latter seemed to have no influence. When residual disease measured <2 cm, 2–6 cm or >6 cm, negative second look rate was 35, 30, 40% respectively. Initial reports from the GICOG of Milan [44] appears to confirm this. In 129 evaluable patients treated with either cis-Platinum alone, cis-Platinum with Cytoxan or Cytoxan, cis-Platinum and Adriamycin, the response rate was 87.5% for residual tumors <2 cm and 78% for tumors residual >2 cm. The latter group included 60/81 patients with residuals >5 cm and 40 of them had masses >10 cm. Although the response rate to platinum containing regimens in all groups is indeed encouraging, analysis of survival in these patients confirmed a negative effect of tumor burden at initiation of therapy. When the residual was microscopic or none, 75% of patients, are alive at 2 years. When bulk was surgically reduced to the size of 1–2 cm, only 32% of patients are alive at 18 months. Survival further decreases with increased residual. An ECOG study analyzing CHAD chemotherapy has also provided interesting data [45]. Whereas they reported an overall 92% response rate in advanced ovarian cancer, survival and time to progression of disease were significantly dependent on bulk of residual tumor after initial surgery. At 2 years follow-up 70% of patients were alive if their residual measured <2 cm. Between 3–10 cm residual, only 50% survived 2 years, and >10 cm, less than 20% achieved a 2-year survival.

Evidence from several clinical trials shows that only 30–50% of patients with advanced ovarian cancer are truely 'debulkable' to tumor size of 2 cm or less, the range is doubtless the result of variable aggressiveness of surgery practiced on a number of centers [20, 35, 41, 42, 46]. Advanced ovarian cancer which cannot be debulked generally appears to be a more aggressive tumor diagnosed at a more advanced stage with further invasion of tissues and thus carries a grave· prognosis. In most recently reported studies attempts at debulking were performed and therefore Stage III and IV patients are divided into two groups by the operability per se. One must continue to question whether debulking these patients alters survival.

Interesting information regarding this subject can be obtained from the results of Parker et al. [47] from Harvard, using CACP combination chemotherapy (Cyclophosphamide, Adriamycin, cis-Platinum). They introduced a 'midtreatment' second debulking surgery after 2–3 cycles of chemotherapy, based on the finding that inoperable cases can result in significant chemical debulking after 1–2 cycles, and when reoperated on, can sometimes be surgically debulked. Of 29 patients who had disease residual <2 cm after initial surgery, followed by chemotherapy, 50% had a negative laparoscopic restaging at completion of therapy. On the other hand, those who were debulked on a second attempt did poorly, only 1 of 9 had a subsequent negative laparoscopy.

This supports the theory that massive tumor at diagnosis carries a grave prognosis, and reducing the tumor size by technical means is not, in itself, a cause for improved survival in these patients.

A thorough review of the impact of tumor mass on drug resistance and survival has been presented by DeVita at the meeting of the Society of Surgical Oncology [11]. With regard to 'debulking' operations as means of improving survival rate, the success is probably limited. Following the Goldie-Coldman hypothesis [12], mutation rate is mass related and therefore when large tumor masses are present upon diagnosis, resistant cell lines are already in existence throughout the tumor when debulking surgery is performed. Therefore the operation may not alter the basic disease biology.

However, it is possible that with improved and aggressive therapy, the response to chemotherapy is enhanced by debulking surgery. While this effect was demonstrated for single agent treatment [42], its contribution may be questioned again when multiagent chemotherapy is used with its presumably greater cell kill.

The final answer to the question of debulking can be obtained from a prospective study in which 'debulkable patients' will be randomized to chemotherapy only vs. surgery followed by chemotherapy. Such a study is probably not feasible. Less satisfactory may be to compare two groups of Stage III patients treated by combination chemotherapy. Those who are diagnosed with disease measuring < 2 cm and require only TAH, BSO, to patients who have large tumor masses but are reduced to < 2 cm residual, by debulking surgery. These two groups have different tumor burdens at diagnosis but the same amount of tumor at the initiation of therapy. Such an evaluation was performed for single alkylating agent by Griffiths and shown identical survival curves for the two groups [41].

It is our opinion that based on multiple clinical trials showing the effect of debulking surgery on response to chemotherapy and, more importantly, on survival, this procedure is justified especially if tumor size can actually be reduced to < 2 cm. Cytoreductive surgery should then be performed as long as it will not delay initiation of chemotherapy. Regrowth of tumor and resistant cell lines can presumably develop in weeks and one has to judge the contribution of the operative procedure in view of this light.

There is still an open question whether with current combinations of greater efficacy, the response to chemotherapy is dependent on residual bulk disease.

4. WHAT IS THE PREFERRED CHEMOTHERAPEUTIC REGIMEN FOR STAGE III, IV OVARIAN CANCER?

The data from clinical trials that has accumulated over the last decade, makes the answer to the above question quite complicated.

Combination chemotherapy appears superior to single agent therapy. Historically, the treatment for this relatively sensitive solid tumor began by studying single alkylating agents as reported by Smith in 1972 [48]. Most commonly studied was Melphalan (L-PAM), and response rates varied at approximately 50%. Other alkylating agents such as cyclophosphamide, chlorambucil, thiotepa or nitrosoureas produced similar response rates when given as initial therapy [33].

Non-alkylating agents have been used, and significant response rates observed, though initially given to alkylating agent failures where results are generally less impressive. Among these are, Hexamethylmelamine, Adriamycin, Methotrexate, 5FU and cis-Platinum. The response to these drugs ranged between 20–30% [49]. Promising results with single agents and the introduction of combination chemotherapy to cancer treatment [50] promoted the use of the latter in ovarian carcinoma.

At the M.D. Anderson Hospital in Houston, the combination of Actinomycin-D, 5 Fluorouracil and cyclophosphamide was compared to melphalan [27]. Although response to combination chemotherapy was better, the overall survival did not improve among the two arms.

An important prospective randomized trial performed at the NCI [51] evaluated the combination of hexamethylmelamine, cyclophosphamide, 5 Fluorouracil and methotrexate (Hexa-CAF) to single agent Melphalan. Eighty patients were randomized and the results showed significant improvement in response (75 vs 54%), complete remission (33 vs 16%) and median survival (29 vs 17 months) for the combination. A similar study by Carmo Pereira et al. [52] was reported showing no difference between the two arms. The Hexa-CAF arm of the latter study utilized lower doses which may have contributed to the different outcome (Abbr: Table 3).

Two drugs were than introduced into the combination trials, – Adriamycin and cis-Platinum. Both agents showing some activity as first and second line treatments [1, 32, 33]. Beginning in the mid-seventies, several clinical trials demonstrated significant improvement in response and survival using platinum containing regimens compared to single alkylating agents or other non-platinum containing regimens. Studies by Decker et al. [53], Sturgeon [54], Vogl [55], and Neijt et al. [56] have all confirmed the advantage of platinum containing combination chemotherapy versus single agent in inducing remissions. Several studies also confirmed prolonged survival and disease free interval when such combinations are used. Others have further shown the improved response to cis-Platinum containing regimens. Sturgeon et al. [54] report a complete response of 30% for PAC vs 19% for HexaCAF. Neijt et al. [56] have shown superiority of CHAP-5 regimen over Hexa-CAF. Omura [57] compared PAC to AC and showed 71% response rate and 46% respectively (p < 0.001). Thus, data is accumulating suggesting the superiority of cis-Platinum containing regimens as first line treatment.

There are however two main difficulties encountered when one attempts to compare the many 'pilot' studies published in the literature. The first is the mode of evaluating response. Intraperitoneal disease is often hard to clinically estimate and follow, and therefore only surgically confirmed responses are of interpretable significance. It has been unusual to find more than 50% of patients to be negative for tumor when undergoing second look operation, after being considered clinically free of disease. The second problem is the design and selection of patients. Randomized trials in which stratification by patients age, performance status, tumor type or grade and bulk disease post operatively, are seldom reported.

We therefore agree with the statement made by Decker [53] who suggested two parameters for the evaluation of chemotherapy in ovarian cancer.

a) Time to progression of disease.

b) Duration of response and overall survival.

The two parameters can be further stratified by the prognostic factors mentioned. In Table 3 we present selected recent studies in which platinum containing protocols were used and sufficient restaging and follow up data is available for evaluation of results. The overall median survival using these combinations is well over 2 years, whereas with alkylating agents alone it was only 10–14 months in unselected series. There are now three principal groups of protocols with either four, three or two drugs, which are commonly used and still evaluated using cis-Platinum as a base [39, 45, 47, 53, 57, 60–66]. Selected regimens are presented in Table 3, with treatment sche-

Table 3. Overall survival and progression free interval (PFI) for Stage III IV treated by platinum containing regimens.

	# Pts	Regimen	Median survival	Median PFI	Abbr.
1. Decker, *et al.* 1983 [53]	21	Cyclophosph. Cis-Platin.	40 mos (projected)	28 mos.	CP
2. Vogl, *et al.* 1983 [45]	26	Cyclophosph. Hexamethyl Adriamycin Cis-Platin.	25 mos.	13 mos.	CHAD
3. Ehrlich, *et al.* 1979, 1983 [58, 59]	56	Cyclophosph. Adriamycin Cis-Platin.	N.A.	33 mos. CR 12.7 mos PR	CAP
4. Parker, *et al.* 1983 [47]	72	Cyclophosph. Adriamycin Cyclophosph. Cis-Platin.	36 mos.	N.A.	CAP
5. Bruckner *et al.* 1983 [39]	20	Adriamycin Cisplatin	25 mos.	21 mos.	AC
	37	Cyclophosph. Hexamethyl Adriamycin Cis-Platin.	27 mos.	25 mos.	CHAP
6. Wernz *et al.* 1983 [60]	31	Cyclophosph. Cis-Platin.	37 mos.	23 mos.	CP

dules separately presented in Table 4. Although some uncertainty remains concerning a clear advantage in survival of cis-Platinum containing combinations over single alkylating agents, the recent randomized study by Decker et al. [53], and the trend in most other studies should put this issue to rest. However, it may be still arguable whether cis-Platinum alone performs equally well. Such a question is quite academic since the toxicity of cis-Platin alone is probably quite equivalent to the combinations. Such a situation may not pertain to the platinum analogues, which we shall discuss further.

The decision as to which combination is preferred is based on common factors:

A. Activity in ovarian carcinoma with high response rate.
B. Reasonable and tolerable toxicity.
C. Simple and safe mode of administration.
D. Reduced treatment time.

The two most active drugs in our opinion are the alkylating agent and cis-Platinum. Based on the observation that there is a dose response curve for cis-Platinum as shown in clonogenic assays as well as in humans [43],

Table 4. Selected platinum containing combination chemotherapy

1. CHAD				
Cyclophosphamide (cytoxan)		600 mg/m^2 i.v. day 1		150 mg/m^2 p.o. day 2–8
Hexamethylmelamine	A	150 mg/m^2 p.o. days 8–22	B	150 mg/m^2 p.o. day 2–8
Adriamycin	(45)	25 mg/m^2 i.v. day 1	(38)	50 mg/m^2 i.v. day 1
Cis-Platinum		50 mg/m^2 i.v. day 1		50 mg/m^2 i.v. day 1
2. PAC				
Cyclophosphamide		750 mg/m^2 i.v. day 1		750 mg/m^2 day 1
Adriamycin	A	50 mg/m^2 i.v. day 1	B	50 mg/m^2 day 1
Cis-Platinum	(58)	50 mg/m^2 i.v. day 1	(50)	20 mg/m^2 i.v. day 1–5
Cyclophosphamide	C	400 mg/m^2 i.v. day 1	D	500 mg/m^2 i.v. d 1&
	(39)		(47)	650 mg/m^2 d 22
Adriamycin		40 mg/m^2 i.v. day 1		45 mg/m^2 i.v. d 1
Cis-Platinum		50 mg/m^2 i.v. day 1		20 mg/m^2 i.v. d 22–28
3. CP				
Cyclophosphamide	A	600 mg/m^2 i.v. day 4	B	1000 mg/m^2 i.v. day 1
Cis-Platinum	(67)	20 mg/m^2 i.v. day 1–5	(53)	50 mg/m^2 i.v. day 1
AP				
Adriamycin		50 mg/m^2 i.v. d 1		
Cis-Platinum	(64)	50 mg/m^2 i.v. d 1		
MP				
Melphalan		0.66 mg/kg p.o. d 1–5		
Cis-Platinum	(46)	50 mg/m^2 i.v. d 1		

246

we have eliminated other drugs from the regimens and tried to maximize the doses of cis-Platinum with Cytoxan. Results of the studies from the Mayo Clinic, our institution as well as preliminary reports from Milan and the Netherlands confirm the efficacy of the two drug combination in inducing remission. At NYU the regimen using cis-Platinum 20 mg/m^2 × 5 for 8 cycles produced 71% per cent response and 68%, 2 year survival. At the Mayo Clinic a similar combination with platinum administered at 50 mg/m^2 × 1 for 12 cycles produced 61.9% 2 year survival.

The results of these trials suggest that a regimen with Cytoxan and cis-Platinum is as good as others which include Adriamycin or Hexamethylmelamine. The toxicity of the latter two drugs can be eliminated, especially in a patient population where advanced age and cardiac disease is so common.

At the present time two drug regimen using cis-Platinum and an alkylating agent has been recommended as initial therapy at the Mayo Clinic, M.D. Anderson, Milan Institute, the Netherlands and others [44, 46, 53, 66]. A different opinion was recently expressed by Bruckner et al. [63] who consider Adriamycin and cis-Platinum combination sufficient for induction. Cyclophosphamide in their opinion was a cause for increased toxicity and reduction in the dose of the two former and active drugs.

While most current regimens include cis-Platinum, the best combination has clearly not been established by randomized trials. Although it appears that combination chemotherapy has increased the rate of complete remission from disease, it is unlikely that further juggling of the known active agents in equivalent dosages will lead to appreciable increase in the survival rate. A search for more active drugs and new approaches for administering the combinations should be sought.

5. WHAT IS THE ROLE OF SECOND LOOK OPERATIONS?

Since the introduction of second-look surgery by Wangensteen in 1949 for intrabdominal malignancy [68], the indications for the operation have varied. Whereas the rationale in the past was part of an aggressive surgical management, our approach today is an integral part of multimodal treatment of ovarian carcinoma. Yet, in both periods the need for second look surgery stems from the inability of physical examination and non-invasive evaluations to determine the extent of disease in the peritoneal cavity. Considerable expectations towards improved evaluation have developed since the introduction of CAT scanning of the abdomen and pelvis, but the results are not promising as discussed in a previous section [9, 10]. A study by Cohen et al. [38] reported of 73 patients undergoing second look after completing various chemotherapeutic regimens, and a negative non-invasive restaging. Only 30 patients (41%) were found to have no evidence of disease upon exploration. Other studies further confirm that only a surgical exploration can establish accurately the response to chemotherapy [43, 69-71].

Laparoscopy can replace a complete reexploration only when the findings are clearly positive. In that situation one can obtain fluid for cytology and inspect as much peritoneal surface as possible by this technique. However, a negative laparoscopic second look does not exclude residual disease in areas not visualized by laparoscopy. In that situation a formal second look laparotomy is required to confirm the complete response to chemotherapy.

The next question is, what is the correlation between findings at second look and the prognosis? Cohen et al. [38] found that 3 years survival decreased from 78% to 47.3% when the disease on second look was none, microscopic or macroscopic respectively. A study from the M.D. Anderson [72] evaluated 83 patients from 1971-1982 in Stage III and IV ovarian carcinoma who had negative second look laparotomies. The 2 and 5 year survival rates are 100% and 85% respectively. When 44 patients with persistent microscopic or cytologic disease at second-look were evaluated [73], the uncorrected 2 and 5-year survival rates were 98% and 78%, respectively. Despite differences in these series it appears that findings at second look surgery are useful in predicting the prognosis. Comparison of response rates in clinical trials using the variety of regimens cannot be properly done without surgical restaging, and therefore survival data has been suggested as sole criteria if second looks are not performed.

Since the newer chemotherapeutic regimens are toxic and hard to tolerate [74, 75] second look surgery is currently the only reliable means of obtaining an indication to stop treatment. However, no matter how much useful information this procedure provides, it may not alter the outcome. The study by Cohen et al. [38] presented data concerning the survival of patients eligible for second look operation. The survival curve for patients who eventually had the operation was identical to that of patients who, by chance, did not undergo second look. Second look surgery can also be part of a multimodal protocol. Such an approach has been reflected in the series of Fuks et al. [34] and Malcolm et al. [76] in which patients receive a full course of chemotherapy prior to second look exploration. According to the findings at the operation, residual tumor is removed, and patients are then treated with total abdominal irradiation according to their protocol. Another multimodal approach has been the use of intraperitoneal instillation of radioisotopes, chemotherapy or immunotherapy, based upon the findings at second look [77].

Finally, recurrence rate after negative second look has been reported to range between 20-50 percent, depending upon the length of follow up [71].

Even when the platinum containing regimens are used, more evidence accumulates that the recurrence rate is significant [59].

We therefore believe that justification for performing second look operations on patients with negative non-invasive evaluation is either in relation to the availability of other treatment modalities or in the context of a clinical investigation. If the patient has reached maximal tolerable doses of chemotherapy, and no other treatment modality is available, the role of second look is of questionable value.

6. CAN WE INCREASE CIS-PLATINUM DOSAGE?

There has been an extensive search in the past years for means to reduce the toxicity of platinum containing combination chemotherapy. Nephrotoxocity has been the major limiting factor in multiple Phase II trials, requiring dose modification. Recording the number of cycles which were delayed or reduced, in our cis-Platinum Cytoxan protocol reveals that in approximately 50% of cycles alteration in the basic schema takes place. At the same time there appears to be a dose response relationship between cis-Platinum and epithelial ovarian cancer [48]. Therefore, a hypothesis to improve results includes attempts to administer higher possible doses of cis-Platinum, without an increase in toxicity.

In order to achieve the goal of high dose and safe administration, several paths have been pursued and are currently being studied. Pre and post treatment hydration with diuresis have been used for some time, and have shown to partially diminish the nephrotoxicity [78, 79]. The use of Furosemide or Mannitol has been common practice in clinical trials [80].

The intraperitoneal administration of chemotherapy in general and cis-Platinum in particular has the advantage of providing higher drug doses to the tumor. Further discussion of this approach is presented further in this chapter.

Sodium thiosulphate has been studied by Howell *et al.* both in animals and in humans [81, 82]. The sulfur containing compound was chosen since previous experiments have shown that the toxic effects of cis-Platinum on the renal tubular epithelium can be rescued by administering the compound concomitantly with cis-Platinum. Binding of cis-Platinum to Sulfur-containing compounds is capable of blocking the formation of cis-Platinum-DNA complexes, and reducing the resulting cytotoxicity and antitumor activity [81]. Animal studies established a significant protection of renal function, but at the same time revealed profound reduction in anti-tumor activity. The latter finding has led to the human trial in which cis-Platinum was administered IP and the thiosulfate systemically [82]. It was shown that

IP administration of cis-Platinum provides high drug concentration in tumor nodules while the systemic thiosulfate provided renal protection. The dose of cis-Platinum was increased to 270 mg/m^2 body surface without any change in serum creatinine. Preliminary reports on 9 patients [83] treated ith combination IP therapy (cis-Platinum, Adriamycin, ARA-C) have shown no nephrotoxicity when thiosulfate was given simultaneously (12 gr/m^2 I.V. over 6 hours).

Litterst [84] and Earhart [85] have studied hypertonic saline as means of reducing nephrotoxicity in animals. Using 4.5% NaCl as vehicle for cis-Platinum administration lethality of the drug to mice was greatly reduced when compared to preparation of the drug in D5W. Antitumor effect was preserved in this setting. The explanation for the role of hypertonic saline is a shift in the cis-Platinum aquation reaction, as a result of high chloride concentration in the renal tubule. The diamminedichloro form is favored, and this compound is less toxic than the aquated species. Earhart [85] in fact demonstrated that low chloride concentrations in the urine result in the re-excretion of this aquated species, and this correlates with nephrotoxicity.

This principale was used by Ozols et al. [86] and others [87, 88] when a high dose cis-Platinum protocol was tested in patients with testicular and ovarian carcinomas who had previously progressed on conventional doses of platinum. A dose of 200 mg/m^2 (40 mg/m^2/d × 5) was given each cycle, I.V., to six patients with ovarian carcinoma who failed previous platinum containing combinations. Only 2 patients had transient renal insufficiency which did not recur with subsequent cycles of high dose – cis-Platinum. Schmoll et al. [90] also report a significant reduction in nephrotoxicity when cis-Platinum was used with hypertonic saline. It is of importance to remind the reader that other toxic effects of the treatment are not significantly altered. Such effects include – nausea and vomiting, diarrhea, ototoxicity, myelosuppression or peripheral neuropathy. Nevertheless, this approach has important clinical applications which should be further studied.

Several analogues of cis-Platinum have been introduced in the attempt to decrease the nephrotoxicity. The drugs which are currently evaluated are JM8 and JM9 (CHIP). Preliminary results with JM8 (carboplatin, CBDCA) from England presented by Wiltshaw [91] and Calvert [92] have shown similar response rates to cis-Platinum, with decreased toxicity when the former is used. When five months of 100 mg/m^2 cis-Platinum followed by five months of 20 mg/m^2 were compared with 10 cycles of 400 mg/m^2 of JM8, the incidence of nephrotoxicity was 74% and 12% respectively. It was also the impression that the JM8 treatment was easier for patients to tolerate. Response rate for both single agent regimens was about 50%. Further information from Phase II, III trials of platinum analogues in advanced ovarian cancer are expected in the next few years and include combination regimens compared with cis-Platinum combinations.

7. IS THERE A ROLE FOR RADIATION THERAPY AFTER INITIAL SURGERY AND CHEMOTHERAPY?

Radiotherapy in ovarian carcinoma has been considered and tried mainly for early Stage I and II disease [1, 33]. In addition minimal residual Stage III patients have also been successfully treated by several centers [93, 94]. These groups will not be discussed in this chapter.

Our discussion concerns patients with poor prognosis, those with advanced ovarian carcinoma which cannot be optimally debulked at initial surgery. Since 75% of patients present in Stage III-IV, and only a quarter of them can be successfully debulked, we are actually dealing with fifty percent of the entire patient population. The prognosis of this group is grave; under 8% survive five years [28, 94]. Most often these tumors have the aggressive characteristics in terms of poor differentiation of type and grade. In addition, the patients are of advanced age and suffer from nutritional and metabolic problems which accompany situations with diffuse peritoneal involvement by large tumors [33]. As mentioned by Smith [27] and Dembo [28], radiotherapy is of little value in this group and has been palliative in a small number of cases.

Since the introduction of highly effective combination chemotherapy with response rates up to 90%, the role of Radiation Therapy is reconsidered. It is now evaluated for two purposes, i.e., consolidation of chemotherapy induced remission, and treatment of small but resistant residual tumor. The logistics of such approaches are to initiate treatment with aggressive chemotherapy. Using available active combinations, effective reduction of tumor mass is commonly observed. Second look surgery is then performed and further debulking is attempted when necessary. Patients with residual disease < 2 cm are then treated by total abdominal radiation for consolidation of response and eradication of microscopic residual tumor. It is of major importance in this treatment to direct the radiation ports to the entire abdomen with specific doses to the para-aortic and diaphragmatic lymphatics [13, 95].

A major problem in this approach stems from the use of radiation therapy of high dose and extended fields, following several courses of combination chemotherapy. The toxicity of these treatments is a significant obstacle in completing the desired scheduled doses. A recent study by Schary et al. [96] reports that in 68.5% of patients treated by total abdominal radiation following chemotherapy, treatment was altered as a result of toxicity mainly thrombocytopenia. In contrast, such side effects occured in 17.6% of patients receiving RT without prior chemotherapy. Rose *et al.* [97] report that of 10 patients who received Total Abdominal Radiation following chemotherapy, seven are NED. However, Radiation Therapy following 8 cycles of chemotherapy was associated with high toxicity, mainly hematologic.

Fuks and Rizel [34] report on their protocol in which patients are initially treated with CHAD combination chemotherapy. Following 6–14 cycles, second look surgery is performed, with cytoreduction attempted. Abdominal radiation is then given to a total dose of 5100 rads to the pelvis, 3000 rads to upper abdomen and 1200 rads to a T shaped field including the para-aortic area and the diaphragms [95]. Actuarial 3 years survival is 40% in this poor prognostic group. Toxicity is high but tolerable in their report. Malcolm *et al.* [76] reported recently on 17 patients treated by consolidation with Total Abdominal Radiation following CHAP chemotherapy for 6 cycles. Residual disease was <2 cm at second look, with eleven patients having only microscopic residuals. Planned RT included 3000 rads to the whole abdomen and a pelvic boost of 1400–2000 rads. Toxicity was severe with myelosuppression altering treatment in 10/17 patients. Six of seven patients who completed treatment with RT, relapsed at a median of 14 months from completion of consolidation. Though they concluded that abdominopelvic radiation is poorly tolerated, those patients who completed treatment had longer disease free intervals. Vogl *et al.* [98] reported on the first 25 patients who entered a protocol of remission induction with CHAD (4–7 cycles) followed by consolidation combining radiation therapy with chemotherapy. After second look surgery, patients were given cis-Platinum (50 mg/m^2 i.v. d 1,) 150 rads whole abdomen $\times 7$ (d 3–11), and HMM (150 mg/m^2 p.o. d 15–28) repeated at 35 days. Of 11 patients with no residual gross tumor at second look, who received this treatment, 5 are free of disease between 13–37 months from consolidation. These numbers are too small to make conclusions about the value of this regimen. However, it is the investigator's impression that radiation and chemotherapy consolidation is less effective when palpable tumor is present at second look.

As has been documented, even cases with completely negative second look operations have recurrence rates of 40–50% [33, 99], and therefore some form of consolidation therapy would be desirable. This preliminary data on radiation therapy as means of consolidation suggests that it is very toxic, but a worthwhile lead. A related lead is combining radiation with a 'sensitizer', although hypoxic sensitizers have been disappointing to date.

Encouraging reports by Dembo *et al.* [100] and Schary [96] provide data on the safety of open field Total Abdominal Radiation. Further clinical experience with longer follow up is required in order to evaluate the role of this modality as adjuvant to chemotherapy in advanced disease.

8. IS THERE A ROLE FOR IMMUNOTHERAPY?

Amplification of response to chemotherapy by immunotherapy has been an approach studied in a small number of trials, and definite answers are not available at this point. Review of the immunobiology of ovarian cancer has recently been published in this series [101].

The theoretical basis for immunotherapy may be directly derived from animal model of murine ovarian cancer. (Though this tumor may actually be a reticulum cell sarcoma of the hystiocytic origin, it is sensitive to active drugs in ovarian carcinoma). Intraperitoneal administration of Corynebacterium Parvum can cure mice that have been inoculated with 10^5 tumor cells. The addition of rabbit heteroantiserum further enhanced antitumor activity [77, 102]. A GOG study reported by Creasman et al. [103] compared Melphalan + C. Parvum, as a non specific immunomodulating agent to a historical control of melphalan alone. Response rate was 29% to Melphalan alone compared to 53% for combined modality treatment. An ongoing GOG prospective study compares the two arms, Melphalan (7 mg/m^2 days 1–5) and Melphalan + C. Parvum (4 mg/m^2 day 7). Patients in both arms are of optimal stage III, and both arms, though not identified, show no difference in survival with projected median of 23 months.

Alberts et al. [104] reported results of the SWOG trial in which Adriamycin, cyclophosphamide with BCG in one arm, were compared to the same chemotherapy without BCG. Response rate was 53% vs 36% respectively. Survival was 23.5 months (median) for chemoimmunotherapy compared to 13.1 months for chemotherapy alone (p<0.004).

Bast and Knapp [72, 102] report on intraperitoneal administration of C. Parvum following initial surgery and full course of chemotherapy with CAP (6–13 months). Of 11 evaluable patients 5 (45%) had an objective response confirmed by surgery. Complete response in two patients lasted five and twelve months. Evaluation of tumoricidal activity of peritoneal cells showed significant increase in activity during treatment with C. Parvum. Intraperitoneal injection of C. Parvum is accompanied by peritonitis, fever and abdominal pain. As a result of these complications the team is now using recombinant leukocyte A Interferon for immunostimulation, following initial reports on interferon by Gutterman et al. [105] and Einhorn et al. [106] but data has not been published yet.

The group from Johns Hopkins is currently investigating the combination of chemotherapy and Human-Ovarian-Anti-Tumor-Serum (HOATS) derived from immunized New Zealand white rabbits [107]. In fourteen patients, treated by this modality, no significant toxicity was noticed, and chemotherapy was not altered. The role of immunotherapy as an enhancing factor in patients who respond to chemotherapy is not defined as yet. More randomized studies with non-specific immunotherapy with longer follow-up are required in order to assess that modality.

New therapeutic possibilities are currently being investigated using specific monoclonal antibodies. The possibility of attaching radionuclides, cytotoxic drugs or toxins directly to tumor specific antibody and thus directing the drug only to tumor cells, is the goal of the research [26, 27, 101]. A recent *in vitro* study of monoclonal antibodies, raised against ovarian carcinoma cell line, had shown reactivity of the antibody with six of six serous ovarian tumors, five of five non ovarian tumors and with normal endometrial and endocervical tissue [108, 109]. Although the technique may be of value in the near future for diagnostic purposes and non invasive follow up, as a treatment modality, it is still at the basic research phase.

9. IS THERE ADVANTAGE TO INTRAPERITONEAL CHEMOTHERAPY?

An effort to improve the initial response to chemotherapy, which is a documented way to prolong survival [43], has led to the investigation of intraperitoneal administration of chemotherapy. To date, no randomized prospective trial evaluating this mode of therapy has been reported. Nevertheless, the approach has biologic and pharmacokinetic basis to rationalize its use in treatment investigation. 1) Ovarian carcinoma has a prolonged phase of intraperitoneal disease without dissemination outside the peritoneal cavity. Even in the most terminal phases of disease, tumor burden is often solely intra-peritoneal with resultant anatomic and metabolic complications. 2) *In vitro* and *in vivo* studies indicate that there is a dose response relation between cytotoxic agents and malignant ovarian cells. Systemic drug administration is however limited by bone marrow, gastrointestinal and renal toxicity. Therefore attempts should be made to reduce the toxicity in order to administer high doses of drugs. 3) The peritoneal cavity has a specific pharmacokinetic advantage since the clearance of many molecules from that space is slower than that from the systemic circulation. By direct intraperitoneal instillation higher concentrations of drugs can be obtained in the peritoneal cavity, delivered directly to tumor nodules, without significantly increasing the systemic toxicity. The clearance of drugs from the peritoneal cavity mainly depends upon molecular weight and lipid solubility of the various compounds. In addition, these drugs have different direct effect on the peritoneal surfaces. These variables individually alter the clinical pharmacologic characteristics of each compound.

Although the peritoneal cavity has been used for the treatment of malignant disease over twenty years ago, recently published studies, have carefully evaluated the dynamics of intraperitoneal administration of cytotoxic agents in animals and humans. Several important studies have been performed at the NCI [110–112]. Two technical principles have been used in these investigations. The first was the use of semi-permanent Tenckhoff dialysis catheter as means for repeated cycle treatment administration and evaluation of peritoneal cytology [113]. The second was the administration of large volume (2 liters) of fluid with the cytotoxic drugs [114]. These modifications are based on studies by Dedrick et al. [115] in which the pharmacologic advantage for intraperitoneal chemotherapy was predicted to depend upon repetitive administration of a drug in a large volume of fluid. The latter provides for uniform distribution of drug throughout the peritoneal cavity.

Studies conducted by Ozols et al. [112], Speyer et al. [111], Pfeifle et al. [116], Howell et al. [82, 83], Pretorius et al. [117] and Casper et al. [118] have all shown that with the evaluated compounds, concentrations in the peritoneal cavity were markedly larger than that in the systemic circulation, ranging up to 3 log concentration gradient, as shown in Table 5.

Administration of drugs into the peritoneal cavity is limited by two side effects which are added to those encountered when systemic therapy is utilized. These problems are chemical peritonitis resulting from irritation of peritoneal surfaces by the drug, and bacterial peritonitis for which there is increased risk when chronic indwelling foreign body is present in the peritoneal cavity. Whereas the latter is usually not common when proper tech-

Table 5. Results of intraperitoneal chemotherapy, (Phase I, II) given to previously treated ovarian cancer patients

	# Pts	Dose	Objective response	Chemical peritonitis	Mean concentration peritoneal fluid/plasma
Methotrexate (111) (MTX)	5	7.5–50 μM	0	Common	23*
5–FU (111) (5Fu)	5	1–8 μM	2	None	298**
Adriamycin (112) (ADR)	10	9–55 μM	3	Common	343***
Cis-Platinum (80)	7	90–270 mg/m²	1	None	10–1000
(117)	4		4	None	
Ara-C (116)	10	1000 μM	2	None	450–1250
Ara-C+		100–100 μM	Minimal		
Cis-Platinum + (83)	4	100–200 mg/m²	3		
Adriamycin		18 μM			

* 50 μM MTX
** 4 mM 5FU
*** 55 μM ADR

nique is used, and commonly controlled with antibiotics [113, 119], the former can cause severe symptomatology and limit the use of these drugs [110]. Peritoneal dialysis has been well tolerated in the reported studies, and has produced minimal complications that did not require cessation of therapy, even for bacterial peritonitis. With Adriamycin and possibly with Methotrexate, chemical peritonitis was dose limiting.

Evaluation of the response to therapy and effect on survival is hard to appreciate at the present time. The group of treated patients, in these studies, has a notably poor response rate to any form of therapy since they have all failed previous therapy with single or combination chemotherapy. Preliminary results are shown in Table 5. It should be emphasized that these Phase I and some Phase II studies were aimed at clinical pharmacological evaluation of the modality itself and the resultant toxicity.

Observations in ovarian carcinoma have shown that half the patients who obtain clinical complete response with systemic chemotherapy, are found to have residual microscopic or minimal disease at second-look surgery. In addition, salvage treatment for recurrent previously treated, disease has shown very limited success in the multiple small clinical trials [43]. Preliminary data from these intraperitoneal trials is encouraging. The approach appears to be safe and tolerable while the pharmacologic advantage is obtained. Even combination chemotherapy [83] has been tried and tolerated. However, intraperitoneal chemotherapy is still clearly in the domain of clinical investigation and is not recommended outside of clinical trials.

Prospective clinical trials using the intraperitoneal approach for initial therapy should be able to provide data and answers to the above presented quetion. Such a trial is being conducted at the National Tumor Institute in Milan, Italy, in which patients are randomized after initial surgery to one of two arms: intraperitoneal cis-Platinum and systemic Cyclophosphamide or both drugs given systemically. Other centers including our own are now evaluating the advantage of intraperitoneal administration of first line therapy, and within 2–3 years more conclusive information should be available.

SUMMARY

1. The staging system for ovarian epithelial cancer is useful but has limitations. Further division of patients by grade and bulk (prior to and post debulking surgery) should provide better prognostic information and improved comparability for clinical trials.
2. With the limited effectiveness of chemotherapeutic regimens in advanced disease – maximal debulking at the time of primary surgery still

256

appears to be a worthwhile goal. Further information from trials with better prognostic information or better therapy could alter this.

3. The preferred chemotherapy or duration of therapy for advanced disease is not certain. Whenever possible chemotherapy should include cis-Platinum and an alkylating agent. Other drugs may or may not add to the efficacy and/or toxicity of these regimens. Further 'juggling' of currently available drugs and regimens is unlikely to result in significant survival benefit.

4. The survival and time to progression are the best determinants of the efficacy of a regimen in this disease. Restaging laporotomy is by far the most accurate way to measure response and check for residual disease. The 'second look laporotomy' is appropriate in clinical trials where determination of response must be made or when the outcome will have meaningful impact on subsequent therapeutic decisions.

5. Total abdominal radiation as part of aggressive combined modality therapy with surgery and chemotherapy may provide additional benefit. The approach is still investigational and has considerable morbidity.

6. Meaningful progress in ovarian cancer must now come from new avenues of research. There are interesting leads from immunotherapy with IP C. parvum and an antiserum directed at ovarian cancer cells. Monoclonal antibody technology may provide a whole family of new agents or radiocolloids with increased specificity.

7. New agents are eagerly awaited. There is great interest in the new platinum analogue in term of efficacy and possible decreased toxicity.

8. Finally there are ongoing efforts to improve the delivery of currently available agents. The results of further clinical trial with chloride loading or blocking agents to decrease platinum toxicity and improve the therapeutic index are eagerly awaited. Intraperitoneal chemotherapy has been established as a safe workable system for delivery of high concentrations of drug to the abdominal cavity with much lower systemic exposure. Controlled clinical trials using this therapy early in the course of patients with small bulk disease are now being conducted to determine if the route of delivery will alter the survival of these patients.

ACKNOWLEDGMENTS

We gratefully acknowledge helpful comments by Drs. E.M. Beckman, G.W. Douglas, and F.M. Muggia, and manuscript preparation by Peggy Nixdorf.

This study was supported in part by Cancer Center Grant CA 16987 and the Lila Motley Fund and LILAC.

REFERENCES

1. DiSaia PJ, Creasman WT: Advanced epithelial ovarian cancer. In: Clinical gynecologic oncology. St. Louis, CV Mosby Co. 253–320, 1981.
2. Musumeci R, Banfi A, Bolis G, et al.: Lymphangiography in patients with ovarian epithelial cancer. Cancer 40:1444–1449, 1977.
3. Cochrane WJ, Thomas MA: Ultrasound diagnosis of gynecologic pelvic massess. Radiology 110:649–654, 1974.
4. Samuels BI: Usefulness of ultrasound in patients with ovarian cancer. Semin Oncol 2:229–233, 1975.
5. Lewis E, Zornoza J, Jing BS, et al.: Radiologic contributions to the diagnosis and management of gynecologic neoplasms. Semin Roentgen 17:251–268, 1982.
6. Johnson RJ, Blackledge G, Eddleston B, Crowther D: Abdomino-Pelvic computed tomography in the management of ovarian carcinoma. Radiology 146:447–452, 1983.
7. Mettler FA, Christie JK, Crow NE, et al.: Radionuclide bone scan, radiographic bone survey, and alkaline phosphatase. Studies of limited value in asymptomatic patients with ovarian carcinoma. Cancer 50:1483–1485, 1982.
8. Mettler FA, Christie JH, Crow NE, et al.: Utility of radionuclide liver/spleen scanning and serum enzyme level in detecting hepatic metastases from ovarian carcinoma. Cancer 50:909–911, 1982.
9. Stern J, Buscema J, Rosenshein N, Siegelman S: Can Computed tomography substitute for second-look operation in ovarian carcinoma? Gynecol Oncol 11:82–88, 1981.
10. Brenner DE, Grosh WW, Jones HW, et al.: An evaluation of the accuracy of computed tomography in patients with ovarian carcinoma prior to second look laporotomy. Proc Am Soc Clin Onc 2:581, 1983.
11. DeVita VT, Jr: The relationship between tumor mass and resistance to chemotherapy. Cancer 51:1209–1220, 1983.
12. Goldie JH, Coldman AJ: A mathematical model for relating the drug sensitivity of tumors to their spontaneous mutation rate. Cancer Treat Rep 63:1727–1733, 1979.
13. Fuks Z, Bagshaw MA: The rationale for curative radiotherapy for ovarian carcinoma. Int J Roentgen 1:21–32, 1975.
14. Piver MS, Barlow JJ, Lele SB: Incidence of subclinical metastasis in Stage I and II ovarian carcinoma. Obstet Gynecol 52:100–104, 1978.
15. Rubin P: Understanding the problem of understaging in ovarian cancer. Semin Oncol 2:235–243, 1975.
16. Day TE, Smith JP: Diagnosis and staging of ovarian carcinoma. Semin Oncol 2:217–222, 1975.
17. Knapp RC, Friedman EA: Aortic lymph node metastasis in early ovarian cancer. Am J Obstet Gynecol 119:1013–1017, 1974.
18. Delgado G, Chun B, Caglar H, Bepko F: Paroaortic lymphadenectomy in gynecologic malignancies confined to the pelvis. Obstet Gynecol 50:418–423, 1977.
19. Creasman WT, Abu-Chazaleh S, Schmidt HJ: Retroperitoneal metastatic spread of ovarian cancer. Gynecol Oncol 6:447–450, 1978.
20. Wharton JT, Herson J: Surgery for common epithelial tumors of the ovary. Cancer 48:582–589, 1981.
21. Tobias JS, Griffiths CT: Management of ovarian carcinoma: Current concepts and future prospects. N Engl J Med 294:818–822, 1976.
22. Rosenoff SH, DeVita VT, Hubbard S, Young RC: Peritoneoscopy in the staging and follow up of ovarian cancer. Semin Oncol 2:223–228, 1975.
23. Fisher RI, Young RC: Advances in the staging and treatment of ovarian cancer. Cancer 39:967–972, 1977.

258

24. Benson MD, Lurain JR, Newton MX: Ovarian tumor antigens. J Reprod Med 28:17-23, 1983.
25. Knauf S, Urbach GI: A study of ovarian cancer patients using a radioimmunoassay for human ovarian tumor associated antigen OCA. Am J Obstet Gynecol 138:1222-1223, 1980.
26. Liebel SA, Klein JL, Sgagias M, et al.: The integration of tumor associated antigens in cancer management. Semin Oncol 8:92-102, 1981.
27. Smith JP, Day TG: Review of ovarian cancer at the University of Texas Systems Cancer Center, M.D. Anderson Hospital and Tumor Institute. Am J Obstet Gynecol 135:984-993, 1979.
28. Dembo AJ, Bush RS: Choice of postoperative therapy based on prognostic factors. Int J Radiation Oncology Biol Phys 8:893-897, 1982.
29. Beller U, Bigelow B, Beckman EM, et al.: Epithelial carcinoma of the ovary in the reproductive years, clinical and morphological characterization. Gynecol Oncol 15:422-427, 1983.
30. Ozols RF, Garvin AJ, Costa J, et al.: Histologic grade in advanced ovarian cancer. Cancer Treat Rep 63:255-263, 1979.
31. Ozols RF, Garvin AJ, Costa J, et al.: Advanced ovarian cancer. Correlation of histologic grade with response to therapy and survival. Cancer 45:572-581, 1980.
32. Katz ME, Schwartz PE, Kapp DS, et al.: Epithelial carcinoma of the ovary: Current Strategies. Ann Intern Med 95:98-111, 1981.
33. Young RC, Knapp RC, Perez CA: Cancer of the ovary. In: Cancer. Principles & Practice of Oncology. DeVita VT, Hellman S, Rosenberg SA (eds). Philadelphia: J.B. Lippincott Company 884-913, 1982.
34. Fuks Z, Rizel S, Anteby SO, Biran S: The multimodal approach to the treatment of stage III ovarian carcinoma. Int J Radiation Oncology Biol Phys 8:903-908, 1982.
35. Homsley HD: The appropriate extent of bulk resection in advanced ovarian cancer. In Gynecologic Oncology. Controversies in Cancer Treatment. Ballon SC (ed), Boston: GK Hall Medical Publishers, 321-322, 1981.
36. Malkasian G, Decker D, Webb M: Histology of epithelial tumors of the ovary: clinical usefulness and prognostic significance of the histologic classification and grading. Semin Oncol 2:191-201, 1975.
37. Hernandez E, Rosenshein NB, Parmley T, et al.: Tumor cell heterogeneity in epithelial ovarian cancer. Proc Amer Soc Clin Onc 2:586, 1983.
38. Cohen CJ, Goldberg JD, Holland JF, et al.: Improved therapy with cisplatin regimens for patients with ovarian carcinoma (FIGO Stages III and IV) as measured by surgical end-staging (second-look operation). Am J Obstet Gynecol 145:955-967, 1983.
39. Bruckner HW, Cohen CJ, Goldberg JD, et al.: Cisplatin regimens and improved prognosis of patients with poorly differentiated ovarian cancer. Am J Obstet Gynecol 145:653-658, 1983.
40. Goldhirsch A, Davis B, Greiner R: Different responses of different histological types of ovarian cancer to a combination of cis-Platinum, Melphalan (L-PAM) and Hexamethylmelamine. Proc Am Soc Clin Onc 2:607, 1983.
41. Griffiths TC: Surgical resection of tumor bulk in the primary treatment of ovarian carcinoma. Natl Cancer Inst Monogr 42:101-104, 1975.
42. Griffiths TC, Parker LM, Fuller A: Role of cytoreductive surgical treatment in the management of advanced ovarian cancer. Cancer Treat Rep 63:235-240, 1979.
43. Young RC, Myers CE, Hamilton TC, et al.: New chemotherapeutic approaches to ovarian cancer. In: Adriamycin in Cancer Treatment, Ogawa M, Muggia FM, Rozencweig M(eds). Tokyo: Excerpta Medica, 1984.
44. Pecorelli S, Bianchi UA, Mangioni C: Radiotherapy following second look laporotomy in

stage III, IV epithelial ovarian cancer treated by chemotherapy: cis-Platinum versus Cyclophosphamide and cis-Platinum versus Cyclophosphamide, Adriamycin and cis-Platinum. Soc Gynecol Oncol Feb 1983.

45. Vogl SE, Pagano M, Kaplan BH, et al.: Cis-Platin Based combination chemotherapy for advanced ovarian cancer. Cancer 51:2024–2030, 1983.
46. Wharton JT, Edwards CL: The role of surgery in the management of gynecologic malignancies. Cancer 51:2480–2484, 1983.
47. Parker LM, Griffiths CT, Janis D, et al.: Advanced ovarian carcinoma: Integration of surgical treatment and chemotherapy with cyclophosphamide Adriamycin and cis-diamminedichloroplatinum. Proc Am Soc ClinOnc 2.599, 1983.
48. Smith JP, Rutledge F, Wharton JT: Chemotherapy of ovarian cancer, new approaches to treatment. Cancer 38:1565–1571, 1972.
49. Young RC, Myers CE, Ozols RF, Hogan WM: Chemotherapy in advanced disease. Int J Radiation Oncology Biol Phys 8:899–902, 1982.
50. DeVita VT, Schein PS: The use of drugs in combination for the treatment of cancer: Rationale and results. N Engl J Med 288:998–1006, 1973.
51. Young RC, Chabner BA, Hubbard SP, et al.: Advanced ovarian carcinoma: A prospective clinical trial of Melphalan (L-PAM) versus combination chemotherapy. N Engl J Med 299:1261–1266, 1978.
52. Carmo-Pereira J, Oliveira-Costa F, Henriques e, Ricardo JA: Advanced ovarian carcinoma: A prospective and randomized clinical trial of cyclophosphamide versus combination cytotoxic chemotherapy (HEXA-CAF). Cancer 48:1947–1951, 1981.
53. Decker DG, Fleming TR, Malkasian GD, et al.: Cyclophosphamide plus cis-Platinum in combination. Treatment program for Stage III or IV ovarian carcinoma. Obstet Gynecol 60:481–487, 1982.
54. Sturgeon JFG, Fine S, Gospodarowicz MK: A randomized trial of Melphalan alone versus combination chemotherapy in advanced ovarian cancer. Proc Amer Soc Clin Onc 1:418, 1982.
55. Vogl SE, Kaplan B, Pagano M: Diamminedichloroplatinum based combination chemotherapy is superior to Melphalan for advanced ovarian cancer. Proc Amer Soc Clin Onc 1:462, 1982.
56. Neijt JP, Ten Bokkel Heinink WW, Burg MEL: Combination chemotherapy with Hexa-CAF and CHAP-5 in advanced ovarian carcinoma: A randomized study of the Netherlands joint study group for ovarian cancer. Proc Amer Soc Clin Onc 2:577, 1983.
57. Omura GA, Ehrlich CE, Blessing JA: A randomized trial of cyclophosphamide plus adriamycin with or without cis-Platin in ovarian carcinoma. Proc Am Soc Clin Onc 1:403, 1982.
58. Ehrlich CE, Einhorn L, Williams SD, Morgan J: Chemotherapy for Stage III-IV ovarian cancer with cis-Dichlorodiammineplatinum (II), Adriamycin, and cyclophosphamide: A preliminary report. Cancer Treat Rep 63:281–287, 1979.
59. Stehman FB, Ehrlich CE, Einhorn LH, et al.: Long term follow-up and survival in stage III-IV epithelial ovarian cancer treated with cis-dichlorodiammine Platinum, adriamycin and cyclophosphamide (PAC). Proc Amer Soc Clin Oncol 2:573, 1983.
60. Wernz JC, Beller U, Speyer JL, et al.: Unpublished Data.
61. Omura GA, Ehrlich CE, Blessing JA: A randomized trial of cyclophosphamide plus adriamycin with or without cis-Platinum in ovarian carcinoma. Proc Amer Soc Clin Onc 1:403, 1982.
62. Carmo-Pereira J, Oliveira Costa F, Henriques E: Cis-Platinum, Adriamycin and Hexamethylmelamine vs. Cyclophosphamide in advanced ovarian carcinoma – a randomized study. Proc Amer Soc Clin Onc 1:144, 1982.
63. Bruckner HW, Cohen CJ, Goldberg J, et al.: Ovarian cancer: Comparison of Adriamycin

and cisplatin + cyclophosphamide. Proc Amer Soc Clin Onc 2:594, 1983.

64. Bruckner HW, Cohen CJ, Goldberg JD, *et al.*: Improved chemotherapy for ovarian cancer with cis-diamminedichloroplatinum and Adriamycin. Cancer 47:2288-2294, 1981.

65. Parker LM, Griffiths CT, Yankee RA, *et al.*: Combination chemotherapy with Adriamcyin – Cyclophosphamide for advanced ovarian carcinoma. Cancer 46:669-674, 1980.

66. Israel L, Aguilera J, Breau JL: Treatment of advanced ovarian cancer with cis-dichlorodiammine platinum in combination with cyclophosphamide. An ECOG pilot study. Am J Clin Oncol 6:85-89, 1983.

67. Wernz JC, Speyer JL, Noumoff JS, *et al.*: Cisplatin/Cytoxan: A high dose regimen for advanced stage ovarian carcinoma. Proc Amer Soc Clin Onc 1:435, 1982.

68. Arhelger SW, Jenson CB, Wangenstein OH: Experience with the 'second look' procedure in the management of cancer of the colon and rectum. Lancet 77:412-417, 1957.

69. Webb MJ, Snyder JA, Williams TJ, Decker DG: Second-look laparotomy in ovarian cancer. Gynecol Oncol 14:285-293, 1983.

70. Raju KS, McKinna JA, Barker GH, *et al.*: Second-look operations in the planned management of advanced ovarian carcinoma. Am J Obstet Gynecol 144:650-654, 1982.

71. Berek J, Hacker N, Lagasse L, *et al.*: Second look laparotomy for epithelial ovarian cancer. Proc Amer Soc Clin Onc 2:613, 1983.

72. Gershengon DM, Copeland LJ, Wharton JT, *et al.*: Surgically-determined complete responders in advanced ovarian cancer. Soc Gynecol Oncol Feb 1983.

73. Copeland LJ, Gershengon DM, Wharton JT, *et al.*: Microscopic disease at second look laparotomy in advanced ovarian cancer. Soc Gynecol Oncol Feb 1983.

74. Einhorn N, Eklund ε, Franzen S, *et al.*: Late side effects of chemotherapy in ovarian carcinoma. Cancer 49:2234-2241, 1982.

75. Chiuten D, Vogl S, Kaplan B, Camacho F: Is there cumulative or delayed toxicity from cis-Platinum? Cancer 52:211-214, 1983.

76. Malcolm AW, Hainsworth JD, Johnson DH, *et al.*: Advanced minimal residual ovarian carcinoma: Abdominopelvic irradiation following combination chemotherapy. Proc Am Soc Clin onc 2:588, 1983.

77. Knapp RC, St John E, Bast RC: A review of intraperitoneal therapy of human ovarian carcinoma. Periton Dialysis Bullet 3:59-62, 1983.

78. Jacobs C, Kalman SM, Tretton M, Weiner MW: Renal handling of cis-Diamminedichloroplatinum (II). Cancer Treat Rep 64:1223-1226, 1980.

79. Lagasse LD, Pretorius RG, Petrilli ES, *et al.*: The metabolism of cis-dichlorodiammineplatinum (II): Distribution, clearance, and toxicity. Am J Obstet Gynecol 139:791-798, 1981.

80. Ostrow S, Egorin MJ, Hahn D, *et al.*: High dose cis-Platin therapy using mannitol versus furosemide diuresis: Comparative pharmacokinetics and toxicity. Cancer Treat Rep 65:73-78, 1981.

81. Howell SB, Taetle R: Effect of sodium thiosulfate on cis-Dichlorodiammineplatinum (II) toxicity and antitumor activity in L1210 leukemia. Cancer Treat Rep 64:611-616, 1980.

82. Howell SB, Pfeifle CL, Wung WE, *et al.*: Intraperitoneal cisplatin with systemic thiosulfate protection. Ann Int Med 77:845-851, 1982.

83. Markman M, Green MR, Pfeifle CE, *et al.*: Combination intracavitary chemotherapy in patients with stage III-IV ovarian carcinoma failing standard treatment regimens. Proc Amer Soc Clin Onc 2:575, 1983.

84. Litterst CL: Alterations in the toxicity of cis-Dichlorodiammineplatinum – II and in tissue localization of platinum as a function of NaCl concentration in the vehicle of administration. Toxicol Appl Pharm 61:99-108, 1981.

85. Earhart RH, Martin PA, Tutsch KD, *et al.*: Improvement in the therapeutic index of cisplatin (NSC 119875) by pharmacologically induced chloruresis in the rat. Cancer

Research 43:1187–1194, 1983.

86. Ozols RF, Deiserroth AB, Javadpour N, *et al.*: Treatment of poor prognosis nonseminomatous testicular cancer with a 'High-Dose' platinum combination chemotherapy regimen. Cancer 51:1803–1807, 1983.

87. Buamah PK, Howell A, Whitby H, *et al.*: Assessment of renal function during high-dose cis-Platinum therapy in patients with ovarian carcinoma. Cancer Chemother Pharmacol 8:281–284, 1982.

88. Barker GH, Wiltshaw E: Use of high-dose cisdichlorodiammineplatinum (II) following failure on previous chemotherapy for advanced carcinoma of the ovary. Br J Obstet Gynecol 8:1192–1199, 1981.

89. Schmoll HJ, Weib J, Diehl V: Cisdiamminedichloroplatinum ultra high dose (DDP-HD) in testicular carcinoma: Toxicity and activity. Fourth International Symposium on Platinum Coordination Complexes in Cancer Chemotherapy. Burlington, VT, June 1983.

90. Wiltshaw E, Evans BD, Jones AC, *et al.*: JM8, successor to cis Platin in advanced ovarian carcinoma? Lancet :587, 1983.

91. Calvert AH, Baker JW, Dalley VM, *et al.*: Phase II trial of cis-diammine-1,1-cyclobutane dicarboxylate platinum II (CBDCA, JM8) in patients with carcinoma of the ovary not previously treated with cisplatin. Fourth International Symposium on Platinum Coordination Complexes in Cancer Chemotherapy. Burlington, VT, June 1983.

92. Dembo AJ, Bush RS, Beale FA, *et al.*: Ovarian carcinoma: Improved survival following abdominopelvic irradiation in patients with a completed pelvic operation. Am J Obstet Gynecol 134:793–800, 1979.

93. Dembo AJ, Bush RS: Radiation therapy of ovarian carcinoma. In: Gynecologic Oncology. Griffiths CT, Fuller AF (eds). Boston: Martinus Nijhoff Publishers 263–298, 1983.

94. Glatstein E, Fuks Z, Bagshaw MA: Diaphragmatic treatment in ovarian carcinoma: A new radiotherapeutic technique. Int J Roentgen 2:357–362, 1977.

95. Schary M, Martinez A, Howes A: Toxicity of whole adbominal irradiation in gynecologic malignancy with and without prior combination chemotherapy. Proc Amer Soc Clin Onc 2:614, 1983.

96. Rose C, Notnick L, Come S, *et al.*: Advanced ovarian carcinoma: Possible role for the sequential use of multi-agent systemic chemotherapy and whole abdominal radiation. Proc Amer Soc of Clin Onc 2:592, 1983.

97. Vogl SE, Seltzer V, Greenwald E, *et al.*: Consolidation radiotherapy and chemotherapy for ovarian cancer after chemotherapy induced remission: Long term remission of initial bulky disease. Proc Am Soc Clin Onc. 2:590, 1983.

98. Kapp DS: The role of the radiation oncologist in the management of gynecologic cancer 51:2485–2497, 1982.

99. Dembo AJ, Bush RS, Beale FA, *et al.*: A randomized clinical trial of moving strip versus open field whole abdominal irradiation in patients with invasive epithelial cancer of ovary. Proc Amer Soc Clin Onc 2:571, 1983.

100. Bast RC, Knapp RC: The immunobiology of ovarian carcinoma. In: Gynecologic Oncology. Griffiths CT, Fuller AF (eds). Boston: Martinus Nijhoff Publishers 187–226, 1983.

101. Bast RC, Berek SS, Obrist R, *et al.*: Intraperitoneal immunotherapy of human ovarian carcinoma with Corynebacterium Parvum. Cancer Res 43:1395–1401, 1983.

102. Creasman WT, Gall SA, Blessing JA, *et al.*: Chemoimmunotherapy in the management of primary stage III ovarian cancer: A Gynecologic Oncology Group Study. Cancer Treat Rep 68:319–323, 1979.

103. Alberts DS, Salmon SE, Moon TE: Chemoimmunotherapy for advanced ovarian carcinoma with Adriamycin – Cyclophosphamide + BCG: Early report of a Southwest Oncology Group Study. Recent Results Cancer Res 68:160–165, 1978.

104. Gutterman J, Fein S, *et al.*: Recombinant human leukocyte interferon (IFL-rA). A phase I

clinical study of pharmacokinetics, single dose tolerance and biologic effects in cancer patients. Ann Inter Med 96:549–556, 1982.

105. Einhorn N, Cantell K, Einhorn S, Strander H: Human leukocyte interferon therapy for advanced ovarian carcinoma. AmJ Clin Oncol 5:167–172, 1982.

106. Pino Y, Torres JL, Bross DS, Hernandes E, *et al.*: Multimodality treatment of patients with advanced ovarian carcinoma. Int J Radiation Oncology Biol Phys 8:1671–1677, 1982.

107. Berkowitz R, Kabawat S, Lazarus H, *et al.*: Comparison of a rabbit heteroantiserum and a murine monoclonal antibody raised against a human epithelial ovarian carcinoma cell line. Am J Obstet Gynecol 146:607–612, 1983.

108. Kabawat SE, Bast RC, Welch WR, *et al.*: Immunopathologic characterization of monoclonal antibody that recognizes common surface antigens of human ovarian tumors of serous, endometrioid, and clear cell types. Am J Clin Path 79:98–104, 1983.

109. Speyer JL, Myers CE: Intraperitoneal chemotherapy of ovarian cancer. in: Recent advances in clinical oncology I, Williams CJ, Whitehouse JMA (eds), Edinburgh: Churchill Livingstone, 181–195, 1982.

110. Speyer JL, Collins JM, Dedrick RL, *et al.*: Phase I and Pharmacological studies of 5-Fluorouracil administered intraperitoneally. Cancer Research 40:567–572, 1980.

111. Ozols RF, Young RC, Speyer JL: Phase I and pharmacological studies of adriamycin administered intraperitoneally to patients with ovarian cancer. Cancer Research 42:4265–4269, 1982.

112. Jenkins JF, Sugarbaker DH, Gianola FJ, Meyers CE: Technical considerations in the ue of intraperitoneal chemotherapy administered by Tenckhoff catheter. Surg Gynecol Obstet 154:858–864, 1982.

113. Jones RB, Collins JM, Meyers CE, *et al.*b: High-volume intraperitoneal chemotherapy with methotrexate in patients with cancer. Cancer Research 41:55–59, 1981.

114. Dedrick RL, Meyers CE, Bungay PM, DeVita VT, Jr: Pharmacokinetic rationale for peritoneal drug administration in the treatment of ovarian cancer. Cancer Treat Rep 62:1–11, 1978.

115. Pfeifle CE, King ME, Howell SB: Pharmacokinetics and clinical efficacy of intraperitoneal cytarabine (ARA-C) treatment of advanced ovarian cancer. Proc Amer Soc Clin Onc. 2:584, 1983.

116. Pretorius RG, Hacker NF, Berek JS, *et al.*: Intraperitoneal cis-Platinum in patients with ovarian carcinoma. Proc Amer Soc Clin Onc 1:437, 1982.

117. Casper ES, Kelsen DP, Alcock NW, Lewis JL, Jr: IP cisplatin in patients with malignant ascites: Pharmacokinetic evaluation and comparison with IV route. Cancer Treat Rep 67:235–238, 1983.

118. Jenkins JF, Hubbard SM, Howser DM: Managing intraperitoneal chemotherapy: A new assault on ovarian cancer. Nursing 12:78–83, 1982.

Index